SAUNDERS TEXT AND REVIEW SERIES

NEUROLOGY

ROBERT C. COLLINS, MD

Professor and Chairman
Department of Neurology
UCLA School of Medicine
Los Angeles, California

W.B. SAUNDERS COMPANY
A Division of Harcourt Brace & Company
Philadelphia London Toronto Montreal Sydney Tokyo

W.B. SAUNDERS COMPANY
A Division of Harcourt Brace & Company

The Curtis Center
Independence Square West
Philadelphia, Pennsylvania 19106

Library of Congress Cataloging-in-Publication Data

Collins, Robert C.

Neurology / Robert C. Collins.—1st ed.

p.   cm.

ISBN 0–7216–5992–6

1. Nervous system—Diseases.   2. Neurology.   I. Title.
    [DNLM: 1. Nervous System Diseases.   WL 140 C712n 1997]

RC346.C567 1997   616.8—dc21

DNLM/DLC   96–48724

NEUROLOGY   ISBN 0–7216–5992–6

Printed in the United States of America.

Last digit is the print number: 9   8   7   6   5   4   3

To
Valerie, Lisa, and Graham
Strength, courage, and imagination
Because . . .

PREFACE

Advances in neurology have come in different stages. The profession's scientific history began in the nineteenth century when anatomical localization of pathological processes was brought to bear on the analysis of patients' symptoms. The deductive science and art of localization remain a cornerstone of clinical practice, now greatly facilitated by neuro-imaging techniques. The discovery of brain and nerve electrical activity in the 1920s led to sensitive methods for measuring and defining pathophysiological events underlying symptoms. With the discovery of abnormalities in dopa metabolism in the etiology of Parkinson's disease in the 1960s, neurology entered the current modern stage of development. Today, as clinicians localize and describe symptoms anatomically and pathophysiologically, they strive to define disease processes in molecular terms whenever possible. Understanding the molecular pathology of a DNA transcript, an ion channel, or a synaptic receptor brings advances in therapy and new hope for patients.

In this book I attempt to integrate the past discoveries and the rapidly expanding fields of neuroscience into a single thesis for the student. The thesis is simple. Physicians must bring a comprehensive and secure knowledge of fundamentals to bear upon disease processes that can destroy the essential qualities of human existence: perception, language, memory, emotion, and movement. Symptoms of neurological dysfunction properly arouse an urgency in physicians for expeditious, intelligent, and compassionate action. Students of all medical disciplines must be prepared for this action on behalf of their patients.

Single-authored books are necessarily incomplete for lack of breadth of expertise and diversity of perspective. I hope that some compensation is provided by a uniformity of exposition and style. Students—medical, graduate, and nursing—and house officers beginning diverse careers should find here an introductory text that provides basic understanding of the fundamentals of neurology on the one hand and the processes of the common neurological diseases on the other. *Section I* provides an overview of the field of neurology and an introduction to the patient. *Section II* is devoted to an analysis of disorders of movement, sensation, homeostasis, and the brain's higher functions. These four chapters should be read with the patient's symptoms in mind—how does the physician approach weakness, dizziness, aphasia, or other symptoms to reach a diagnosis and start therapy? *Section III* contains 10 chapters devoted to the most common disease processes affecting the nervous system. Case studies, often taken from the rich history of the profession, have been added for illustration. Brief expositions of new experimental approaches are given to indicate our changing understanding of diseases. Finally, each chapter includes some current approaches to therapy, acknowledging that treatment changes rapidly as our molecular understanding of disease advances. By necessity and design this book is under-referenced. Each chapter closes with a list of selected readings that are representational rather than citational for the material discussed.

I am grateful to my professional colleagues at UCLA whose neurological expertise and commitment to education proved invaluable in writing this book. Drs. Jeff Cummings, Mike Graves, John Keesey, Charles Markham, Gary Mathern, Jeff Saver, Allan Tobin, Tony Verity, Harry Vinters, Rhonda Voskuhl, Chuck Wilson, and Roger Woods provided particular assitance. A general note of thanks to the many colleagues who granted permission for the reproduction of their illustrations. I ask the indulgence of the scientific community for the many oversights this work contains. Finally, I thank Bill Schmitt for his persuasive vision in this project and Carol Vartanian for her persistent encouragement and attention to detail in bringing this book to print.

ROBERT C. COLLINS, MD

CONTENTS

SECTION I

INTRODUCTION TO NEUROLOGY

1. The Practice of Clinical Neurology 3

2. The Neurological Evaluation 9

SECTION II

THE NEUROLOGICAL BASIS OF SIGNS AND SYMPTOMS

3. Disorders of the Motor System 23

4. Disorders of Sensation 37

5. Disorders of Homeostasis 52

6. Disorders of Higher Functions 65

SECTION III

COMMON NEUROLOGICAL DISEASES

7. Myopathy 85

8. Myasthenia Gravis 96

9. Peripheral Neuropathy 106

10. AMYOTROPHIC LATERAL SCLEROSIS AND THE MOTOR NEURON DISEASES 117

11. PARKINSON'S DISEASE AND THE MULTIPLE SYSTEM ATROPHIES 127

12. HUNTINGTON'S DISEASE AND THE HEREDITARY ATAXIAS 138

13. SEIZURES AND EPILEPSY 148

14. MULTIPLE SCLEROSIS 159

15. CEREBROVASCULAR DISEASE 172

16. ALZHEIMER'S DISEASE AND THE PRIMARY DEMENTIAS 184

INDEX 195

INTRODUCTION TO

NEUROLOGY

These first two chapters introduce the practice of neurology and the methods used to diagnose conditions affecting the nervous system. Chapter 1 provides an overview of the incidence and impact of neurological conditions, the changing attitudes and expectations of patients, and the role played by generalists and neurologists in caring for their patients. Chapter 2 outlines the clinical method in neurology. Emphasis is placed upon taking a complete history, with the neurological examination and laboratory investigations being used to test the hypotheses of a working diagnosis. The determination of precise etiology, the pursuit of specific and supportive treatment, patient education, and long-term care are the cornerstones of the neurological exercise.

CHAPTER ONE

THE PRACTICE OF CLINICAL

NEUROLOGY

THE PATIENT'S PERSPECTIVE 4

EPIDEMIOLOGY OF NEUROLOGICAL DISEASE 4

MEDICAL STUDENT EDUCATION 5

THE ROLE OF THE GENERALIST 6

THE ROLE OF THE NEUROLOGIST 6

FUTURE DIRECTIONS IN NEUROLOGY 6

THE PATIENT'S PERSPECTIVE

Patients with diseases of the nervous system require special attention and care, since these diseases can affect the most precious aspects of human behavior—thought, memory, language, emotion, sensation, and movement. A patient with a stroke, brain tumor, or neurodegenerative disease is categorically different from a patient with a broken arm, myocardial infarction, or systemic disease. Brain dysfunction can alter the capacity to recognize and describe the dysfunction, can cause marked episodic or permanent changes in behavior, and can result in disability disproportionate to the severity of a disease process. Patients and their families are rightfully fearful of these conditions when they first encounter a physician and require skillful and empathic help from the medical profession.

Society has not always been understanding or supportive of patients with neurological illness. People with epilepsy or mental retardation were once confined to custodial institutions and were sterilized to prevent reproduction. Others unable to walk were often confined to home owing to architectural barriers to wheelchairs in public buildings and to transportation. Even members of the medical profession once believed that when an illness invaded the nervous system, such as a metastasis from a systemic cancer, further evaluation and therapy should not be pursued.

These attitudes and practices have largely receded as a result of several events. First, advances in biomedical research have brought new understanding of the causes and consequences of neurological illness, and many therapies are, or are about to become, available. Second, a rapid growth in the number of clinical neurologists has made access to expert diagnosis and care easier for a greater number of people. Third, there has been a remarkable expansion of public education and support for patients with neurological illness. Popular books and films have been devoted to specific illnesses and disabilities. Patients have formed advocacy groups to support families and caregivers and have established networks with physicians, scientists, and politicians to advance research and education. In 1990, the Americans with Disabilities Act was enacted and President Bush signed a congressional declaration making the 1990s the "Decade of the Brain."

Patients now are increasingly aware of the neurological illnesses and are better prepared to work with physicians to achieve a realistic understanding of their disease and disability and to pursue treatment and rehabilitation.

EPIDEMIOLOGY OF NEUROLOGICAL DISEASE

Medical conditions affecting the nervous system and primary neurological diseases are among the most common causes of morbidity in the United States (Table 1–1). Determination of the exact incidence (new cases per 100,000 population per year) or point prevalence (cases in existence at one point in time) is problematic. Determinations depend upon current diagnostic classifications, the skill of physicians, the accuracy

TABLE 1-1. Epidemiology of Common Conditions Affecting the Nervous System

Common Medical Conditions	Incidence per 100,000	Approximate Distribution of Cases	
		Specialist	Generalist
Head trauma	1800	10–20%	80–90%
Headaches	4000	10–20%	80–90%
Lumbosacral spine pain syndromes	1650	10–20%	80–90%
Cervical spine pain syndromes	215	10–20%	80–90%

of laboratory tests, and the ease of accessing medical records. In addition, only a few epidemiology centers in the world study neurological illness, so the characteristics of the population sample must always be kept in mind. In the United States, some of the most accurate data reflect studies performed at the Mayo Clinic on the predominantly white population in Olmsted County, Minnesota, and the prospective study focused on cardiovascular and cerebrovascular diseases collected over many years in Framingham, Massachusetts. Finally, there is likely an underestimation of true morbidity rates owing to patient failure to seek medical attention for common conditions and physician failure to diagnose or properly report certain uncommon illnesses.

Patients often seek medical attention for common medical conditions that affect the nervous system (Table 1–1). Although a small percentage of these might indicate serious neurological illness, the great majority represent simple benign processes such as soft tissue injury or inflammation that generalists are skilled in handling. In cases of head trauma, specialists are consulted when there has been loss of consciousness, a skull fracture, focal signs, posttraumatic amnesia, or encephalopathy. Neurologists are consulted in cases of migraine headache when the diagnosis is uncertain or the treatment plan becomes complicated. Local pain in the neck and low back are among the most common complaints of patients and only rarely indicate serious disease processes. Specialists in neurology, neurosurgery, or orthopedics are consulted when conservative treatment plans fail to relieve chronic symptoms or when there is clinical evidence of impaired neurological function.

Epidemiological studies also indicate that the high incidence of primary neurological illness (Table 1–2) reflects in part the manifestations of common disease processes. Atherosclerosis, hypertension, and diabetes are major risk factors for cerebrovascular disease. Trauma is a significant cause of seizures as well as of spinal cord dysfunction. Diabetes and alcoholism are major causes of peripheral neuropathy. Recent studies indicate that genetic factors are implicated in at least 10% of cases of Alzheimer's disease, the most common cause of dementia, and amyotrophic lateral sclerosis, the most common form of motor neuron disease. Genetic factors also are involved in the autoimmune ab-

TABLE 1-2. Epidemiology of Neurological Disease*

Neurological Disease or Condition	Incidence†	Prevalence‡	Cost§ (billion dollars/year)
Cerebrovascular disease	200	650	18
Seizures and epilepsy	120	650	3
Peripheral neuropathy	100		
Dementia	50	250	113
Parkinsonism	20	200	2.5
Primary tumors	15	65	
Spinal cord disorders	13	90	22.5
Trigeminal neuralgia	4	40	
Multiple sclerosis	3	60	4
Motor neuron disease	2	6	0.3
Muscular dystrophies	1	8	
Hereditary degenerative disorders	1	20	
Polymyositis	0.4	6	
Huntington's disease	0.4	5	
Myasthenia gravis	0.4	4	

*Data modified from Kurtzke, J.F. The current neurologic burden of illness and injury in the United States. Neurology 32:1207–1214, 1982.
†Incidence = new cases/100,000 population/year.
‡Prevalence = number of cases in existence at any one point in time per 100,000 population.
§Cost data, given in approximate 1990 dollars, from The National Foundation for Brain Research, 1992; and NIH Publication No. 88-2957, 1989.

normalities of multiple sclerosis and possibly myasthenia gravis.

When the incidence data in epidemiological studies are sorted by age, sex, race, geography, and other factors, new clues concerning cause and pathophysiology emerge. Aging is a risk factor for many illnesses. Approximately 1% of the population over age 65 will have Parkinson's disease, and perhaps as many as 40% of those over age 80 will get Alzheimer's disease. Elderly men more than women are susceptible to amyotrophic lateral sclerosis and myasthenia gravis. However, there is also a peak incidence of myasthenia among young women. The occurrence of multiple sclerosis is markedly affected by latitude with the incidence for the general population increased over 100-fold at latitudes greater than 45 degrees. Research into the cause of these illnesses makes use of these epidemiological facts to probe biological hypotheses.

The prevalence of neurological illness is the best indicator for determining the real burden of neurological illness, since it takes into consideration the longevity of disease and disability. For example, although many of the degenerative illnesses have a low incidence, patients with these disorders are commonly seen in neurological practice. On a typical day, a neurologist may care for patients with parkinsonism, dementia, a hereditary degenerative disorder, multiple sclerosis, epilepsy, stroke, complicated headache, and a painful spine syndrome as well as for patients presenting with neurological symptoms for diagnosis. The longevity of disease also accounts for the high cost of these illnesses to society when both the direct costs of medical care and the indirect costs of lost wages for both patients and caregivers are considered (Table 1–2).

MEDICAL STUDENT EDUCATION

How much neurology should every medical student learn? The educational dilemma posed by this question is real and likely to endure, as illustrated by the following clinical example. A patient with numbness and weakness of the feet is statistically more likely to have diabetes mellitus than Charcot-Marie-Tooth disease. Medical students should certainly learn about diabetic neuropathy, and all generalists should be comfortable with making the diagnosis and providing care. Yet students should also learn to recognize when a particular constellation of signs and symptoms do not meet the diagnostic criteria of a common disease process so as to seek timely consultation and avoid delay in accurate diagnosis and appropriate treatment. The student's challenge is to acquire a self-learning and practice style that recognizes appropriate limits and boundaries. A medical student may not need to know the details of Charcot-Marie-Tooth disease but does need to know when the clinical findings are not consistent with diabetic neuropathy. A patient with Charcot-Marie-Tooth disease should not be treated with insulin.

Neurologists must be expert in recognizing and treating a great number of uncommon diseases. For example, more than 130 genetic diseases affecting the nervous system have been mapped to chromosomal locations. It would be inappropriate to teach medical students about all these diseases. Yet it would also be inappropriate not to select a few well-studied examples in which new information is revealing entirely new disease mechanisms—information that will likely be important for the future practice of medicine for many common diseases as well as rare conditions. In this context, learning about Charcot-Marie-Tooth disease may be important.

This textbook is aimed at providing what every medical student should know about neurology. Section I provides an introduction to the clinical skills needed for neurology. Section II emphasizes the clinical approach to the common symptoms and signs that patients bring to physicians. Section III discusses common neurological illnesses and selects a few uncommon or even rare conditions in which advances in neurobiology are revealing important new information.

THE ROLE OF THE GENERALIST

Patients with neurological symptoms rarely see a neurologist or neurosurgeon first. This makes it incumbent upon generalists—internists, family practitioners, and pediatricians—to have considerable knowledge and skill in recognizing potentially serious illness and in deciding when to pursue emergency consultation; when and how to proceed with a thorough, comfortable, and efficient evaluation; and how to institute an effective treatment plan. It has been estimated that up to 25% of the complaints with which patients present to their primary care physician are potentially referable to a disease of the nervous system. Twenty percent of hospitalized patients have an illness affecting the nervous system. These considerations, along with an awareness of the increasing incidence of neurological conditions in the aging population, make it important for all physicians to have a fundamental understanding of the practice of neurology.

What kinds of neurological illnesses should generalists be competent to take care of? By historical traditions, this question has been answered differently in different countries; e.g., there are approximately 10 times as many neurologists per capita in the United States as in the United Kingdom. As a result, neurologists in the United States provide care for a greater number of common conditions, but on average they also see fewer uncommon diseases. The rare diseases are shared among the large number of practicing neurologists or concentrated in subspecialty practices at academic medical centers. In the current marketplace of medical practice, this question is also answered differently by physician groups. Some generalists argue that they should provide primary care for all patients with common conditions, particularly headache, neck pain, and low back pain. Some neurologists argue that only professionals devoted to understanding the nervous system and its disorders should provide care for patients with neurological symptoms.

Society has an increasing interest in keeping all clinical exercises as economically efficient as possible. Some think that this will mean curtailing expensive testing done in subspecialty practices. Others argue that generalists unfamiliar with neurological illness and uncertain of their findings order too many diagnostic tests. It seems likely that only a well-designed research study on health care outcomes will determine where patients will get the best and most economical care. Table 1–1 provides an approximation of the current division of patients with neurological symptoms or illness between generalists and specialists.

THE ROLE OF THE NEUROLOGIST

Surveys of the American Academy of Neurology in 1992 indicated that there were 11,300 neurologists in the United States, or approximately 1.6% of American physicians. Work force calculations estimate that this number will increase to 13,000 to 15,000 over the next 30 years before stabilization. Since neurologists need to work closely with generalists and neurosurgeons, most practice in large cities and are affiliated with medical centers. Seventy-five percent are located in metropolitan areas with populations greater than 500,000. Approximately 28% have a full-time academic appointment and spend the majority of their time in clinical or basic research and teaching. An additional 34% have a part-time clinical appointment with a university.

The ratio of neurologists to the U. S. population is 3.7/100,000 with a wide range in distribution from a low of 1.3/100,000 in Wyoming to a high above 7.0 in Massachusetts and Maryland. The number and distribution of physicians are of great concern to health care planners, but there is no consensus on ideal targets at present. Some calculate that when the neurology work force stabilizes at 4.75/100,000 in 2010 there will still be a 35% shortfall. This percentage is based upon assumptions of physician and patient distribution, referral and practice patterns, and rates for training and retirement of clinical neurologists. Training academic neurologists is an important component of future planning, since advances in diagnosis and treatment achieved through research have profound impact on medical practice.

Approximately two-thirds of neurologists have an office practice and perform approximately 37 office and 23 hospital patient visits per week. These numbers are lower than for internists (approximately 64 and 36, respectively) and reflect in part the longer time necessary to perform a comprehensive neurological evaluation. In addition, a high percentage of neurologists perform lumbar punctures and clinical neurophysiological testing, electroencephalography, and electromyography as part of some evaluations. In recent years, there has been a tendency to subspecialize further within neurology with certification processes for pediatric neurology and clinical neurophysiology and somewhat separate and competitive fields for neuroradiology and neuro-ophthalmology. Following 3 years of general neurology training, many neurology residents seek 1- to 2-year fellowships in such areas as epilepsy, neuroimaging, stroke, neuromuscular diseases, rehabilitation, neuro-oncology, and behavioral neurology. Although some authors disparage the fragmentation in continuity of patient care that comes with subspecialization, it has resulted in a remarkable increase in our knowledge of neurological diseases and the successful introduction and validation of many new therapies. All patients with illness of the nervous system require special attention, and all neurologists must be prepared to provide this. The roles of the neurologist are outlined in Box 1–1.

FUTURE DIRECTIONS IN NEUROLOGY

The practice of neurology began to change significantly in the 1970s with the introduction of new imaging technologies (Table 1–3). Today the use of x-ray CT scanning, MRI scanning, PET, and SPECT studies allows relatively easy, noninvasive, high-resolution examination of the anatomical and functional basis of neurological illness. As discussed in Chapter 2, these technologies are used principally to test diagnostic hypotheses generated from a patient's history and examination, to document changes in illness, and to evaluate results of therapy. Used judiciously, these tests add a level of

1. Provides expertise in the evaluation of signs and symptoms of neurological dysfunction while establishing a close rapport with the patient and family.
2. Creates a plan of laboratory investigation when necessary that is goal oriented, economical, and comfortable for the patient.
3. Initiates a plan of treatment that considers pharmacological, surgical, physical, occupational, and social aspects of therapy.
4. Responds emergently to acute neurological illnesses when delay in time can result in further damage, such as in head injury, stroke, and coma.
5. Provides special awareness of the behavioral and psychological aspects of neurological illness and works closely with psychiatrist, social workers, and other health care professionals to achieve the best patient care and support for the family.
6. Maintains long-term care for patients with primary neurological illnesses and has a special capacity for dealing with increasing disability as seen in dementia, Parkinson's disease, muscular dystrophy, etc.
7. Establishes close working relationships with other physicians and health care professionals to provide and request expert consultation for patients.
8. Provides education on neurological illnesses and treatment for patients, lay groups, students, and other professionals.
9. Performs or supports research on the nervous system, its diseases, and treatment so as to advance the welfare of patients.
10. Provides expertise to society for organizing health care delivery that provides the best care for patients with neurological illness.

objectivity and quantification to the neurological evaluation.

Research in neuroimaging will continue to provide new technologies for patient care in the future. New strategies using MRI allow the visualization of changes in blood flow in response to changes in functional activation of the brain. This offers the potential for mapping the human brain noninvasively, without radioactivity, in almost any patient. Other strategies directed at studying diffusion of water allow visualization of the earliest phases of cerebral infarction. This technique will help guide the use of new early-intervention therapies in cerebrovascular disease. MR spectroscopy is a technique that allows measurement of select metabolites in brain *in vivo*, including phosphate, ATP, creatine, *N*-acetylaspartic acid, and lactate. Determining how these compounds are changed by different disease processes will bring a new diagnostic tool to clinical neurology.

Advances in molecular biology will have a significant impact on clinical neurology owing to the discovery that over half of all human genes are expressed in the brain. Research in molecular genetics is providing new ways of classifying several neurological illnesses. For example, Duchenne and Becker type muscular dystrophy, once thought to be different diseases, are now known to be allelic, and both reflect alterations in the structure and level of dystrophin. Recent studies indicate the possibility of different deletions in different families resulting in similar clinical pictures. Genes for Charcot-Marie-Tooth disease lie on chromosomes X, 1, and 17. Alterations in mitochondrial genes can have profound effects on nervous tissue and muscle, but the classification of these diseases is not yet clear. For example, it is possible to have an identical deletion at position 3243 of the transfer RNA for leucine in mitochondrial DNA in different families that results in entirely different clinical pictures, e.g., the MELAS syndrome, progressive external ophthalmoplegia, or diabetes with hearing loss (Chapter 7). Molecular studies of the rare "prion" degenerative diseases (Creutzfeldt-Jakob, kuru, and scrapie) have revealed pathogenetic mechanisms that can be both inherited and transmissible (Chapter 16).

These advances in molecular genetics have added complexity to the principles of simple Mendelian inheritance. For some diseases, it will be important to know not only whether a disease gene has been transmitted but also what the exact magnitude of the genetic defect

TABLE 1-3. Advances in Neuroimaging

Imaging Technique	Basic Principle	Clinical Application
CT scan (computerized axial tomography)	Tissue attenuation of x-rays	Acute trauma and cerebral hemorrhage
MRI scan (magnetic resonance imaging)	Differential behavior of tissue protons in magnetic fields	High resolution of brain structure, localization and elucidation of pathological processes
MRA scan (magnetic resonance angiography)	Special pulse sequences for blood	Visualization of blood vessels for abnormalities or lesions
Functional MRI (fMRI)	Ultrafast images of blood oxygenation	Changes in local blood flow during functional activation, research in brain mapping
MRS (magnetic resonance spectroscopy)	Behavior of protons in different chemical compounds	Regional changes in brain metabolites during disease processes
PET scan (positron emission tomography)	Localization of positron-emitting radionuclides	Epilepsy surgery, dementia, degenerative diseases, research in brain mapping
SPECT scan (single-photon-emission computed tomography)	Localization of gamma-emitting radionuclides	Localization of blood flow changes in dementia, epilepsy, degenerative diseases, and cerebrovascular diseases

is in order to understand the potential severity and age of onset of the disease process. For example, for neurogenetic diseases caused by the excess repetition of a sequence of triplet base pairs (e.g., fragile X syndrome, myotonic muscular dystrophy, Huntington's disease), the onset and severity of the clinical course are partly dependent on the number of excess triplets (Chapter 12). In addition, in some diseases it is also important to know whether the disease gene comes from the mother or father—a condition called imprinting—since a different phenotypic expression may ensue (e.g., the Prader-Willi and Angelman syndromes), or the offspring may be more severely affected by inheritance from one parent rather than the other (e.g., myotonic dystrophy).

From the diagnostic point of view, there now exist prenatal *in utero* screening tests to guide genetic counseling for many neurogenetic diseases. These genetic tests can also be used to identify presymptomatic carriers, raising an ethical dilemma for many patients and families about whether the test is useful or harmful when no therapy is available for those who test positive. Nevertheless, since the pace and severity of neurogenetic diseases are almost always influenced by environmental factors, it will be scientifically important to identify and study some presymptomatic carriers to identify therapeutic strategies. Advances in molecular genetics will likely lead to the chromosomal identification of many inherited neurological conditions as well as major new insights into the pathophysiology of the disease process.

In addition to anticipated advances in brain mapping on the one hand and gene mapping on the other, the field of neurology will continue to experience advances in therapeutics with the introduction of major new rational treatments. Continuing basic science studies of membrane channels will likely lead to new analgesics, anesthetics, and anticonvulsants. Since the early

experiments on dopamine and its role in Parkinson's disease, additional studies on catecholamine transmission have led to new therapies for migraine, manic depressive illness, schizophrenia, and movement disorders. Further research into the complexity of neurotransmitter release and reuptake and the mechanisms of multiple receptor subtypes will lead to further insights for new drugs. The recent discovery and elucidation of the biology of the growth factors have already led to clinical trials for neurodegenerative diseases. Progress in molecular neuroimmunology is introducing entirely new strategies to the treatment of multiple sclerosis, myasthenia gravis, and the immune-mediated neuropathies.

The remarkable growth in basic and clinical neuroscience research over the past 20 years is now bringing new therapies to the bedside and into the clinic. The next 20 years will bear witness to an era of new therapy for diseases of the nervous system.

Selected Readings

Cohen, M. S., and S. Y. Bookheimer. Localization of brain function using magnetic resonance imaging. Trends Neurosci 17:268–276, 1994.

Gilman, S. Advances in neurology. N Engl J Med 326:1608–1616 and 1671–1676, 1992.

Kurtzke, J. F. The current neurological burden of illness and injury in the United States. Neurology 32:1207–1214, 1982.

Kurtzke, J. F., M. M. Murphy, and M. A. Smith. On the production of neurologists in the United States: An update. Neurology 41:1–9, 1991.

Ringle, S. P., T. L. Rogstad, and the Human Resources Subcommittee of the American Academy of Neurology. Neurologists—1991 to 1992. Neurology 43:1666–1672, 1993.

Rowland, L. P. The first decade of molecular genetics in Neurology: Changing clinical thought and practice. Ann Neurol 32:207–214, 1992.

Scherokman, B., K. Cannard, J. Q. Miller, and the American Academy of Neurology Undergraduate Education Subcommittee. What should a graduating medical student know about neurology? Neurology 44:1170–1176, 1994.

CHAPTER TWO

THE NEUROLOGICAL EVALUATION

OVERVIEW 10

THE NEUROLOGICAL HISTORY 11

   Anatomic Localization 13

   Pathophysiology 13

THE NEUROLOGICAL EXAMINATION 14

   The Mental Status Examination 14

   Station and Gait Examination 15

   Cervical and Lumbar Spine Examination 15

   Cranial Nerve Examination 15

   Motor Examination 16

   Sensory Examination 16

   Reflex Examination 17

   Summary and Formulation 17

THE SCREENING NEUROLOGICAL EXAMINATION 17

LABORATORY INVESTIGATION 18

   CT Scans 18

   MRI Scans 18

   Lumbar Puncture 19

   DNA Diagnostic Studies 19

SUMMARY 19

OVERVIEW

How does a physician make a neurological diagnosis? In many ways, the process is no different from making any other diagnosis in clinical medicine. The physician must (1) locate the patient's symptoms and signs anatomically, (2) interpret temporal features in terms of pathophysiological events, and (3) explore these ideas during an examination and laboratory investigation in order to uncover pathological processes. Taken altogether, these steps lead to the formulation of an etiological hypothesis. The hypothesis is tested by further history and examination and occasionally laboratory investigation. Once there is a likely etiology, a treatment plan can be formulated. This is the clinical method in neurology (Figure 2–1). As John Hughlings Jackson, one of the founding fathers of British neurology, wrote in 1873,

In the investigation of the Epilepsies, or any kind of case of nervous disease we have three lines of investigation. We have: (1) To find the organ damaged (localization). (2) To find the functional affection of nerve tissue. (3) To find the alteration in nutrition. There is, in brief, (1) anatomy, (2) physiology, (3) pathology in each case.

—Hughlings Jackson. On the anatomical, physiological and pathological investigation of the epilepsies. The West Riding Lunatic Asylum Medical Reports III:315, 1873.

Today the accurate diagnosis of neurological illness is not difficult in the majority of cases. A clinician can usually be right 60% of the time by "pattern recognition" alone. Of course, the physician cannot afford to be wrong 40% of the time. There must be an accurate, step-by-step clinical methodology that does not fail.

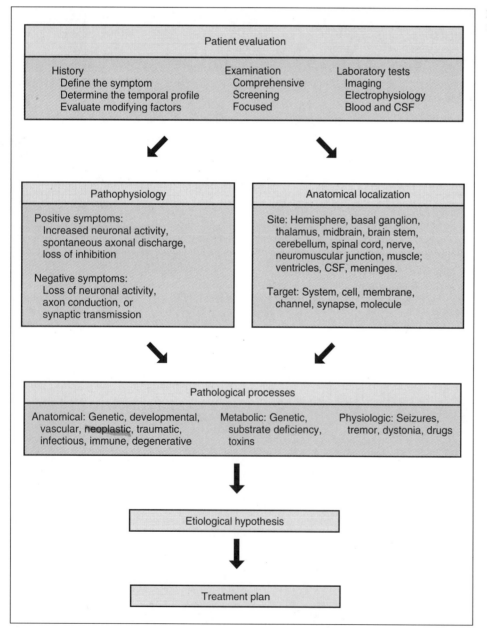

FIGURE 2–1. The clinical method in neurology.

The diagnosis of pathological conditions in the nervous system implies the determination of the site of disease, the recognition of the manner in which the pathological disorders function, and the nature of the pathological lesion. Localization is a matter of stating in terms of anatomy the parts of structures involved, and therefore requires the knowledge of anatomy; determination of the manner in which dysfunctions are disordered naturally necessitates an acquaintance with the physiology or functions of the diseased organ, and recognition of the nature of the lesion depends on the knowledge of morbid factors which involve the nervous system and the mode of its reaction to them.

—Gordon Holmes. *Introduction to Clinical Neurology.* 1946.

Making a neurological diagnosis thus involves answering the following three questions. *Where is the lesion? What is the pathophysiological basis of abnormal signs and symptoms? What is the pathological process?* Clinicians who practiced before the 1970s used the patient's history and examination alone to reach conclusions in most cases. Today's physician has the help of potent tools of laboratory investigation—neuroimaging, electrophysiology, and molecular analysis of genes and biochemical analysis of blood and spinal fluid. Nevertheless, these tools remain supplemental to the primary diagnostic exercise. A careful history and examination are the foundation of neurological practice.

THE NEUROLOGICAL HISTORY

The neurological history is the most important component in making a diagnosis. Not only is the content of the history vital information, but the behavior of the patient and family members during the taking of the history also provides important clues.

The neurological examination actually begins when the physician greets the patient in the waiting room and escorts him or her into the office. During the history taking, a patient's difficulty in understanding questions may reflect a focal problem with language comprehension or a more global problem with dementia. Lack of facial expression might indicate depression or parkinsonism. Asymmetric movement of a limb or one side of the body would suggest a focal lesion in the motor system to be tested further during examination. These *indirect* observations of behavior are often more important than the direct observations obtained during the formal neurological examination.

Patients tell stories. Something happens to them, or some strange feeling begins inside that is foreign to their sense of well-being. They usually mark its onset and follow its time course with an internalized narrative. Taking a good history is simply drawing out the patient's narrative, eliciting details, asking for clarification, and interjecting an occasional question to test an idea. The skill is that of a good detective. Physicians know that if they have an hour to spend with a patient, then 30–40 minutes will often be spent in taking the history. Skilled physicians are skilled listeners and observers. Conversely, many diagnostic mistakes result

from impatience, from too eager a leap from a patient's first complaint to an etiological hypothesis. The diagnostic process must follow sequential steps to reach a secure conclusion, without an unnecessary waste of time or extravagant use of unnecessary tests.

There are three tasks to accomplish while taking a history (see Figure 2–1). The first is to define the symptom. The physician must interact with the patient and the family to clarify the exact nature of the problem. It is best to do this before pursuing the time course of the narrative so as to provide a primary focus.

What Is It? The physician should help the patient be precise. A 65-year-old man says, "Doc, I'm dizzy." This vague statement could reflect fainting (cardiovascular problem?), spinning and imbalance (vestibular problem?), continuous lightheadedness (anemia?), or even a psychogenic problem. The physician should ask the patient to define "dizziness" in other terms. "Well, Doc, you know, I feel like the world is spinning and I'm going to fall down. Almost like the time I was seasick." This is helpful information. Using his own words, the patient has helped translate "dizziness" into a spinning sensation, or vertigo, suggesting dysfunction of vestibular, brain stem, or cerebellar systems. The physician is now prepared to track the narrative in anatomical systems.

What Is It Not? The symptom complex can often be defined better by eliminating irrelevant issues. One technique is to "suggest the ridiculous." The physician might ask this patient, "By 'dizziness' do you mean that you feel you are going to faint?" He may reply, "No, Doc, that's ridiculous. I feel like I'm going to vomit." In this case, 'dizziness' is *not* faintness. Cardiac disease and other causes of syncope can be removed from this patient's symptom complex with some assurance. Spinning and nausea together reinforce considerations of vestibular and brain stem functions. The physician can now track the narrative in physiological systems.

The second task is to determine the temporal profile of the condition. This is achieved by plotting the time versus intensity course of the symptom. The most important point is to be certain about when and how it started.

What's First? Patients often choose the most dramatic episode in their narrative as the focal point for analysis. For the physician it is more important to focus on the very first example of dysfunction even if it proves to be subtle or transient. This will give clues about where the problem started and how it progressed. Try to ask an open-ended question such as, "Have you ever had anything like this before?" The patient may not recollect previous episodes, and a family member may provide better information. If this pattern occurs throughout the history taking, it may suggest memory problems and perhaps dementia as well as dizziness. This patient might say, "Oh yes, Doc, come to think of it I did have an episode of dizziness and vomiting several months ago. It must have been something I ate." Although the patient has explained away this brief episode as a digestive problem, a physician will consider it as the first event in a recurring, episodic pathophysiological process within a neuroanatomical system.

How Did It Happen?   Details are important. What were the circumstances surrounding the onset? What was the patient doing? Did anyone witness the episode who could describe the patient's appearance and behavior? This patient's wife might recall, "I remember he had difficulty speaking clearly at the time, as if he had been drinking too much. But it was only for a few minutes." This is key information. Spinning and vomiting are now coupled with slurred speech, or dysarthria. Thinking in neuroanatomical terms, the physician would now conclude that the problem could *not* be confined to the vestibular system alone but would have to involve motor pathways subserving speech, most likely in the brain stem. By way of contrast, if the wife recalled that the patient had complained of difficulty hearing in one ear during the episode, then the process could very well be confined to the vestibular and auditory functions subserved by the eighth nerve. Symptoms indicate anatomical locations.

The exact sequence of the first symptoms should be explored. Did the dizziness come before the vomiting, or was it a delayed consequence? When did the dysarthria occur? How long did it last—seconds, minutes, hours? Patients overcome by neurological symptoms rarely time events by the clock, but usually they can estimate time crudely by reference to common daily events, such as the length of a television program (half-hour) or a series of television commercials (2–3 minutes). In this type of analysis, the physician is exploring the speed of events against known temporal profiles of disease processes (Figure 2–2).

What's Next?   One of the most important tasks in taking a history is to construct a time-intensity profile of the clinical events. This is done by having the patient describe a symptom as mild, moderate, or severe over a period of time. Alternatively, the accumulation of different symptoms over time can be used to construct a temporal profile. At the conclusion of the history, it should be possible to draw a graph representing one of the curves in Figure 2–2, thus giving strong clues about the pathophysiological process. The history of the elderly man with dizziness indicates recurrent episodes of acute vertigo with nausea and dysarthria, lasting 5–15 minutes, without other neurological symptoms and with complete recovery after each occasion. The anatomical localization of the symptoms, coupled with the time-intensity profile, would suggest recurrent transient ischemic attacks within the vertebrobasilar arterial supply of the brain stem. Further patient evaluation would be directed at exploring this hypothesis.

The third task in taking a history is to search for possible modifying variables. There are several types of questions that can yield important clues about underlying pathological processes.

What Makes the Symptom Better or Worse?   Asking open-ended questions to search for a variety of factors that can influence neurological diseases or conditions often yields important information. Musculoskeletal pain of the spine is usually aggravated by certain movements or postures. The symptoms of multiple sclerosis are made worse by hot weather. Caffeine can trigger migraine headaches. Alcohol can reduce essential tremor. Some types of seizures occur during sleep; others are more frequent upon awakening.

Are There Any Risk Factors?   These can be identified by probing several areas. A family history of a similar condition could indicate a genetic disease or predisposition as a risk factor. Personal habits such as smoking, alcohol intake, and recreational drug or medicine use should always be queried. A history of employment and hobbies may reveal exposure to neurotoxins. Finally, a careful review of medical systems can reveal important systemic risk factors. The neurological history of the elderly man with dizziness sug-

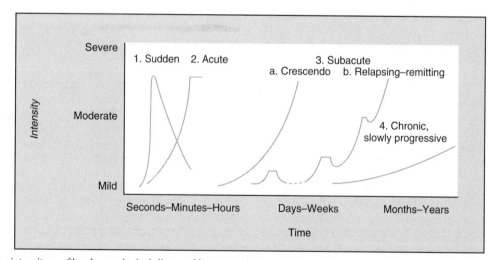

FIGURE 2–2. Time-intensity profile of neurological disease. Many neurological diseases cause characteristic temporal profiles. 1. Sudden: Onset in seconds or minutes followed by more gradual improvement. This implies a paroxysmal disorder such as epilepsy (seconds), or a brief vascular phenomenon (minutes) such as a transient ischemic attack. 2. Acute: Onset in minutes or hours with or without recovery. This occurs with vascular phenomena (e.g., ischemia, migraine) and some infections. 3. Subacute: (a) Crescendo. The onset occurs over days to weeks with progressive worsening. This is seen with expanding mass lesions such as a tumor or abscess and with intracranial infections. (b) Relapsing-remitting courses are seen with recurrent strokes and multiple sclerosis. 4. Chronic. Slowly progressive deterioration over months and years is seen with the degenerative diseases such as Parkinson's and Alzheimer's.

gested the possibility of vascular disease. It would be necessary to probe for risk factors of hypertension, diabetes, cardiac disease, and smoking.

Anatomical Localization

During the taking of the history, physicians should ask *themselves* several types of questions relevant to the anatomical localization of the symptoms (Figure 2–1).

What Is Inside the Lesion?   What anatomy *must* be involved to explain the dysfunction? A patient with monocular blindness must have a unilateral lesion somewhere between the cornea and the optic chiasm. A patient with an absent tendon reflex must have a lesion somewhere in the relevant afferent and efferent reflex arc. A patient with true vertigo must have a lesion somewhere within the vestibular system. The task is to determine the location and size of the anatomic lesion that will explain the symptoms.

What Is Outside the Lesion?   This is a question of refinement. For the patient with spinning, nausea, and dysarthria, there likely is dysfunction in brain stem pathways. If the patient denies weakness, descending corticospinal tracts can be excluded from the lesion. Absence of double vision during the episodes would likely eliminate oculomotor pathways, and absence of facial numbness or weakness would exclude pathways of the fifth and seventh cranial nerves as well. If all these pathways in the neighborhood of the lesion are functioning normally, then the lesion must be small enough or distant enough not to affect them. By determining normal functions in the history, the physician defines what is outside the lesion and begins to delineate its three-dimensional size and location.

What Is the Site?   In the analysis of some symptoms such as weakness or numbness, it is best to use a systematic approach to determine the site of the abnormality. Weakness can be the result of a disease process at one of many sites, yet each one will yield slightly different historical features and different signs of abnormality on examination. It is useful to explore these symptoms in the history by conceptually moving from peripheral to central structures, e.g., muscle, neuromuscular junction, peripheral nerve, or spinal cord. For example, patients with leg weakness from a central lesion will often note that their legs "jump" when they lie down at night—a sign of spasticity. This sign does not occur in patients with weakness due to abnormalities of peripheral nerves or muscle.

After many years of practice, clinical neurologists become highly skilled in localizing the anatomic site of lesions from the history and the examination. Generalists should be comfortable in localizing lesions to regional anatomic areas as indicated in Figure 2–1. The clinical importance of regional anatomic localization lies in its implications for further workup. For example, a patient with weakness due to a spinal cord lesion should usually be evaluated emergently, while weakness due to peripheral neuropathy can be evaluated routinely.

In an increasing number of diseases, the concept of localization can be carried further to cellular and biochemical levels. Weakness localized to a muscle disease might be further localized to a muscle membrane ion channel. Changes in cognition that reflect a diffuse hemispheric dementing illness might be further localized to abnormal metabolism of specific cytoskeletal proteins. This reductionist approach ultimately reveals the chemical pathophysiology of disease processes and suggests strategies for specific treatments.

What Is the Type?   There are four types of lesions: focal, multifocal, diffuse, and systemic. From the history alone, it should be possible to hypothesize whether a single focal lesion explains all the symptoms. This situation is common following a stroke and with the presentation of a primary tumor. A multifocal process is inferred by determining that more than one distinct lesion must exist to explain different constellations of symptoms. This situation can occur with multiple cardiac emboli, multiple metastases, and symptoms of multiple sclerosis. Diffuse processes affect the brain widely and produce symptoms in many categories, disrupting integrated behavior. Infectious, metabolic, and dementing illnesses are examples. Finally, there are several disease processes that usually affect particular pathways. For example, the dorsal columns and corticospinal tracts of the spinal cord are preferentially damaged in vitamin B_{12} deficiency—a process aptly called subacute combined degeneration. Other pathways in the cerebellum, brain stem, and spinal cord can be preferentially damaged by hereditary degenerative diseases, such as the olivopontocerebellar atrophies. The exact cause of many of these system degenerations is unclear. Future research will likely reveal whether a particular genetic abnormality, biochemical process, or antigenic site within these pathways makes them selectively vulnerable to particular diseases.

Pathophysiology

Finally, during the analysis of symptoms it is important for physicians to consider the type of pathophysiological events that are occurring. Traditionally, symptoms and signs have been categorized as positive or negative events. For example, a focal seizure is a positive symptom reflecting the active discharge of neurons in a seizure focus and its circuits that results in behavioral convulsions. Perhaps less obvious, tingling paresthesias in the fingertips are positive symptoms that can reflect spontaneous discharges in demyelinated sensory pathways. On the other hand, the numbness associated with injury to sensory pathways is considered a negative symptom because there is loss of function. Other examples of negative symptoms include weakness, aphasia, and visual loss.

There are "positive" symptoms and signs whose pathophysiology is complex and does not simply reflect an abnormal excessive discharge of neurons. A simple example is spasticity, in which there is an increase in muscle tone and reflexes. These changes result from a net decrease in inhibition of the spinal stretch reflex mechanism following damage to the corticospinal tract. The rigidity and tremor seen in parkinsonism is another, more complex example. In this case, changes in the balance of neuronal activity in sequential inhibitory circuits in the basal ganglia alter the initiation and control of movement.

The clinical utility of analyzing symptoms in this way lies not only in reaching conclusions about the underlying pathology but also in considering potential therapies. Many important pharmacological agents work at excitatory and inhibitory synapses and can be used to provide symptomatic relief from positive and negative symptoms even when the primary disease process cannot be cured.

At the conclusion of taking a neurological history, the physician should have reached clear hypotheses regarding the location of the lesion, the temporal profile of symptoms, and the basic type of pathological process. These hypotheses remain tentative, however, until tested further during the neurological examination and, if necessary, by laboratory investigation. It is always important to maintain some uncertainty, since the history may be incomplete or unreliable, or the patient may present new or unusual issues beyond a physician's current knowledge or understanding. In either case, the physician must generate a plan of action to fill in gaps in the story that prevent reaching a clear diagnostic conclusion. This may include selecting aspects of the neurological examination for particular emphasis, performing a few laboratory tests, consulting a colleague for advice, or searching the literature for additional information.

THE NEUROLOGICAL EXAMINATION

The neurological examination is performed to localize the site of damage to neuroanatomical structures that cause the signs and symptoms of neurological disease. There are several different strategies for using examination techniques to achieve this goal. First is the notion of the "complete" neurological examination—a sequence of tests that explore all neurological functions. While clinical neurologists come to know a great number of these examination techniques, they rarely need to use all of them on any one patient. Rather, the "complete" neurological examination is best thought of as a reference set of skills to be used selectively in individual circumstances. A "screening" neurological examination (see below) should be used quickly and efficiently as part of a general physical examination for the purpose of providing assurance that no major abnormalities of neurological function exist. Such a screening examination is a brief survey of the performance of most parts of the nervous system. All generalists should be able to perform a competent screening neurological examination. When neurological symptoms are present, certain components of the neurological examination are elaborated to explore and define subtleties of dysfunction in one or more systems. In these situations, a detailed "focused" neurological examination is used by the neurologist. In all situations, the neurological examination is an interactive exercise between the physician and the patient, who must work together to elicit, explore, and define abnormalities. This requires that the physician gain the confidence and cooperation of the patient at the outset. Examinations are most successful when their purpose is fully explained, when potentially misunderstood procedures are first demonstrated by the physician, and when the patient's own observations are encouraged and verified when abnormalities are found.

The neurological examination begins upon first contact with the patient. Indirect observation is important. The physician should note the patient's ability to give a clear history as well as any abnormalities of cognition, language, speech, or memory; how the patient walks, sits, and holds himself or herself during conversations; the symmetry of the face and body positions; the emotional range as illustrated on the face and in the voice; peculiarities of movement or lack of movement; and behavioral manifestations of pain in the face or posture. The patient's neurological behavior *before the examination* is an integral part of the examination.

During the early years of clinical practice, it is often best to perform the neurological examination according to a routine sequence of steps. A top-to-bottom approach is useful. Parts of the examination are performed in the vertical, sitting, and supine positions. The neurological examination described below should be viewed as an introductory outline. The best method for learning these skills is to practice them with an experienced neurologist. Subsequent chapters will expand upon examination techniques when relevant topics are discussed.

The Mental Status Examination

A patient's performance on a mental status examination is always in part a reflection of nondisease variables such as age, level of education, cultural background, employment history, and language. A skilled physician will modify specific questions to take these factors into account. If the patient has difficulty in giving a clear history, a thorough evaluation of mental status must be performed. Occasionally, a patient may feel insulted or embarrassed by mental status testing. For this reason, it is best to explain to the patient that these are standard tests used to measure specific skills.

1. Attention and concentration. An impairment in attention mechanisms can obscure all other aspects of the mental status examination. It is therefore important to test it first. Can the patient answer questions rapidly and accurately? If not, test one or more of these functions directly.

   a. Digit span. A patient should be able to repeat 7 ± 2 numbers forward and give 5 ± 1 numbers in reverse.

   b. The "A" test. The patient is asked to lift his or her hand every time he or she hears the letter "a" when being given a series of random letters. Failure to do so indicates impairment of attention.

   c. Serial sevens. Have the patient count backward from 100 by 7s.

2. Orientation. A patient should give the correct day, date, season, location, and circumstances surrounding the visit.

3. Language. Abnormalities in understanding speech (comprehension deficit), or in communicating clearly (expressive aphasia or dysarthria) are usually evident in the history taking. These observations can be further explored by direct testing.

a. Comprehension. Ask the patient to perform tasks of increasing complexity, e.g., hold up one hand; point to the ceiling, then to the door.

b. Observe the length of the patient's sentences in spontaneous speech for fluency, rhythm, and tonalities of language.

c. Naming. Ask the patient to name simple and then more uncommon objects, e.g., coat, collar, sleeve, buttonhole, watch, stethoscope.

d. Repetition. Ask the patient to repeat simple phrases, e.g., "no ifs, ands, or buts about it," "the third riding cavalry regiment." Observe for errors (paraphasia) in words or in sounds.

e. Reading. Ask the patient to read a simple magazine text, noting fluency and comprehension.

4. Memory. The test is organized to be certain that the patient can register, store, and recall *new* information. Recall of old information that can be verified is noted during history taking. Tell patients you will test their memory by asking them to remember three unrelated items. Say the items, e.g., "Mississippi river boat, Santa Monica fishing pier, Los Angeles Dodgers." Ask them to repeat these three items to be certain the items are registered. Five minutes later, ask them to recall the three items.

5. Cognitive skills. It is important to test a variety of intellectual skills and aptitudes to determine whether there are global problems with mental functions (suggesting a diffuse process) or isolated difficulties with a subset of functions such as memory, language, or reading (suggesting a focal lesion).

a. Calculations. $5 \times 7 - 19$, etc.

b. Verbal skills. Spelling "world" forward and backward.

c. Right versus left orientation of body parts and external objects, e.g., the examiner's hands and fingers.

d. Visual-constructive abilities. Ability to draw a clock and set a time; ability to copy a three-dimensional cube.

e. Word generation. How many animals can be named in 60 seconds (normal, 18 ± 6)? How many words beginning with the letter "s" can be named in 60 seconds (normal, 15 ± 5)?

f. Serial motor sequences. Ask the patient to copy the instructor's hand movements, e.g., slap, fist, scissors.

g. Shifting sequences. Test the patient's ability to alter performance with altered instructions, e.g., the patient is asked to tap once when the examiner taps twice, and twice when the examiner taps once.

h. Abstraction. Ask the patient to interpret simple proverbs, e.g., people who live in glass houses shouldn't throw stones.

Station and Gait Examination

1. Carefully observe the patient as he or she arises from the chair in the waiting room, walks into the examination office, and sits down. Is this action performed smoothly without hesitation and without problems of balance? Is there a full arm swing on both sides, with the feet slightly everted on a narrow base? Can the patient perform a tandem walk (heel-to-toe) without swaying; with eyes closed? Can the patient walk on heels and toes; hop on each foot independently; do a deep knee bend?

2. Stance and posture. Can the patient stand with heels and toes together, eyes closed, and not sway? Does the patient lose balance if pushed slightly?

3. Examine the pattern of the gait for common clinical abnormalities. The cerebellar gait is the drunken ataxic sailor. The parkinsonian gait shows a stooped, simian posture with short, shuffling steps. The steppage gait is characterized by exaggerated hip flexion to overcome a foot drop. Spastic hemiplegia shows unilateral circumduction of the leg and a flexed arm and wrist. Spastic paraplegia causes a scissor gait. The waddling gait is due to proximal muscle weakness. Dystonic/choreoathetotic gaits are interrupted by involuntary abnormal movements.

Cervical and Lumbar Spine Examination

Pain and limitation of motion in the neck and low back are common complaints, and these areas should be examined routinely. While the patient is standing, test the mobility of the head on the spine in flexion, extension, lateral rotation, and lateral bending. Test these same movements at the waist. Palpate and percuss the spine. With the patient in the recumbent position, perform the straight leg raising test to evaluate tightness of the hamstring muscles, low back mobility, and tenderness of the sciatic nerve.

Cranial Nerve Examination

I. Olfactory nerve. It is not important to test smell routinely. In patients suffering head trauma, there may be injury to these nerves. Test each nostril for detection of common odors such as coffee, cinnamon, etc.

II. Optic nerve.

a. Funduscopic examination: Inspect the clarity of the disk margins. Look for hemorrhages, exudates, and pigment.

b. Visual acuity. Test each eye alone with and without glasses.

c. Visual fields. Use the method of confrontation with unilateral and bilateral simultaneous stimulation.

d. Pupillary light reflex. Observe for direct and consensual pupillary constriction to a bright light.

III. Oculomotor nerve; IV. Trochlear nerve; VI. Abducens nerve.

a. Eye movements. Inspect the eyes to see if they are conjugate, and ask the patient about seeing double. Have the patient follow your finger through the six cardinal fields of gaze.

b. Smooth pursuit. Have the patient follow your finger to observe continuous tracking without interruption.

c. Saccades. Have the patient look quickly from one fixation point to another, 45 degrees apart.

V. Trigeminal nerve. The three zones of the sensory division of the fifth cranial nerve can be tested for appreciation of touch and pain. Compare side to side, using the same intensity of stimulus. When there is facial numbness, the corneal reflex is tested by applying a wisp of cotton at the edge of the cornea to observe for a bilateral blink response. The motor division of V is tested by observation of symmetric jaw opening and side-to-side movement. The jaw reflex is tested by percussion of the physician's finger against a half-open jaw.

VII. Facial nerve. The facial musculature is first tested by observation of spontaneous movements during the history taking. Simple inspection of the width of each palpebral fissure, the symmetry of the nasolabial folds, and the corners of the mouth will provide clues about subtle facial weakness. The speed and ultimate success in performing full facial movements are tested directly. Ask patients to raise their eyebrows, open and close their eyes, close their eyes tightly (bury their lashes), puff their cheeks, purse their lips, screw up their nose, and show their teeth.

VIII. Vestibular/acoustic nerve. Hearing can be simply tested by holding a 512-Hz tuning fork next to the patient's ear until the sound disappears. Compare the patient's hearing with your own. If there is diminution of hearing, inspect the ear canals for obstruction. Appreciation of air conduction should be better than bone conduction if the canals are unobstructed. Vestibular dysfunction is manifested by imbalance and nystagmus. Special maneuvers can be used to elicit vestibular signs (Chapter 5).

IX. Glossopharyngeal nerve; X. vagus nerve. Difficulty with speaking clearly or swallowing or a hoarse voice may indicate abnormalities of these nerves. The patient should be able to elevate the palate and the uvula in the midline when saying "ahhh." The patient should be able to appose both vocal cords to phonate a high-pitched sound ("eee"). The gag reflex tests IX and X.

XI. Accessory nerve. The sternocleidomastoid muscles are tested for strength by having the patient rotate the head laterally against resistance. The muscle is seen and felt. Shoulder shrug tests the upper portions of the trapezius muscles. Head flexion versus resistance is also a useful test.

XII. Hypoglossal nerve. The tongue is inspected in the mouth for symmetry of mass and the absence of any adventitious movements. Protrusion in the midline and rapid side-to-side movements of the tongue are inspected.

Motor Examination

The motor system is tested bilaterally for muscle mass, tone, and power versus resistance. Movements are tested for coordination and fine movement skills. Note any involuntary movements: tremor, myoclonus, chorea, etc.

1. Muscle mass. When there are symptoms of weakness, the muscle mass of the relevant area should be inspected, palpated, and compared against the other side or against normal. Inspect carefully for fasciculations.

2. Muscle tone. Move the upper and lower extremities through motions of flexion and extension to feel passive resistance. Determine if there is increased or decreased tone in an extremity, on one side, in the legs versus the arms.

3. Power. Subtle weakness can often be appreciated by observing a patient's movements independent of direct testing, such as a decrease in arm swing while walking. In addition, upper extremity weakness can be revealed by the presence of downward drift and pronation of a patient's outstretched arms, or by difficulty in manipulating a small object such as a coin in the hand. The muscles of the extremities are tested directly for strength against the examiner's resistance, primarily for movement around joints. If there is weakness, some clinicians find it useful to assign a grade of strength using the British system:

0 = No contraction
1 = Trace of contraction
2 = Active movement with gravity eliminated
3 = Active movement against gravity
4 = Active movement against resistance
5 = Normal power

4. Coordinative movements. Each extremity is tested for the ability to perform rapid, rhythmic, alternating movements. Ask the patient to tap the hand against the leg, alternating the palm and back side of the hand, or to rapidly rotate the outstretched hands, or to rapidly tap the first finger against the thumb. Lower extremities can be similarly tested with the patient tapping the floor or tapping the examiner's hand. Speed and accuracy of movements can be tested with the finger-to-nose test in the upper extremity and with the heel-to-knee-to-shin test in the lower extremity. These functions can also be tested for the muscles of articulation in speech by having the patient give rapid repetition of labial ("bbbb"), lingual ("lalala"), and pharyngeal muscles ("kakakaka").

5. Fine movements. Fine movements are best tested in each hand by rapid manipulation of a coin or by rolling a small piece of paper between the fingers. Testing the toes for the ability to wiggle them independently or to cross them over is also useful. These are the best tests of subtle lesions of the pyramidal system.

Sensory Examination

If there are no complaints of sensory loss (numbness, tingling), a simple "screening" examination is usually sufficient. Attention is directed primarily to the fingers and toes because these are supplied by the longest nerves, which are the most susceptible to injury or disease. The fingers and toes should be tested on each side for appreciation of pinprick, position sense, and vibration. It is often best to reassure the patient about the pinprick test by demonstrating it on your own hand. Use a clean, fresh pin on each patient. Instruct the patient to discriminate between a sharp touch and a dull touch. Test for appreciation of sharpness at the distal end of the extremities compared with more proximal sites. Test for the ability to feel a 128-Hz tuning fork in the fingers and toes until the vibration extinguishes. Test for appreciation of threshold of movement and direction of movement in the fingers and toes using small, slow joint displacements. Attention should be paid to right side versus left side differences as well as to distal versus proximal differences.

If sensory loss is a possibility, the affected region must be examined carefully. It is best to test sensory loss early in the sequence of the examination to gain the patient's full attention and cooperation. Does the zone of sensory loss relate to the distribution of a peripheral nerve or a spinal root? Is there a sensory level (spinal cord)? Is there a neglect of sensory stimulation when the patient is distracted (parietal cortex)? Temperature sensation is tested by a patient's appreciation of warm and cold by comparing a warm versus a cold branch of a tuning fork. "Cortical sensation" is tested by a patient's capacity to identify objects placed in the hand, to discriminate between two points placed closely on the skin, or to distinguish between rough and smooth textures.

Reflex Examination

Muscle stretch reflexes are tested with the percussion hammer and observations made concerning the strength of the reflexes compared to normal, side-to-side, and upper versus lower extremities. A grading scale is helpful.

Segmental Reflexes	Graded Response
Jaw jerk (V)	0 = no response
Brachioradialis (C5–C6)	1 = low normal
Biceps (C5–C6)	2 = normal
Triceps (C6–C7)	3 = brisk reflexes, not necessarily abnormal unless asymmetric
Finger flexors (C7–C8)	
Knee jerk (L2–L4)	4 = hyperactive and pathological, often associated with clonus
Ankle jerk (S1–S2)	

Superficial reflexes are tested on the abdomen by scratching above and below the umbilicus and observing for local contraction of the abdominal musculature. In males, the cremasteric reflex (L1 and L2) is tested by stroking the anterior medial thigh, observing for elevation of the testes. The anal reflex (cauda equina) is tested with a pin by touching the perianal area and observing for sphincter contraction.

The plantar reflex is tested for movement of the great toe in response to nociceptive (pain) stimulus of the plantar side of the foot (S1). An abnormal response is extension of the big toe and fanning of the smaller toes (the Babinski sign).

Summary and Formulation

At the end of the neurological examination a note is written succinctly summarizing the history for its chief complaint and time-intensity course. The abnormalities are summarized so as to lead to an anatomical localization of the abnormality. With these data it is possible to propose a differential diagnosis for the type of pathological process at an anatomical site. This summary leads to one or a few specific etiological hypotheses that can be tested by more history, additional examination, or laboratory tests.

The summary and formulation of each case are of critical importance. If insufficient time is devoted to this exercise, important data may be overlooked or diagnostic hypotheses not considered. The inclusion of lists of diagnostic possibilities and tests to be performed or of drawings in the note is often useful. A good note conveys the best thinking of the examining physician and serves historically as a marker in an evolving disease and therapeutic process.

THE SCREENING NEUROLOGICAL EXAMINATION

Generalists should be able to perform and describe a screening neurological examination—one that is brief, precise, and efficient (Box 2–1). This should be part of a general physical examination in the office or hospital or prior to surgery when there are no neurological symptoms requiring more detailed testing by a neurologist. Such recorded observations, even if they are entirely normal, provide an important reference point for the future. This is especially critical in the elderly, since the incidence of neurological illness increases rapidly with age.

BOX 2-1 The Normal Screening Neurological Examination

1. The patient gives a cogent history and answers questions rapidly and accurately without any clear evidence of difficulty with language, memory, or cognition, exhibiting an appropriate range of emotional expression.
2. Station, gait, and tandem gait are normal.
3. The face, tongue, and palate are symmetric at rest and during movement. Vision is normal bilaterally. Hearing is normal bilaterally. Extraocular movements are full without nystagmus.
4. The motor system is normal for mass, tone, power, and fine rapid movements in the upper and lower extremities.
5. The sensory system is normal for appreciation of pinprick and position sense at the fingers and toes.
6. Reflexes are normal at the biceps, triceps, knees, and ankles. There are no pathological reflexes.

LABORATORY INVESTIGATION

At the conclusion of the neurological history and examination, the physician determines whether laboratory tests will aid in the diagnosis and management of the neurological illness. The decision to perform a test, the choice of test, and the speed of performing the evaluation are critical factors. In cases of severe trauma or suspected intracranial hemorrhage, neuroimaging tests should be done emergently, often preempting the completion of a detailed history and examination if the patient will be best served by rapid transfer to the operating room. Common clinical conditions such as headache or neck or low back pain rarely require laboratory evaluation despite the realization that a test could rule out a rare lesion. Clinical judgment must weigh the costs of the tests, the possible discomfort and inconvenience to the patient, as well as the use of potential results on patient treatment and management.

The laboratory tests available to clinicians for studying diseases of the nervous system are some of the most potent in medicine. Neuroimaging studies can detect abnormalities at the millimeter level of resolution. Electroencephalography (EEG) can detect abnormal cortical discharges in patients with unusual spells, leading to a diagnosis of epilepsy and appropriate treatment. Electromyography (EMG) and nerve conduction studies are invaluable in diagnosing and classifying abnormalities of peripheral nerve and muscle. The uses of neuroimaging tests are described below, and examples are given throughout the book in relation to specific conditions. The use of EEG is described fully in Chapter 13 and of EMG and nerve conduction studies (NCS) in Chapter 3.

CT Scans

During a CT (computerized tomographic) scan of the brain, the patient lies on his or her back on a table and is advanced in small steps through a gantry that contains focused x-ray beams and photon detectors. As x-rays pass through the head, they are attenuated (deflected or absorbed) in proportion to the density of the tissue, with bone having the greatest density, water and cerebrospinal fluid (CSF) intermediate, and air least. Gray and white matter densities lie in between those of bone and CSF. The x-rays are passed through the tissue from a variety of angles, and the emergent intensity is measured by the detectors. The amount of x-ray attenuation for any volume unit (voxel) is assigned a relative absorption value, which is then digitally displayed on a black and white scale in a two-dimensional cross-section of the head. By convention, high-density structures such as bone are white, air and CSF are black, and brain tissue is revealed in shades of gray (Figure 2–3A). From these principles, it can be appreciated that when tissue becomes calcified, as with certain tumors, there will be an increase in density or whiteness. Similarly, there is increased whiteness in areas of acute hemorrhage owing to the presence of hemoglobin. Conversely, when tissue edema occurs there is a decrease in density owing to the increase in tissue water content. The diagnostic use of intravenous contrast agents containing iodine causes increased density in blood vessels as well as in areas where there is a breakdown in the blood-brain barrier around tumors, infections, or infarcts.

CT scanning is useful in the emergency evaluation of trauma and suspected intracranial bleeding because it is rapid and the patient can be observed fully during the test. It is also helpful in diagnosing and following hemispheric lesions such as primary or metastatic tumors. Although its resolution is not as good as that of the MRI scan in this situation, the CT scan is less expensive. While the CT scan shows relatively poor resolution of brain structures next to bone, such as around the pituitary, base of the brain, posterior fossa, and craniocervical junction, it is excellent for the examination of bones themselves.

MRI Scans

During an MRI (magnetic resonance imaging) scan of the brain, the patient lies on the back within a powerful magnetic field. The magnetic field causes the protons in the tissue to align themselves within this field. A radiofrequency pulse is then introduced into the field that causes the protons to move out of their original alignment. When the pulse is turned off, the protons fall back into their original magnetic alignment and give off their own radiofrequency signal, which is measured. This signal can be processed similarly to a CT scan to give an image of the brain.

The different signals given off by tissue depend on the density of protons and the time it takes for them to give off their signal upon relaxation. This relaxation time has two major components, called T1 and T2. The T1 decay time reflects protons giving off their energy to surrounding tissue, which is rapid in tissues of low water content. By convention, in T1-weighted images, CSF appears black while white matter pathways appear relatively more white (Figure 2–3B). The T2 relaxation curve depends on the rate of spin of the protons and the time it takes for them to become out of phase owing to the effects of neighboring protons. By convention, in T2-weighted images, CSF and water appear white (Figure 2–3C). Although the anatomic resolution of the T2 scan is not as good as that of the T1 scan, it is more sensitive to pathological changes because of the disruption of local proton environments. T1 and T2 scans are done as part of a single MRI brain scan sequence.

MRI scans are useful in the evaluation of almost all neurological conditions. Because conventional MRIs are slower than CT scans, however, they are not as useful clinically in emergency situations, in children or patients who cannot hold still for a long time, or in patients with implanted metallic devices such as cardiac pacemakers or aneurysm clips. In addition, MRI scans can cost 1.5 to 2 times as much as a CT scan. The field of MRI research continues to advance rapidly with the introduction of new strategies for pulse sequences and measurements, assays and imaging of other magnetic nuclei besides hydrogen, and the use of paramagnetic contrast agents.

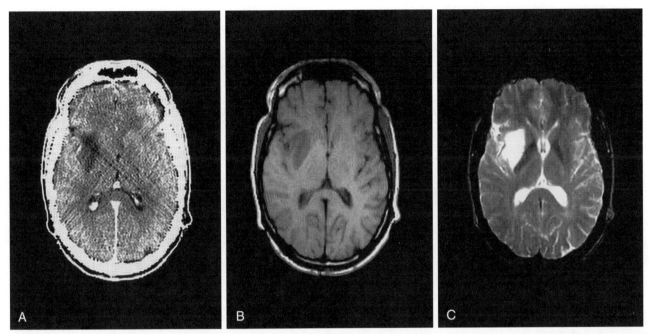

FIGURE 2–3. Co-registered images of a patient with a lesion in the right temporal lobe extending into the sylvian fissure and putamen. *A,* CT scan. *B,* T1-weighted MRI scan. *C,* T2-weighted MRI scan. The images indicate that the density of the lesion is the same as that of CSF. The smooth edges of the lesion, lack of distortion of surrounding tissue, and absence of edema indicate that it is likely a benign cyst. (Provided, with permission, by J. M. Fitzpatrick as part of the project "Evaluation of Retrospective Image Registration." National Institutes of Health, Project No. 1RO1NS33926-01. Principal Investigator, J. Michael Fitzpatrick, Vanderbilt University, Nashville, Tennessee.)

Lumbar Puncture

The indications for performing a lumbar puncture as part of a patient evaluation have decreased in recent years following the introduction of CT and MRI scans. The principal indication is to aid in the diagnosis of infectious meningitis, when patients present with fever, headache, stiff neck, and confusion. The goal is to obtain CSF for measurement of glucose and protein as well as microscopic and bacteriologic analysis. Even in this case, however, it is often wise to obtain a CT scan before proceeding if there is time. A posterior fossa brain abscess, although less common than meningitis, can present with the same symptoms. The mass effects of the abscess can cause herniation with brain stem compression following release of pressure with a lumbar puncture.

Lumbar punctures are also useful in the diagnosis of carcinomatous and lymphomatous meningitis and should be performed in suspected cases when brain imaging is normal or inconclusive. In positive cases, it is often important to give intrathecal chemotherapy via a lumbar puncture. Examination of the CSF can be useful in the evaluation of multiple sclerosis where there is usually evidence of increased production of immunoglobulin in the brain by finding raised IgG levels or oligoclonal bands (Chapter 14). Finally, lumbar punctures are indicated in the evaluation of normal pressure hydrocephalus as well as pseudotumor cerebri after appropriate indications are obtained from imaging studies.

The data from laboratory investigations usually will confirm, refine, or refute a diagnostic hypothesis. When studies are normal, they are important educationally for

the physician and occasionally for the patient who is overly concerned about a serious pathological process. Nevertheless, excessive use of costly tests in normal situations must be avoided.

The neurological history and examination, supplemented by results from appropriate laboratory tests, lead in most cases to the generation of a single etiologic hypothesis. In cases in which this cannot be achieved, at least the pathological process is almost always identified, such as infectious or degenerative, etc. (Figure 2–1). An appropriate treatment plan is initiated after education of the patient and the family on the results of the evaluation.

DNA Diagnostic Studies

Techniques for determining the presence of genetic abnormalities are now available in most medical centers as well as commercial laboratories. Analysis of DNA from white blood cells, muscle biopsy specimens, or fetal amniotic cells collected from amniocentesis during pregnancy often provides a specific diagnosis. Genetic counseling is part of the procedure to ensure that patients and the family are fully cognizant of the implications of possible results before a test is performed. Genetic tests are commonly done in evaluation of cases of myopathy (Chapter 7), peripheral neuropathy (Chapter 9), suspected Huntington's disease and the ataxias (Chapter 12), and occasionally for members of families with hereditary amyotrophic lateral sclerosis (Chapter 10) or Alzheimer's disease (Chapter 16).

SUMMARY

The diagnosis of neurological disease requires a complete history, a careful examination, and appropriate laboratory procedures. This exercise identifies the location of the lesion, provides understanding of the pathophysiology of the signs and symptoms, and identifies the cause in almost all cases. Patient education is an integral part of every step to ensure patients' cooperation and enlist their support in developing a plan of treatment. Diagnostic errors occur most commonly from failure to appreciate and fully explore the significance of a particular symptom or from too quick a leap from a common symptom to a supposed etiology before all possibilities are considered.

Selected Readings

Adams, R. D., and M. Victor. *Principles of Neurology*, 4th ed. New York, McGraw-Hill Book Co., 1989.

Duus, P. *Topical Diagnosis in Neurology*, 2nd ed. New York, Thieme Medical Publishers, 1989.

Weisberg, L. A., R. L. Staub, and C. A. Garcia. *Decision Making in Adult Neurology*, 2nd ed. St. Louis, Mosby, 1993.

SECTION II

THE NEUROLOGICAL BASIS OF SIGNS AND SYMPTOMS

Patients bring symptoms to physicians, who translate them into anatomical loci, pathophysiological events, and abnormal molecules in order to discover cause and cure. In neurology, this exercise proceeds by an orderly, step-by-step process based on an understanding of basic principles. These four chapters divide the domain of symptoms into four areas: abnormalities of the motor system, sensation, homeostasis, and higher brain functions. Patients' symptoms in these areas reflect abnormal molecular events at specific sites and times. Most patients are acutely aware of their abnormalities although their descriptions require careful analysis on the part of the physician. Other patients, however, may be unaware of a deficit that is obvious to family and friends. Clinicians must be prepared to recognize and evaluate the rich and diverse phenomenology that patients bring to them. In neurology, the disease changes the organ of behavior, a factor that challenges while it informs clinicians in their quest to help.

CHAPTER THREE

DISORDERS

OF THE

MOTOR SYSTEM

INTRODUCTION 24

ANATOMY AND PHYSIOLOGY 24

LOWER MOTOR NEURON SYSTEM 25

UPPER MOTOR NEURON SYSTEM 27

CORTICAL SYSTEMS 30

BASAL GANGLIA 31

    Hypokinetic Movement Disorders 32

    Hyperkinetic Movement Disorders 32

CEREBELLAR SYSTEMS 33

OCULOMOTOR SYSTEM 35

SUMMARY 36

INTRODUCTION

Weakness, slowness, fatigue, stiffness, incoordination, and abnormal movements are common disorders of the motor system that lead people to seek medical attention. Occasionally the symptoms reflect isolated, focal problems such as unilateral facial weakness or footdrop, while other symptoms reflect problems of complex integrated functions of the motor system such as difficulty in speaking or walking. The physician's job is to translate such symptoms into anatomical terms in order to localize the site of the abnormality, and to determine the temporal profile and clinical characteristics of the disorder in order to develop etiologic hypotheses (Chapter 2).

ANATOMY AND PHYSIOLOGY

The human nervous system devotes a large portion of its anatomy to the maintenance of posture and the performance of movement (Figure 3–1). The act of hitting a tennis ball serves as an example. The visual system gathers exteroceptive information and guides the movement of the body, arms, and legs in preparation for the swing at the oncoming ball. The vestibular and proprioceptive systems gather interoceptive information relative to the body's changing position and provide compensatory feedback to maintain balance and keep the eye on the target. The cerebellar system analyzes actual versus intended performance, making adjustments that provide smooth control of the temporal sequence and range of the movements. Cortical-subcortical loop circuits through the basal ganglia and thalamus continuously monitor ongoing changes in the magnitude and speed of movements and provide directives for subsequent action. The cerebral cortex becomes bilaterally activated in analyzing all this information, moving the body appropriately to receive the ball, assembling an internal program for the execution of the swing, and then driving the ball hard down the line or dropping it softly just over the net. Throughout this action, ongoing cortical decisions are projected through descending pathways to the anterior horn cells of the spinal cord and out this final common pathway to muscle. It is remarkable to think that all these events

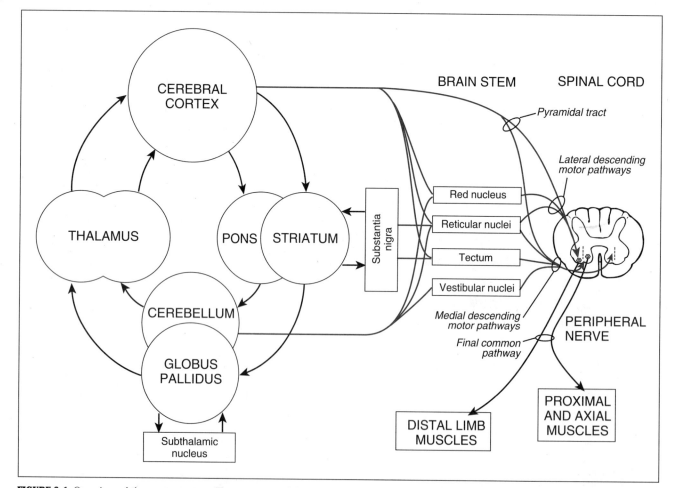

FIGURE 3–1. Overview of the motor system. The structures of the motor system are involved in the planning and execution of movement and the maintenance of posture. The initiation of movement and the maintenance of speed and accuracy are the functions of the hemispheres and the loop circuits through the basal ganglia–thalamus (striatum and globus pallidus) and cerebellum-thalamus. The execution of movement is projected from the hemispheres through medial and lateral descending pathways to brain stem and spinal cord motor neurons, which are the final common pathway for action.

are accomplished by simple changes in the sequence and firing rate of individual neurons throughout these integrated systems.

In the above example, it can be appreciated that a disorder of the visual, vestibular, or somatosensory system would impair the final swing of the racket. This fact emphasizes the integrated nature of the nervous system's component parts in the execution of movement, as well as the arbitrary choice of assigning certain structures and not others to the motor system. Nevertheless, there is clinical utility in defining and dividing the motor system into component parts. Diseases within these parts cause characteristic signs and symptoms of weakness and movement, providing clues for pathophysiology as well as etiology. This chapter provides an overview of the dysfunction that occurs from abnormalities in the lower motor neuron system, upper motor neuron system, cortex, basal ganglia, cerebellum, and oculomotor system.

LOWER MOTOR NEURON SYSTEM

The motor unit is defined as an anterior horn cell, its axon, neuromuscular junction, and innervated muscle fibers. The innervation density is a few muscle fibers per anterior horn cell in the extraocular muscles where fine control is essential. It is several thousand fibers per anterior horn cell in the extensor, antigravity muscles of the leg where strong contractions are important to maintain posture. The α-motor neurons of the brain stem and spinal cord determine the physiological and biochemical properties of their innervated muscle fibers. These range from slow twitch, oxidative, tonically contracting units (type 1, red fibers) to fast twitch, glycolytic, phasic motor units (type 2a and b, white fibers). When these fibers are stained for specific enzymes, a mosaic pattern is seen that reflects the interdigitation of motor units within the muscle (Figure 3–2A).

The state of contraction of a muscle at rest is called muscle tone. It is determined by the action of the muscle spindle, which monitors muscle length, and the Golgi tendon organ, which senses muscle tension. When a muscle is stretched, the muscle spindle fires impulses at high velocity through type 1A myelinated afferents to the spinal cord (Figure 3–2B). Through a monosynaptic reflex, the α-motor neurons then fire a volley back down to the muscle, causing a contraction that shortens the muscle, thus correcting for the stretch in length (Figure 3–2C). γ-Motor neurons innervate the muscle spindle itself to maintain appropriate tension. This servomechanism constantly maintains muscle length and tone in preparation for changing posture or the initiation of movement.

Testing this spinal cord reflex gives valuable information about both the lower and upper motor neuron system. The reflex is tested in two ways. First, by passively flexing and extending a patient's limb across a joint, the degree of tone in the stretched muscle can be appreciated. For example, by extending a patient's arm at the elbow, the tone of the biceps muscle is tested. A slight resistance is normally felt in a relaxed patient. Second, percussing a muscle tendon with a reflex hammer causes a quick mechanical stretch of the muscle that forcefully activates the spindles. The result is a highly synchronized discharge into the spinal cord to the motor neurons of the muscle and its agonists and then back down to the muscle, causing a synchronized muscle jerk, called the **tendon jerk**. Diseases that affect the motor unit cause weakness, a decrease in muscle tone, and a decrease in or loss of reflexes. These are the hallmarks of the lower motor neuron syndrome. By contrast, diseases affecting descending motor pathways above anterior horn cells cause weakness, an increase in muscle tone, and an increase in reflexes—hallmarks of the upper motor neuron syndrome (Table 3–1).

The exact site of the disease process within the four components of the motor unit can often be inferred from additional clinical signs. Disease of the anterior horn cell (e.g., motor neuron disease, amyotrophic lateral sclerosis) can cause **fasciculations**. These are spontaneous discharges of one or more motor units that are manifested as visible twitches of muscle fibers. However, they are not strong enough to cause a movement. Chronic disease of the anterior horn cell or its axon results in loss of the nerve's trophic influence on its muscle, causing atrophy of the muscle. For example, when a motor nerve is severed, up to 80% of the muscle will atrophy within 3 months.

Disease at the neuromuscular junction does not cause loss of reflexes or atrophy except in advanced

TABLE 3-1. Lower and Upper Motor Neuron Syndromes

	Lower Motor Neuron	Upper Motor Neuron
Structures involved	Anterior horn cell, root, nerve, neuromuscular junction, muscle	Cerebrum, brain stem, spinal cord
Muscles affected	Individual muscles	Groups of muscles
Wasting	Present, often marked	Absent
Fasciculations	Present	Absent
Tone	Flaccidity	Spasticity
Tendon reflexes	Decreased or absent	Hyperactive
Clonus	Absent	Present
Plantar responses	Flexor	Extensor (Babinski sign)
Superficial abdominal and cremasteric reflexes	Present	Absent
Electromyography (EMG)	Abnormal	Normal

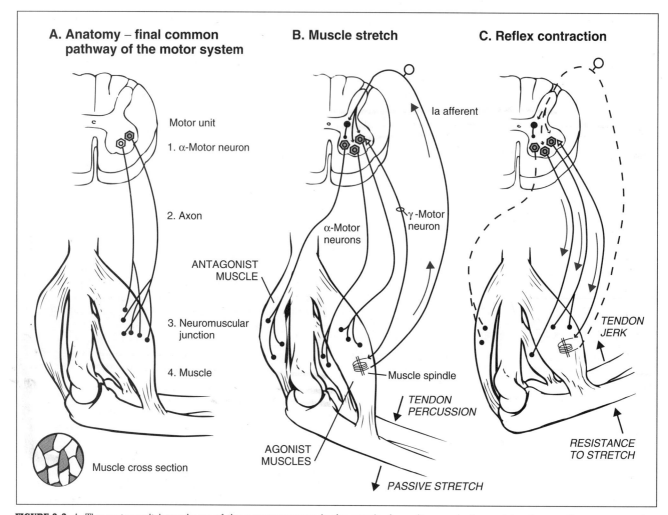

A. Anatomy – final common pathway of the motor system

Motor unit

1. α-Motor neuron

2. Axon

3. Neuromuscular junction

4. Muscle

Muscle cross section

B. Muscle stretch

Ia afferent

γ-Motor neuron

α-Motor neurons

ANTAGONIST MUSCLE

Muscle spindle

TENDON PERCUSSION

AGONIST MUSCLES

PASSIVE STRETCH

C. Reflex contraction

TENDON JERK

RESISTANCE TO STRETCH

FIGURE 3–2. *A,* The motor unit is made up of the α-motor neuron in the anterior horn, its axon in the peripheral nerve, the neuromuscular junction, and the innervated muscle fibers. Through trophic factors, the α-motor neurons determine the biochemical and physiological properties of muscle fibers such that a muscle is a mixture of different fiber types (cross section). *B,* The stretch reflex of muscle occurs when the muscle is either slowly stretched when the examiner tests muscle tone, or rapidly stretched following percussion of a tendon with a reflex hammer. The muscle spindle senses the stretch of the muscle and fires into the spinal cord to synapse on α-motor neurons that supply the muscle, as well as on adjacent agonist motor units. The stretch reflex inhibits adjacent antagonist motor units through an inhibitory interneuron. γ-Motor neurons innervate the muscle spindle to keep it taught and sensitive to stretch. *C,* Upon slow activation, motor units discharge into muscle to maintain tone; and upon synchronous activation their discharge produces the tendon jerk reflex. Damage to any element of the stretch reflex results in a decrease in tone and loss of the tendon reflex. Descending pathways above each brain stem and spinal cord segment synapse upon interneurons that modulate the stretch reflex. If these descending pathways are interrupted, the stretch reflex becomes disinhibited and there is an increase in muscle tone and hyperactive reflexes.

cases. The characteristic clinical feature of disease processes here is fatigability. Muscle power diminishes with repetitive use but recovers with rest owing to dynamic changes in the acetylcholine receptor (Chapter 8). Disease of muscle is associated with weakness that is most prominent in proximal muscles around the pelvic or shoulder girdle. This finding distinguishes muscle disease clinically from neurogenic weakness, which is most prominent distally. Neurogenic weakness (e.g., Guillain-Barré syndrome) often starts in the feet, reflecting the vulnerability of the longest axons to disease processes affecting peripheral nerves.

Laboratory tests are important in identifying the exact site of the lesion within the components of the motor unit, in determining the distribution of the disease throughout the body (e.g., local versus diffuse, upper versus lower extremities, proximal versus distal), and in providing information on the nature of the disease process (e.g., traumatic, degenerative, inflammatory, genetic). **Electromyography** (EMG) involves inserting a fine recording electrode into a muscle to record spontaneous activity and measure the effect of voluntary contraction. In normal muscle, there is little spontaneous activity during insertion of the electrode and none when the muscle is at rest. Mild voluntary contraction results in the discharge of individual motor units that are 0.5–1.0 mV in amplitude and 5–10 msec in duration. The amplitude of the motor unit discharge reflects the number of fibers activated by an axon. Maximal voluntary contraction causes a full interference pattern on EMG (Table 3–2).

EMG in neurogenic weakness shows characteristic

TABLE 3-2. Electromyographic Findings in Cases of Weakness*

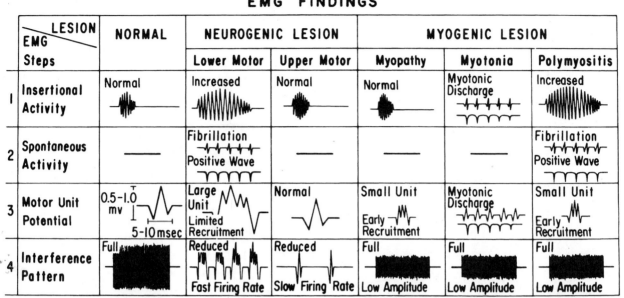

*Reproduced, with permission, from J. Kimura. *Electrodiagnosis in Diseases of Nerve and Muscle: Principles and Practice,* 2nd ed. Philadelphia, F. A. Davis, 1989.

abnormalities that contrast with muscle disease. There is often increased insertional activity and spontaneous muscle discharges at rest. These are called **fibrillations** and represent abnormally excitable muscle membranes. In contrast to fasciculations, they do not cause visible muscle fiber contractions. Mild voluntary contraction reveals large polyphasic units on EMG in neurogenic disease. This finding is characteristic of a neuropathic process in which both denervation and reinnervation occur. Large polyphasic potentials are caused by motor neurons that have added muscle fibers to their motor unit by reinnervating adjacent denervated muscle fibers. With advanced denervation, EMG records a reduction in maximal voluntary contraction. In contrast to neurogenic disease, muscle disease causes dropout of muscle fibers without any reinnervation. EMG records very small motor unit potentials. With maximal voluntary contraction, the interference pattern usually remains full but of lower amplitude in muscle disease than in neurogenic disease.

Nerve conduction studies are important for determining the presence, location, and type of a neuropathic process. The technique involves stimulating a peripheral nerve at a particular point and measuring the evoked compound muscle action potential and the sensory action potential (Figure 3-3). The velocity of the conduction and the amplitude are measured. Demyelinating disease (e.g., Guillain-Barré syndrome) is characterized by slow nerve conduction, since loss of myelin leads to loss of saltatory conduction. Conditions that primarily affect axons (e.g., toxins) result in a depression of the amplitude of the recording, since the number of fibers is diminished. Axonal damage occurs first at the distal end and proceeds as a "dying back" process. The velocity of conduction remains near normal in axonal neuropathies because myelination of the remaining fibers is preserved.

UPPER MOTOR NEURON SYSTEM

The upper motor neuron syndrome is characterized by weakness and **spasticity**, the latter defined as increased muscle tone, increased tendon reflexes, and abnormal reflexes (Table 3-1). Examples of the latter include the spread of reflexes to distant muscles when testing individual tendon jerks (e.g., the contralateral leg adductors contract when testing the knee jerk), clonus (e.g., the rhythmic contraction of agonist and antagonist muscles across the ankle when sustained pressure is applied to dorsiflex the foot), and the Babinski sign (Chapter 2). The cause of spasticity is the net loss of descending inhibitory influences on the spinal cord stretch reflex of the motor unit. As a result, for any given stretch of muscle there is an abnormally large reflex contraction. This results in increased muscle tone, especially in the flexors of the arms and the extensors of the legs, giving a characteristic posture to patients with severe spasticity. Arms become tonically flexed at the elbow and wrist, while the legs become tonically extended, resulting in circumduction during walking if one leg is involved and a scissors gait if both are involved. With mild spasticity, patients experience stiffness when standing up and walking and slow, awkward, effortful movements of the extremities. Patients occasionally comment that their hands or legs are more "disobedient" than they are weak. When testing muscle strength, an examiner will appreciate that a patient's effort is slow but that the patient can often achieve nearly full power. By contrast, in the lower motor neuron syndrome, flaccid weakness is characteristic.

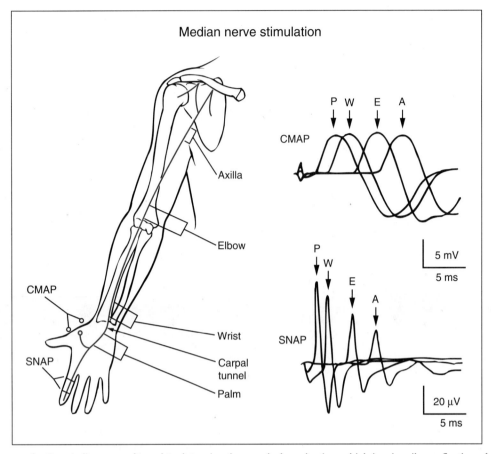

FIGURE 3–3. Nerve conduction studies are performed to determine the speed of conduction, which is primarily a reflection of myelination; and the amplitude of the response, which is primarily a reflection of the number of units that are activated synchronously. Motor nerves can be studied by measuring the compound muscle action potential (CMAP) using surface electrodes. Sensory nerve action potentials (SNAPs) are measured over small areas on the skin. The delay between the peaks of the motor and sensory potentials can be used to calculate the velocity of the nerve segment between two points. Normal values for nerve conduction velocities are above 55 m/s for most nerves. (Adapted, with permission, from J. Kimura, M. Machida, T. Ishida, et al. Relation between size of compound sensory or muscle action potentials and length of nerve segment. Neurology 36:647, 1986. Used with permission of Lippincott-Raven Publishers.)

The exact pathways involved in causing spasticity remain uncertain. It was once thought that lesions of the motor cortex or pyramidal tract were responsible, but experimental lesions in monkeys and rare small strokes in humans disproved this notion. Lesions in the medullary pyramid primarily cause *hypo*tonic weakness of the distal extremity. Lesions affecting the motor system outside the pyramidal tract, the so-called extrapyramidal system, play a role in causing spasticity, although the validity of this notion has changed in recent years. Modern studies of neuroanatomical pathways have shown that the concept of separate pyramidal and extrapyramidal systems is too simplistic. First, corticospinal fibers that travel within the pyramid give off collaterals to the basal ganglia, thalamus, red nucleus, and reticular systems as they move toward the spinal cord, thus directly influencing all the extrapyramidal centers (Figure 3–4). Second, fibers leaving the basal ganglia and the cerebellum project primarily onto the thalamus and hence back to the cortex to modulate the pyramidal system. Thus, the two systems are highly integrated and commonly travel together. Lesions in humans that are associated clinically with spasticity affect pathways which contain both long pyramidal fibers and shorter cortical-subcortical, striatal, thalamic, or cerebellar loop circuits. Small strokes in the internal capsule or pons causing spastic weakness are good examples.

The motor system can be more easily understood from the clinical perspective as comprising cortical, basal ganglial, and cerebellar systems that project into the spinal cord through medial and lateral systems (Figure 3–1). The medial system contains projections from the superior colliculus (tectospinal pathway), brain stem reticular nuclei (reticulospinal pathway), and vestibular nuclei (vestibulospinal pathway), which together receive modulating input from cortex, basal ganglia, and cerebellum. The medial system projects upon the medial aspect of the spinal cord through polysynaptic excitatory and inhibitory interneurons synapsing upon α-motor neurons. Motor neurons in the medial cord project upon paraspinal and proximal extremity muscles for the control of posture and midline body movements. The lateral system is composed primarily of corticospinal and rubrospinal projections upon interneurons in the lateral part of the spinal cord. A small percentage of pyramidal tract fibers end monosynapti-

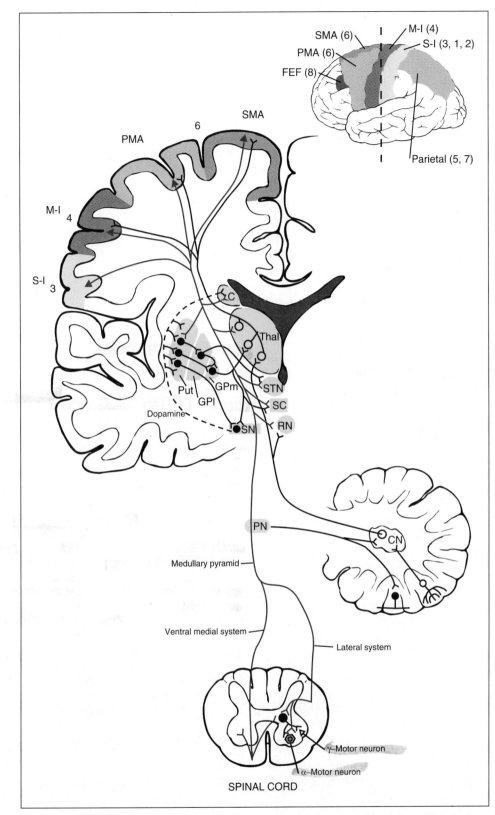

FIGURE 3–4. The pyramidal system. Corticospinal fibers that travel within the medullary pyramid originate primarily from the cortical motor areas: primary motor cortex (area 4), premotor cortex (area 6 laterally), and the supplementary motor cortex (area 6 medially). The primary sensory cortex (area 3) and parietal cortex (areas 5 and 7) contribute fewer fibers. The pyramidal system's primary projection is through the crossed lateral descending system onto anterior horn cells that project to the distal muscles of the limbs. There is also a medial uncrossed descending system that synapses both ipsilaterally and contralaterally on medial anterior horn cells projecting upon proximal and axial muscles. In their course down through the cerebrum, the corticospinal fibers send collaterals into the striatum, thalamus, midbrain, pons, and brain stem reticular nuclei, thus influencing other descending systems. The basal ganglia and cerebellum feed back upon the cortical motor areas to influence the pyramidal system. C, caudate; CN, cerebellar nuclei; FEF, frontal eye fields; GPl, globus pallidus lateral segment; GPm, globus pallidus medial segment; M-I, primary motor cortex; PMA, premotor cortex; PN, pontine nuclei; Put, putamen; RN, red nucleus; S-I, primary sensory cortex; SC, superior colliculus; SMA, supplementary motor cortex; SN, substantia nigra; STN, subthalamic nucleus; Thal, thalamus.

cally on α-motor neurons. Motor neurons in the lateral cord project upon the distal musculature of the limb for the execution of fine, coordinated movements.

The lateral and medial systems work synchronously during movement. To again use the example of hitting a tennis ball, the lateral system makes fine adjustments of the angle and speed of the racket, while the medial system executes large movements of the body and limbs to change position and maintain balance. Disease processes can differentially affect the lateral and medial systems, producing different types of symptoms. Diseases of corticospinal neurons caused by strokes of the motor cortex and internal capsule primarily affect the lateral system and disrupt fine, fractionated movements of the extremities. For example, patients typically exhibit slow, awkward movements when attempting to manipulate small objects, such as rolling a coin. As they put more effort into the performance, overflow contraction of proximal muscles occurs, causing abnormal posturing of the arm. Occasionally, other muscles are activated during effortful movements of the hand, such as the mouth and tongue, or the contralateral hand may exhibit "mirror" movements. By contrast, diseases of subcortical structures primarily affect the medial descending systems. The syndrome of progressive supranuclear palsy (Chapter 16) results from degeneration of neurons in the midbrain tectum and is associated with midline axial rigidity and difficulty with maintenance of posture.

Acute lesions of the upper motor neuron systems can initially cause hypotonic weakness that later evolves into spasticity. This is typical of spinal cord trauma, in which a state of areflexic flaccidity of the legs called spinal shock lasts for days or weeks before spasticity develops. This condition can be quite severe following spinal cord transection, and both extensor and flexor spasms can develop. The latter can be caused by stimuli arising from sores on the skin, such as bed sores, and are characterized by strong repetitive contractions of the legs and abdominal muscles.

Following damage to the motor system in the cerebral hemispheres, there is usually some recovery of function over time. Ipsilateral projections to proximal muscles from each hemisphere take on a major role when the other hemisphere is damaged. PET studies in patients recovering from stroke to one hemisphere indicate that the ipsilateral projections from the undamaged hemisphere become active during unilateral movements. Patients learn new strategies and sequences of movements to accomplish old tasks. For example, patients who have difficulty walking following

a stroke will improve by exercising on a treadmill. This process can be facilitated by suspending the patient in a harness to remove body weight and antigravity reflexes during the early phases of retraining. Doing so allows the emergence of intrinsic pattern generators for walking in the spinal cord and midbrain. Physical and occupational therapy are important in retraining submerged motor patterns as well as teaching new ones.

In considering the treatment of specific upper motor neuron symptoms, considerable attention has been given to the pharmacologic treatment of spasticity. However, in mild cases of spasticity, the increase in tone can provide useful stability to a weak leg, allowing the patient to stand and walk. In this situation, spasticity should not be treated. With severe spasticity, increased tone and extensor spasms impair function. The goal of therapy in this event is to relieve spasticity without unduly compromising strength. Useful agents are indicated in Table 3–3.

CORTICAL SYSTEMS

In its broadest definition, the motor cortex includes three large areas (Figure 3–4). The **primary motor cortex** lies along the precentral gyrus (Brodmann's area 4) and is characterized histologically by the high density of giant corticospinal Betz's cells in layer V. The primary motor cortex receives proprioceptive (muscle spindle and joint afferents) and cerebellar information from the thalamus as well as input from the other motor cortical areas. Electrical stimulation of primary motor cortex causes focal muscle contractions on the contralateral side. The **premotor cortex** (lateral part of area 6) lies anteriorly and receives input from thalamus and posterior association cortex. The **supplementary motor cortex** is located on the medial aspect of the hemisphere as an extension of area 6. It receives strong input from the basal ganglia relayed through the thalamus. Stimulation of premotor and supplementary motor cortex cause patterned movements rather than focal muscle contractions, but strong currents are required. The supplementary motor cortex projects ipsilaterally as well as contralaterally to the spinal cord so that bilateral movements occur with stimulation.

The broad design of the motor cortex was discovered by a neurosurgeon, Wilder Penfield, using surface-stimulating electrodes in awake patients during operations for epilepsy. Penfield found an orderly sequence of body movements when he stimulated along the central sulcus. The leg is located on the medial aspect of the hemisphere, the hand in the middle of the motor

TABLE 3-3. Pharmacologic Treatment of Spasticity

Drug	Mechanism of Action	Dosage*	Side Effects
Diazepam	Enhances GABAergic inhibition	5–50 mg/d	Sedation
Baclofen	? Blocks glutamate	10–80 mg/d	Drowsiness, nausea, weakness
Clonidine	Is α-adrenergic agonist	0.2–0.6 mg/d	Hypotension
Dantrolene	Dissociates excitation-contraction coupling in muscle	25–100 mg/d	Weakness, diarrhea

*Treatment is initiated with low doses, which are increased slowly over weeks and months. Cessation of treatment is by gradual withdrawal.

strip, and the face at the bottom of the precentral gyrus adjacent to the sylvian fissure. The body parts on the cortex fit together in a figurine called a homunculus. Small strokes and tumors can differentially affect these areas, primarily causing focal weakness of the contralateral site.

Intracortical stimulating and recording electrodes have revealed considerable complexity within this homuncular design of the motor system. For example, although neurons within individual cortical columns for the hand seem to be preferentially targeted on individual muscles, they also send input to other muscles involved in synergistic hand and arm movements. Thus, each muscle receives input from several cortical columns in different areas and each column influences several muscles in addition to its main target. The fine details of cortical organization for movement are arranged within a mosaic, or "fractured somatotopy," within large cortical domains for the leg, arm, and face. There is sensory feedback to these columns from the movement produced by stimulating the column. Thus, the motor system is highly integrated and behaves operationally as a sensorimotor, tactile, kinesthetic unit. In addition to the status of sensory input, the use of any particular combination of columnar outputs during action is conditional upon the past experience or training of the person, as well as momentary attentional and intentional (motivational) factors. Studies using functional MRI scanning in humans indicate that the pattern of activation of motor cortex during hand movement is unique for each movement, but there is at least 50% overlap among the various patterns. In essence, rather than viewing the motor cortex as a hard-wired homuncular map for muscles, the metaphor of a piano keyboard is more appropriate. Combinations of different notes, forever changing in tempo and strength, are called upon under different situations to produce the rich melodies of movement.

Recent studies with PET scans reveal that different parts of the motor cortex become differentially activated in preparing for and executing a movement. The supplementary motor cortex becomes activated before a movement. All three areas are active during a movement. The premotor cortex becomes strongly activated during imagining a movement. In addition, the anterior cingulate gyrus (areas 24 and 32) plays an important role in new movements requiring attention, and the parietal cortex (areas 5 and 7) becomes active in movements when the arms are directed toward specific targets in space.

Disease processes within these areas produce different effects upon movement. In general, lesions anterior to the cortical motor areas in prefrontal and cingulate cortex result in a general decrease in movement, especially with bilateral lesions. Patients appear apathetic. Although individual movements can be produced normally on command, the poverty of movement during everyday life reflects lack of attentional or motivational input into the motor system. Some have called this condition "motor neglect." Lesions located posteriorly in parietal cortex result in a lack of attention and movement into contralateral space. Patients do not turn their heads or eyes toward new stim mistakes in reaching toward targets. Th contralateral somatic stimuli. This con... times called "sensory neglect." Lesions here can disrupt the smooth execution of movements, particularly in relation to external objects. Despite the relative absence of weakness or sensory abnormalities, patients have difficulty with learned behaviors such as using a key to open a lock or folding a letter and putting it in an envelope. Such difficulty with learned motor skills is called **apraxia**. Bilateral lesions are particularly potent in causing apraxia, such as occurs in Alzheimer's disease.

BASAL GANGLIA

The basal ganglia include the striatum (caudate and putamen), globus pallidus, subthalamic nucleus, and substantia nigra and their projections into midbrain and thalamus (Figure 3–5). Nearly all neocortical areas project upon the striatum, indicating that the basal ganglia participate in cognitive, sensory, and motiva-

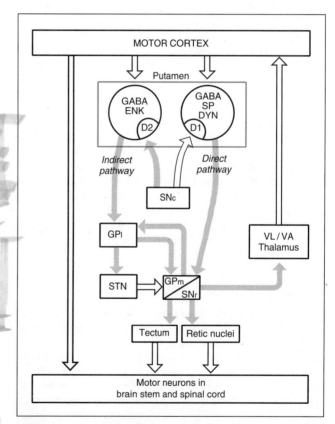

FIGURE 3–5. The functional anatomy of the basal ganglia has been examined by neuropharmacological studies of neurotransmitters and receptors as well as by electrophysiological studies of changes in neuronal firing rates following lesions. The diagram represents a simplification of ongoing work that allows testing of new therapies for disorders of the basal ganglia. Solid arrows indicate inhibitory connections. Open arrows indicate excitatory connections. D1 and D2, dopamine receptors; DYN, dynorphin; ENK, enkephalin; GABA, γ-aminobutyric acid; GPl and GPm, lateral and medial segments of the globus pallidus; SNc, substantia nigra, pars compacta; SNr, substantia nigra, pars reticulata; SP, substance P; STN, subthalamic r cleus; VL/VA, ventrolateral and ventroanterior thalamic nuclei.

tional processes as well as motor functions. For example, the prefrontal cortex projects upon the head of the caudate and subsequently upon a restricted portion of the substantia nigra, pars compacta. It receives input from the anterior and the dorsomedial thalamic nuclei, maintaining a separate but parallel cortical-basal ganglion cognitive loop similar to the motor system loop. Disorders within this circuit cause changes in cognitive and emotional behavior (Chapter 6).

The motor, sensory, and parietal cortical areas project upon the putamen where a somatotopy of body parts is maintained. The corticostriatal projection is glutamatergic, synapsing on neurons within a matrix that surrounds histological structures called striosomes. The matrix projects to the globus pallidus. The striosomes primarily receive input from the limbic system and project to the substantia nigra. Currently it is unclear whether there is integration between these functional systems within the putamen.

There are two projection pathways out of the putamen for the motor system (Figure 3–5). The direct pathway projects upon the medial, or internal, segment of the globus pallidus and the substantia nigra, pars reticularis. These structures subsequently project to thalamus and thence to supplementary motor cortex. Discharges from the corpus striatum through this pathway have the net effect of stimulating movement by decreasing inhibitory input upon thalamus. By contrast, discharges through the indirect pathway to the lateral, or external, segment of the globus pallidus have the net effect of inhibiting movement. This occurs when the subthalamic nucleus becomes disinhibited and fires strongly upon the medial globus pallidus. The result is increasing inhibitory input upon the thalamus. The physiological and pharmacological experiments that revealed these pathways have allowed classification of clinical disorders by the site of the lesion and the neurotransmitters involved. This information has allowed rational choice of pharmacological and surgical therapy for some basal ganglia disorders (Chapters 11 and 12).

Hypokinetic Movement Disorders

Parkinson's disease is the prime example of the hypokinetic movement disorders of diseases affecting the basal ganglia (Chapter 11). It is characterized by rigidity of muscle tone, decreased movements (bradykinesia and akinesia), and resting tremor. *Rigidity* is different from *spasticity*. When an examiner tests muscle tone in a patient with rigidity, there is increased resistance in all directions of movement and often a ratcheting, or cogwheel, characteristic to the resistance. Muscle tendon jerks remain normal, and there are no pathological reflexes with rigidity. Voluntary control of movement and muscle strength are preserved but greatly slowed. **Bradykinesia** is manifested as decreased speed in both involuntary and voluntary movements. There is a decrease in facial expression, strength of voice, speed of chewing and swallowing, and associated movements, such as swinging the arms while walking. The gait is characterized by slow, short, shuffling

steps. Postural mechanisms become impaired in basal ganglia diseases, resulting in frequent falls in advanced cases.

In Parkinson's disease, there is degeneration of the dopaminergic nigrostriatal pathway, and the symptoms of the hypokinetic movement disorder correlate with depletion of dopamine in the putamen. For much of the illness the symptoms can be largely reversed by giving patients L-dopa medications that restore the magnitude and balance of activity in the direct and indirect pathways. In cases in which tremor or rigidity dominates, surgical lesions of the medial globus pallidus or its projections into the thalamus can provide some relief. Such lesions are thought to interrupt the inhibitory influence of the basal ganglia upon thalamocortical projections. PET studies of patients who have had this operation show a return of functional activity to the motor cortex.

Hyperkinetic Movement Disorders

Huntington's disease is the prime example of the hyperkinetic movement disorders of basal ganglia diseases and is characterized by abnormal involuntary movements (Chapter 12). Traditionally a variety of different names are used to describe these movements depending upon their magnitude, speed, and duration. **Chorea** is a rapid, dancing movement. In Huntington's disease, it can occur in the muscles controlling the face, eyes, limbs, and torso. In the early, or mildest, phase of the disease a patient may blend a choreic movement into a gesture, such as wiping the brow when a choreic movement jerks the hand upward. In advanced cases, chorea takes over the entire body, producing a grotesque dance of continuous contortions. The cause of these movements is thought to result from degeneration of medium spiny stellate cells in the striatum that project through the indirect pathway to the lateral globus pallidus (Figure 3–5). The net effect is to decrease the inhibitory output of the basal ganglia upon the thalamus, thus accentuating thalamic stimulation of the motor cortex.

Athetosis is a descriptive term for movements that are slower and more writhing than chorea, but the two terms are often combined as in **choreoathetoid** movements. Such movements are characteristic of children with cerebral palsy who have suffered neonatal hypoxia-ischemia of basal ganglia structures. **Dystonia** is characterized by sustained contractions that hold the limbs or body in tonic postures that change very slowly. The site of the abnormality in dystonia is unknown. The dystonia can be focal, and writer's cramp is considered such an example, or generalized, as in the inherited dystonias. Dopamine-responsive dystonia is a disorder that has been localized to chromosome 14, and generalized torsion dystonia has been localized to 9q34. Advances in molecular genetics will provide insight into the pathophysiology of the dystonias.

Hemiballismus is a rare but very specific abnormality of movement characterized by wild flailing of one arm. The cause in most patients is a small stroke of the subthalamic nucleus. It is proposed that this lesion decreases the inhibitory output of the basal ganglia upon the thalamus. The condition subsides slowly over several weeks. The use of high doses of a dopamine-blocking drug such as haloperidol can be beneficial in treating hemiballismus. Dopamine blockers can also be occasionally helpful in other patients with hyperkinetic movements of dystonia and chorea.

Spasmodic torticollis is an unusual movement disorder characterized by intermittent contraction of sternocleidomastoid and trapezius muscles, twisting the head and pulling the ear toward the shoulder. The site of the lesion and the nature of the abnormality are unknown. Interestingly, many patients discover that simply touching their face lightly will restrain the movements for a few moments. Systemic medicines, psychotherapy, and ablative surgery have proved ineffective. Current therapy uses controlled injections of botulinum toxin to destroy neuromuscular endings in the offending muscles. The goal is to decrease the force of spasms without producing undue weakness. In experienced hands, the treatment is effective. Botulinum toxin is also effective in treating blepharospasm, hemifacial spasms, and some cases of focal dystonias and tics.

CEREBELLAR SYSTEMS

The cerebellum can be divided transversely into three anatomical and functional components (Figure 3–6). The phylogenically oldest part (***archaeocerebellum***) is the flocculonodular lobe buried inferiorly and posteriorly under the main body of the cerebellum. An extension of the vestibular system, it is primarily involved with maintenance of head, eye, and body position in response to changes in head position. Lesions of the structure occur with childhood medulloblastomas that characteristically cause **titubation**, an instability of the body in the sitting and standing position, and nystagmus (see below).

The anterior lobe of the cerebellum receives input from spinocerebellar pathways and is primarily concerned with gait (***paleocerebellum***). The spinocerebellar pathways project into the midline cortex of the cerebellum, into both the vermis and paravermal zones, which contain somatotopic organizations both anteriorly and posteriorly. Visual and auditory representations are found between the two body representations (Figure 3–6). These midline zones seem to be primarily concerned with analyzing proprioceptive input from the limbs and body for the control of balance, coordinated movement, and walking during ongoing action. Alcoholism causes toxic degeneration of the anterior lobe and vermis of the cerebellum and results in a wide-based, ataxic gait and tremor of the arms.

The large hemispheres of the cerebellum constitute the posterior lobe and are phylogenically the most recent addition (***neocerebellum***). They receive input from the cerebral cortex via the pontine nuclei—the crossed corticopontocerebellar system (Figures 3–4 and 3–6). The cerebellar cortex of the hemispheres projects upon the dentate nuclei, which in turn project primarily upon contralateral red nucleus and the ventrolateral

thalamic nucleus—the dentatorubrothalamic tract. This nucleus relays cerebellar information to the primary motor cortex, exerting a direct influence of the cerebellum upon fine movements. Cerebellar outputs from the deep nuclei also project to the reticular and vestibular nuclei in the brain stem, which along with the red nucleus project through descending systems into the spinal cord. PET studies demonstrate that the cerebellar hemispheres and deep nuclei become activated during imagined as well as real movements, and during conditional learning paradigms such as the classical eye-blink response.

Lesions of the cerebellum cause incoordination of movements, or ataxia. Gordon Holmes, a British neurologist who studied gunshot wounds to the cerebellum in World War I soldiers, proposed that the basic abnormality was a decrease in muscle tone. This can be appreciated in the acute stage of injury, such as following an infarct of the superior cerebellar artery to the cerebellar hemisphere. The loss of tone is thought to be due to a decrease in descending cerebellar stimulation on the γ-motor neuron and muscle spindle. Hypotonia causes pendular tendon jerk reflexes and the phenomenon of rebound. The latter is tested by having the patient hold out his or her arms in a fixed position and then striking them both downward. The arm on the side of the cerebellar lesion will fail to check, travel farther, and then rebound farther upward as it attempts to recover. This oscillation of movement about an intended target also characterizes the **intention tremor**, or **dysmetria**, seen on the finger-to-nose and heel-knee-shin tests with cerebellar lesions. This same type of abnormality can also be seen during eye movements. The eyes will overshoot the target, then overshoot on rebound, and only slowly oscillate to the fixation point, an abnormality called **saccadic dysmetria**. During rapid alternating movements, such as supination-pronation of the arms, the movements quickly decompose, a sign called **dysdiadochokinesia**. Speech can also be affected. The smooth sequence of delivery is broken up by unintended pauses, as though the patient were reading poetry.

In contrast to the parkinsonian tremor, which occurs at rest and disappears with movement, **cerebellar tremor** appears with movement and is absent at rest. Characteristically occurring at 2–3 Hz, it can be of large amplitude, making coordinated movements such as eating and drinking impossible. There is no good medical treatment at present. In severe cases, surgical lesions placed in the ventrolateral thalamic nucleus provide relief.

Benign familial tremor occurs as a rhythmic, 6- to 8-Hz, to-and-fro movement that can affect the head, voice, and upper extremities. It is also called **essential tremor** or **senile tremor**. The site of the neurological abnormality is unknown. Catecholamines play a role in this tremor, since β-blockers (e.g., propranolol) provide some relief. Primidone can also be useful. Certain metabolic conditions (e.g., hyperthyroidism, alcohol withdrawal, lithium toxicity, and anxiety) are associated with an **action tremor**, which

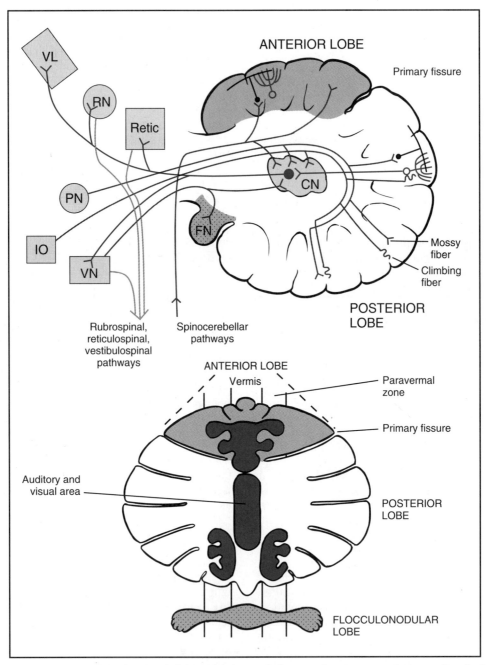

FIGURE 3–6. Cerebellar systems. The three functional divisions of the cerebellum can be seen on sagittal as well as horizontal views. The flocculonodular lobe (dotted) receives input from the vestibular system. The anterior lobe (shaded) receives its main input from the spinocerebellar pathways, which also project to the midline vermis and paramedian vermal zones along the longitudinal axis of the cerebellum. The cerebellar hemispheres (posterior lobe) receive their principal input from the cerebral cortex via the mossy fibers in the pontine nuclei. Each fiber influences many Purkinje cells. The climbing fibers from the inferior olive also innervate the cerebellum, synapsing individually on the Purkinje cell. All cerebellar afferents innervate the deep nuclei as well as the cortex. The output of the deep nuclei projects upon the ventrolateral thalamic nucleus for feedback to the motor cortex; and upon the red nucleus and vestibular and brain stem reticular nuclei, which send fibers to brain stem and spinal cord motor neurons. CN, cerebellar nuclei; FN, flocculonodular lobe; IO, inferior olive; PN, pontine nuclei; Retic, reticular nuclei; RN, red nuclei; VL, ventrolateral thalamic nucleus; VN, vestibular nuclei.

is an accentuation of normal physiologic tremor at 8–12 Hz.

OCULOMOTOR SYSTEM

The oculomotor system in the brain stem is composed of the cranial motor nuclei to the eye muscles (III, IV, and VI), the lateral gaze center in the parapontine reticular formation, the vertical gaze center in the midbrain, and the interconnecting pathways between these sites (Figure 3–7). Input from the vestibular system plays a continuous role in keeping the eyes steady during head movements—the vestibulo-ocular reflex (Chapter 5). Input from the superior colliculus links visual input from the retina to the oculomotor system for tracking objects in central vision (smooth pursuit), and for the quick jerk response of the eyes (saccades) to the appearance of new stimuli in peripheral vision. Superimposed upon these lower motor neuron systems are the cortical systems that volitionally modulate both smooth-pursuit movements from the posterior hemisphere and saccadic eye movements from the frontal eye fields.

Lesions within the oculomotor system produce characteristic abnormalities of eye movement that reflect the site of the lesion (Table 3–4). Clinicians experi-

FIGURE 3–7. The oculomotor system. The third, fourth, and sixth cranial nerve nuclei to the eye muscles are integrated into a functional unit by subcortical and cortical systems to maintain vergence of the eyes and unitary vision in all directions of gaze. Input from the vestibular system maintains fixation of gaze during movements of the head, called the vestibulo-ocular reflex (VOR). There is a "lateral gaze center" in the parapontine nucleus adjacent to the sixth nerve nucleus. It coordinates horizontal gaze to the same side through the sixth nerve (abduction) and the contralateral third nerve (adduction) via the medial longitudinal fasciculus. A "vertical gaze center" in the midbrain serves to coordinate both third nerve nuclei in up-and-down gaze. The midbrain tectum also coordinates the light reflex (Edinger-Westphal nucleus) and near reflex for both eyes. The cortex controls volitional gaze by descending pathways to the centers in the tectum and brain stem. FEF, frontal eye field; MLF, medial longitudinal fasciculus; PPRF, parapontine reticular formation.

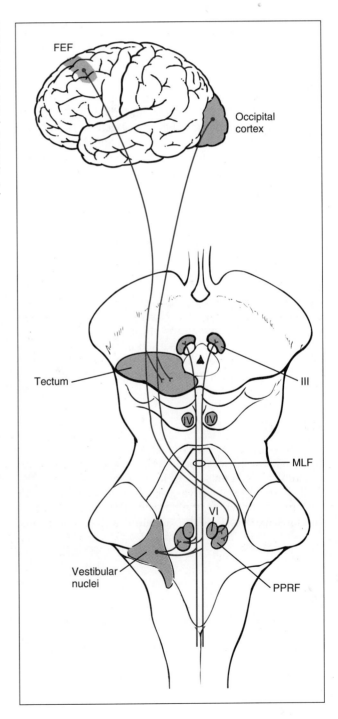

TABLE 3-4. Disorders of the Oculomotor System

Site	Example	Clinical Findings
Eye muscle	Kearns-Sayre mitochondrial myopathy	Progressive external ophthalmoplegia
Neuromuscular junction	Myasthenia gravis	Fatigue on upgaze, ptosis, diplopia due to fluctuating weakness
Third nerve palsy	Diabetes	Ptosis, diplopia due to weak adduction, pupil usually normal
	Aneurysm	Ptosis, diplopia due to weak adduction, pupil usually dilated and nonreactive
Sixth nerve palsy	Intracranial pressure	Diplopia due to weak abduction
Midbrain tectum	Pinealoma	Weak upgaze, dilated nonreactive pupils, nystagmus on upgaze and convergence (Parinaud syndrome)
Medial longitudinal fasciculus	Multiple sclerosis	Internuclear ophthalmoplegia: diplopia due to weak adducting eye, with nystagmus of abducting eye
Lateral brain stem	Stroke	Ipsilateral gaze palsy
Frontal cortical eye field	Stroke	Contralateral gaze palsy
Basal ganglia	Parkinson's disease	Slow (cogwheel) pursuit movements, hypometric saccades

enced in identifying and testing for these abnormalities bring expertise in localization and diagnosis of many nervous system abnormalities. Inspection of the eye positions at rest and during saccadic and pursuit movements reveals much information about the nervous system. The light reflex and near vision reflex (convergence) test the oculomotor nuclei in the midbrain. The presence of **nystagmus** provides important clues regarding the site and etiology of disease. This sign is a quick involuntary jerk of the eyes that is named for the direction of the fast component, such as left, right, clockwise, vertical, and so on. Nystagmus can occur at rest or with eye movements (gaze-direction nystagmus). In the latter event, there are often other signs of brain stem or cerebellar dysfunction indicating a central cause for the nystagmus. Nystagmus can also be induced by quick movements of the head, which is usually accompanied by the sensation of vertigo, or spinning. In these cases, there are usually abnormalities of the vestibulo-ocular pathways either peripherally or centrally (Chapter 5).

SUMMARY

The motor system extends from the cerebral cortex to individual muscle fibers. Responsible for involuntary postural adjustments as well as planned acts of great skill, it receives modifying input from all other brain systems. It provides the functional output by which humans express thought, emotion, and intention and

discover it in others. Disorders of the component parts of the motor system cause characteristic changes in balance and movement that reflect the site and etiology of the abnormality. Experienced clinicians come to recognize these abnormalities by carefully listening to the details of patients' symptoms and observing the telltale signs of site-specific dysfunction. Careful physical examination of muscle mass, tone, strength, speed, and dexterity during willed, involuntary, and reflex-induced movements provides the necessary additional information for formulating an anatomical and etiological hypothesis to be further tested in the laboratory.

Selected Readings

Chollet, F., V. DiPiero, R.J.S. Wise, et al. The functional anatomy of motor recovery after stroke in humans: A study with positron emission tomography. Ann Neurol 29:63–71, 1991.

Decety, J., D. Peranl, M. Jeannerod, et al. Mapping motor representations with positron emission tomography. Nature 371:600–602, 1994.

Deiber, M.-P., R. E. Passingham, and J. G. Colebatch. Cortical areas and the selection of movement: A study with positron emission tomography. Exp Brain Res 84:393–402, 1991.

Graybiel, A. M., T. Aosaki, A. W. Flaherty, et al. The basal ganglia and adaptive motor control. Science 265:1826–1831, 1994.

Houk, J. C., and S. P. Wise. Distributed modular architectures linking basal ganglia, cerebellum, and cerebral cortex: Their role in planning and controlling action. Cereb Cortex 2:95–110, 1995.

Sanes, J. N., J. P. Donoghue, V. Thangaraj, et al. Shared neural substrates controlling hand movements in human motor cortex. Science 268:1775–1777, 1995.

Young, R. R. Spasticity: A review. Neurology 44(suppl. 9):S12–S20, 1994.

CHAPTER FOUR

DISORDERS

OF

SENSATION

INTRODUCTION 38

SENSORY LOSS 38

PAIN 41

    Peripheral Nerve Pain 43

    Trigeminal Neuralgia 43

    Headache 43

    Neck Pain 46

    The Low Back Syndrome 46

VISUAL LOSS 47

HEARING LOSS 50

SUMMARY 51

INTRODUCTION

Sensory systems are organized to perceive light, sound, and odor in the outside world and to sense changes on the surface of the body and within its internal milieu. The visual, auditory, and olfactory systems detect and analyze stimuli at a distance, while specialized somatosensory endings and pathways sense changes in touch, pressure, movement, heat, and pain. All systems share characteristic features. There is a threshold for activation for peripheral receptors which signal that *something new* has just happened. There is specificity in peripheral fibers and central pathways for the different types of modality of stimuli, such as touch versus temperature on the skin, or different frequencies of sound or light. These labeled lines of communication identify *what* has just happened. The frequency of firing of sensory nerves conveys the *intensity* of the event. The location of the sensory endings on the skin or in the retina faithfully convey *where* the event is localized on the body or in external space by preserving topographic relationships in body maps and visual field maps in central stations.

Sensory pathways are almost everywhere only one synapse away from motor pathways so that the two systems operate as an integrated functional unit in everyday life. Occasionally the new information is of such a type, location, or intensity that a primitive reflex is automatically and instantly invoked, such as flexion withdrawal of the hand from a sharp object, the saccadic jerk of the eyes toward a large, dark shadow that intrudes into a peripheral field, or a jump of the entire body upon a sudden loud sound. Such sensations arouse behavior to a state of vigilance, turn the head and eyes toward the stimulus, and prepare the body for fight or flight. At the other behavioral extreme, sensory stimuli can be silently and dispassionately observed, collected, analyzed, and stored for future reference. This act requires focused attention, suppression of body movement, and the exercise of well-developed cognitive skills.

Disorders of sensation can occur as isolated clinical problems, since the systems are partially separated from other neuroanatomical systems as they travel from the periphery to the cortex. For example, a common clinical malady such as stroke can cause pure sensory loss of the arm with infarction of the thalamus, or complete visual loss in one eye with ischemia of the retina. In addition, certain disease processes selectively affect sensation owing to the specificity of epitopes on proteins, such as the immune-mediated sensory loss associated with small cell carcinoma of the lung or with Sjögren's syndrome.

Clinicians should be adept at eliciting disorders of sensation, recognizing that patients commonly use terms that must be translated from one disorder to another, such as mistaking numbness for weakness, or dizziness for visual blurring. A tingling sensation (**paresthesia**) can be instructive, usually indicating highly localized information about abnormalities within a particular nerve, root, or central pathway. Humans are able to detect the spontaneous discharge of a single sensory axon. Injured as well as regenerating nerves are often supersensitive (**hyperesthesia** and **hyperalgesia**) to mechanical stimuli from touch and pressure as occurs with change in body position. Patients often report such heightened sensations when a critical area is examined. However, patients with tingling paresthesias may have no detectable sensory loss. In this situation, patients are the best observers of their own sensations and such subjective complaints are frequently the first indication of a disease process. In contrast, patients with lesions of central pathways may neglect or even deny their sensory loss. For example, the loss of pain sensation from a lesion of the spinothalamic pathways may go unappreciated until a skin ulcer is seen. Strokes of the parietal cortex can cause a syndrome in which patients ignore contralateral somatosensory stimuli even when they witness the examiner touch them. The physician should be skillful in examination techniques for documenting the existence, type, location, and degree of sensory abnormalities for choosing appropriate laboratory tests.

SENSORY LOSS

The first step in analyzing sensory loss is to determine its location. Compression of a peripheral nerve (Chapter 9) gives a different distribution of abnormality from the dermatomal pattern of loss that results from compression of nerve roots (Figure 4–1). In addition, a nerve lesion causes relatively sharp boundaries of localization compared with root lesions where there is considerable overlap of dermatomes on the skin. Loss of sensation below a certain level on the body is characteristic of a spinal cord disorder, whereas regional sensory dysfunction of an entire limb or side of the body indicates a lesion in the thalamus or cortex.

The second step is to determine the type of sensory loss. Here it is clinically useful to consider two categories of somatic sensation: the dorsal column "touch-pressure" system and the anterolateral "pain-temperature" system (Table 4–1 and Figure 4–2). These two categories can be largely separated peripherally by modality, fiber size, and degree of myelination; and centrally by their different pathways of projection to the brain stem, thalamus, and cortex. Whereas this information is clinically useful, refined experiments indicate some overlap and redundancy among these features.

Disease processes can differentially affect one or the other system. Often this can be appreciated in the clinical history. For example, patients who complain of numbness due to peripheral neuropathy will note difficulty in feeling the temperature of bath water when small, unmyelinated (γ) or thinly myelinated (Aδ) fibers of the pain-temperature system are involved. This situation occurs in diabetic and amyloid neuropathy. In contrast, highly localized numbness without loss of thermal sensation suggests abnormalities of large, well-myelinated fibers as occurs in demyelinative neuropathies (Chapter 9).

The sensory examination is used to refine the localization and further characterize the type of dysfunction. It is essential to enlist patients' cooperation in this exer-

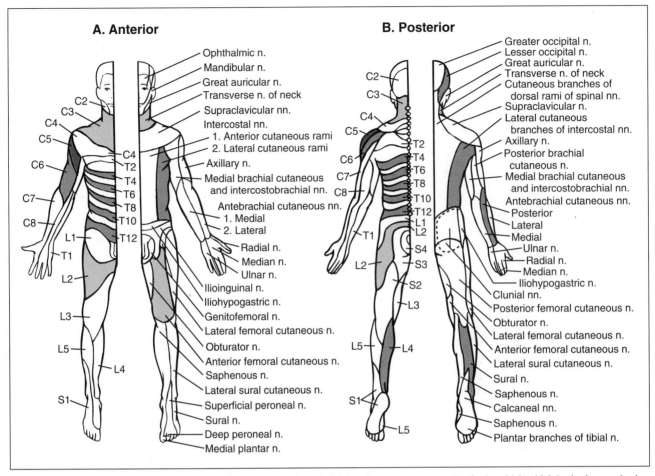

A. Anterior

Ophthalmic n.
Mandibular n.
Great auricular n.
Transverse n. of neck
Supraclavicular nn.
Intercostal nn.
1. Anterior cutaneous rami
2. Lateral cutaneous rami
Axillary n.
Medial brachial cutaneous
and intercostobrachial nn.
Antebrachial cutaneous nn.
1. Medial
2. Lateral
Radial n.
Median n.
Ulnar n.
Ilioinguinal n.
Iliohypogastric n.
Genitofemoral n.
Lateral femoral cutaneous n.
Obturator n.
Anterior femoral cutaneous n.
Saphenous n.
Lateral sural cutaneous n.
Superficial peroneal n.
Sural n.
Deep peroneal n.
Medial plantar n.

B. Posterior

Greater occipital n.
Lesser occipital n.
Great auricular n.
Transverse n. of neck
Cutaneous branches of
dorsal rami of spinal nn.
Supraclavicular nn.
Lateral cutaneous
branches of intercostal nn.
Axillary n.
Posterior brachial
cutaneous n.
Medial brachial cutaneous
and intercostobrachial nn.
Antebrachial cutaneous nn.
Posterior
Lateral
Medial
Ulnar n.
Radial n.
Median n.
Iliohypogastric n.
Clunial nn.
Posterior femoral cutaneous n.
Obturator n.
Lateral femoral cutaneous n.
Anterior femoral cutaneous n.
Lateral sural cutaneous n.
Sural n.
Saphenous n.
Calcaneal nn.
Saphenous n.
Plantar branches of tibial n.

FIGURE 4–1. Anterior and posterior view of dermatomes (left side) and peripheral cutaneous nerve distribution (right side) in the human body. n, Nerve; nn, nerves. (Reproduced, with permission, from A. M. Burt. *Textbook of Neuroanatomy.* Philadelphia, W.B. Saunders Co., 1993, pp. 122–123.)

cise, since their subjective response constitutes the data. The patient should be relaxed and comfortable and instructed to be neither overresponsive nor overdiscriminating. The physician should take the time to show the patient the type of stimulus to be used (e.g., cotton wisp, pin, tuning fork) and demonstrate the test on an area of normal skin with the patient watching. During the actual examination, the patient should not see the area being tested and should be instructed to respond very simply, e.g., "touch," "sharp," "up," or "down" in response to cotton wisp, pin, or joint movement. It is often important to have the patient compare the left and right sides as well as distal and proximal sites. In this way, an abnormal area can be compared with the patient's own control area.

In addition to determining the type and localization of sensory loss, an examiner occasionally needs to confirm whether there is a *dissociated sensory loss,* such as occurs with spinal cord lesions. In this situation, there will be loss of one system, e.g., pain-temperature,

TABLE 4–1. Somatosensory Systems

	Dorsal Column System	Anterolateral System
Peripheral fibers	Aα and Aβ	Aδ and C
	Heavily myelinated	Thinly myelinated and unmyelinated
	Fast conducting	Slow conducting
Clinical modalities	Fine touch	Crude touch
	Position sense	Pain
	Vibration	Temperature
Reflexes	Monosynaptic	Polysynaptic
	Muscle stretch	Flexion withdrawal
	Tendon jerk	Autonomic and endocrine
Neurological diseases	Demyelinating neuropathy	Diabetes, amyloid neuropathy
	Vitamin B_{12} deficiency	Spinal cord ischemia
	Syphilis	Syringomyelia

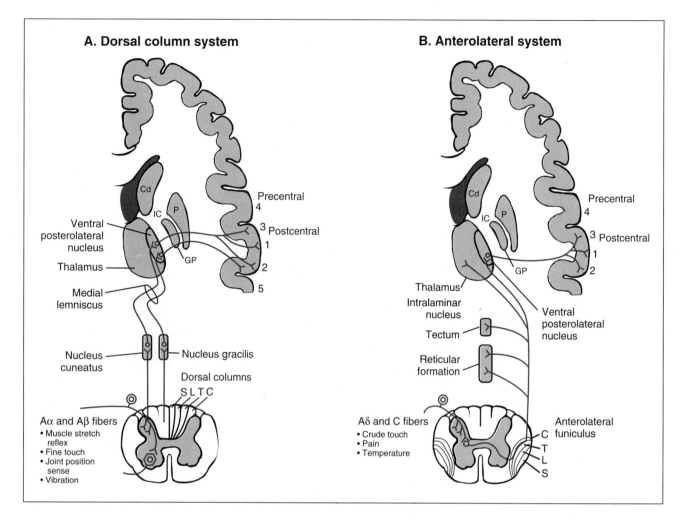

A. Dorsal column system

Cd

IC

P

Precentral
4

3 Postcentral
1

2

5

Ventral
posterolateral
nucleus

GP

Thalamus

Medial
lemniscus

Nucleus
cuneatus

Nucleus gracilis

Dorsal columns

S L T C

Aα and Aβ fibers
• Muscle stretch
  reflex
• Fine touch
• Joint position
  sense
• Vibration

B. Anterolateral system

Cd

IC

P

Precentral
4

3 Postcentral
1

2

GP

Thalamus

Intralaminar
nucleus

Tectum

Ventral
posterolateral
nucleus

Reticular
formation

Aδ and C fibers
• Crude touch
• Pain
• Temperature

Anterolateral
funiculus

C

T

L

S

FIGURE 4–2. Somatosensory pathways. *A,* Heavily myelinated peripheral sensory nerves (Aα and Aβ) serve the stretch reflexes for muscle by synapsing on anterior horn cells (Figure 3–2) and convey information concerning fine touch, joint movement, and vibration to the thalamus. The major pathway for fine touch, joint movement, and vibration is in the dorsal columns that project to the gracile and cuneate nuclei and ventral basal thalamus and from there to the postcentral gyrus. *B,* The thinly myelinated Aδ fibers and unmyelinated C fibers enter the cord and branch within Lissauer's tract for several spinal segments before synapsing in the dorsal gray (see Figure 4–3). These fibers convey sharp, well-localized pain (Aδ fibers) and dull, poorly localized, aching pain (C fibers) as well as thermal sensation. Second-order neurons cross the midline and project within the anterolateral funiculus to the brain stem reticular formation, tectum, and thalamus. C, cervical; Cd, caudate; GP, globus pallidus; L, lumbar; IC, internal capsule; P, putamen; T, thoracic; S, sacral. *C,* The cortical representation of the body surface along the postcentral gyrus (areas 3, 1, 2) is shown for the macaque. Note that the lips and digits occupy the greatest amount of cortical area relative to body surface area because they are concerned with fine spatial resolution. CS, central sulcus; D_{1-5}, digits of hand (medial) or foot (lateral); UL, upper lip; LL, lower lip; FA, forearm; OCC, occiput; PCS, postcentral sulcus; WR, wrist. (*Part C* is reproduced, with permission, from T. P. Pons, P. E. Garraghty, C. G. Cusick, and J. H. Kaas. The somatotopic organization of area 2 in macaque monkeys. J Comp Neurol 241:445–466, 1987. Copyright 1987 by John Wiley & Sons, Inc. Reprinted by permission of John Wiley & Sons, Inc.)

Illustration continued on opposite page

with preservation of the other, i.e., touch-pressure. Ischemia or infarction of the anterior part of the spinal cord from occlusion of the anterior spinal artery will affect the pain-temperature, anterolateral system. Patients will have weakness and loss of pain and temperature sense below the segmental level of the lesion (called a "sensory level") but relatively normal joint position and vibratory sensation in the feet because of preservation of the dorsal columns (Figure 4–2). Similarly, in syringomyelia, a disease of the cervical spinal cord that causes dilation of the central canal, there is loss of pain and temperature sensation in the hands

owing to disruption of the pain fibers as they cross the cord toward the anterolateral funiculus. There is relative preservation of joint position sense in the fingers because the dorsal columns are unaffected. In contrast, when the dorsal columns become demyelinated in vitamin B_{12} deficiency, there is preferential loss of position and vibratory sense with preservation of pain and temperature modalities.

Lesions of the heavily myelinated touch-pressure system in the dorsal columns, lateral lemniscus, thalamus, thalamic radiations, or primary sensory cortex cause a distinctive type of sensory loss. The most dra-

C. Postcentral gyrus

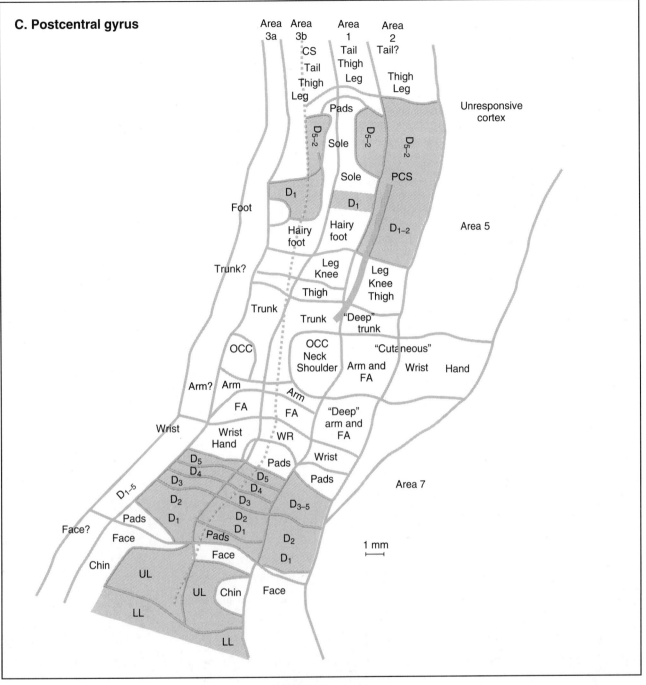

FIGURE 4–2 *Continued*

matic change is in the hand. There is elevation of the touch threshold, a decrease in two-point discrimination, a decrease in joint position sense, and a decreased ability to detect movement across the skin. In addition to these changes in individual modalities, the functions that depend upon these separate sensations acting together are impaired. Patients have difficulty in identifying numbers or letters drawn on the palm (**agraphesthesia**), distinguishing textures, and manipulating and identifying small, familiar objects placed in their hand while their eyes are closed (**astereognosis**). A patient with lesions in this system often neglects so-

matic sensation and appears unconcerned or even unaware of the loss.

PAIN

The sensation of pain signals destruction of tissue from mechanical, thermal, or chemical factors causing discharges of nociceptive fibers. Sharp, relatively well localized nociceptive stimuli are carried to the central nervous system by small, thinly myelinated Aδ fibers (5–30 m/s). Dull, aching, poorly localized nociception is carried by unmyelinated γ fibers (0.5–2 m/s). When a finger is pricked with a pin, the sharp sensation commonly is followed quickly by an automatic reflex withdrawal of the hand and then by a dull aching sensation. The flexion withdrawal is a localized spinal cord nociceptive reflex. It may be accompanied by more widespread nociceptive reflexes including changes in heart rate, blood pressure, posture, movement, facial expression, and endocrine function. These reflexes do not require the cerebral cortex and can be seen in comatose patients. The human experience of pain and suffering requires an intact cerebral cortex.

Nociceptive fibers terminate in the superficial layers of the dorsal horn (primarily Rexed's layers I, II, and V), making synapses upon excitatory and inhibitory interneurons as well as projection neurons. The last cross the spinal cord to form the anterolateral funiculus, which sends endings into the brain stem reticular formation, midbrain tectum, and thalamus (Figure 4–2). The pain system does not become integrated with the touch-pressure system until both are projected upon somatosensory cortex. Here there are four parallel sensory maps in areas 3a, 3b, 1, and 2. Integration among these areas as well as with parietal cortex posteriorly and motor cortex anteriorly results in identification of an object's size, texture, and weight as well as qualities of pain and temperature.

Extensive research has been devoted to the local circuitry and neuropharmacology of the dorsal horn where there is extensive modulation of incoming pain signals (Figures 4–2 and 4–3). First, there is interaction between the touch-pressure system and pain sensation upon entry of fibers into the cord. Pain signals can be dampened by afferent activity in large, heavily myelinated somatosensory fibers. Although exact mechanisms are unknown, it is thought that activity in somatosensory afferents stimulates an interneuron that is inhibitory upon the pain projection neurons, closing a "gate" for the entry of painful stimuli. A common illustration of this principle is the observation that shaking and rubbing a pricked finger diminishes the pain sensation. Similarly, intermittent electrical cutaneous stimulation is used therapeutically in treating some cases of chronic pain. Conversely, diseases of myelinated fibers seem to leave the "gate" open, causing or contributing to chronic neuropathic pain.

Second, nociceptive afferents release substance P (and probably glutamate) as neurotransmitter. Capsaicin is a chemical that is absorbed by sensory endings on the skin, is transported centrally by axoplasmic transport, and depletes substance P in pain fibers at their synaptic ending in the spinal cord. It is used as a topical ointment in the treatment of postherpetic neuralgia. Third, some local inhibitory interneurons use enkephalin or dynorphin as neurotransmitter acting upon mu (μ) receptors. The local, intrathecal infusion of morphine can be used to block spinal pain locally, thus avoiding morphine's CNS depressive effects. Fourth, descending serotonin and norepinephrine pathways from

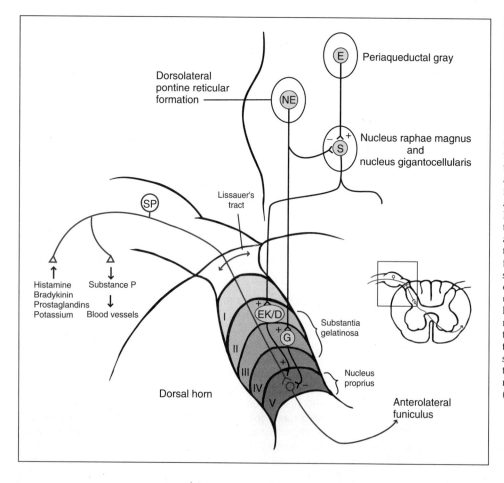

FIGURE 4–3. Neuropharmacology of pain pathways. Transmission of pain signals in the spinal cord is modulated by descending pathways that synapse on interneurons. Endorphin-containing neurons (E) in the periaqueductal gray stimulate neurons in the nucleus raphae magnus and nucleus gigantocellularis. Neurons here contain serotonin (S) and peptides and project upon interneurons in the substantia gelatinosa (Rexed's layers II and III) of the dorsal horn. Serotonin fibers stimulate enkephalin and dynorphin interneurons (EK/D), which inhibit pain fibers through primary depolarization of axoaxonic synapses. This prevents the release of substance P (SP) from pain fibers. A second descending system from the dorsolateral pontine reticular formation uses norepinephrine (NE) to stimulate GABA (G) inhibitory interneurons in the dorsal horn. These interneurons directly inhibit projection neurons in the anterolateral system. Discovery of these neurotransmitter systems has led to a rational approach for treating pain (see Table 4–3).

the brain stem inhibit afferent nociceptive stimuli in the dorsal horn. Drugs that potentiate these neurotransmitters can provide some analgesia. Finally, central opioid peptide systems located in the midbrain periaqueductal gray project upon and disinhibit brain stem serotoninergic systems, providing additional analgesia. Interestingly, electrical stimulation of the periaqueductal gray causes analgesia through this pathway, a response that can be blocked by naloxone, an opioid antagonist.

Peripheral Nerve Pain

Damage to peripheral nerves causes pain. Clinically, this pain is of several different types. Burning, tingling, dysesthetic pain occurs with small-fiber polyneuropathy that is felt on the skin within the distribution of the damaged peripheral nerves. This type of pain is common in the feet of patients with diabetic neuropathy, or along the dermatome of skin affected by post-herpetic neuralgia. There is increased irritability and spontaneous firing of damaged and regenerating nociceptive fibers.

Deep, aching, poorly localized pain usually indicates damage to nerve trunks and discharge of the small nervi nervorum. It occurs in brachial plexus neuritis, where there is severe deep, aching pain in the shoulder. Compression of the sciatic nerve roots or trunk causes pain in the low back and buttocks that is often deep and aching. Occasionally the pain is localized to the lateral part of the leg or foot, suggesting L5 or S1 root compression. Stretching the sciatic nerve in the straight leg raising test can initiate or accentuate this pain.

The sympathetic nervous system can become involved in chronic pain syndromes following peripheral nerve injury. S. Weir Mitchell was the first to describe these painful syndromes in soldiers injured during the Civil War. For example, within a few weeks to months after a gunshot wound to the arm, changes in cutaneous blood flow, sweating, and nutrition occur in the hand. The skin becomes blanched with increased sweating, indicating overactivity of the sympathetic fibers. In severe cases, bone resorption can occur. This is called reflex sympathetic dystrophy or causalgia. It is one of the most painful conditions known. The sympathetic component and much of the pain responds to anesthetic blockade of the cervical sympathetic ganglion.

Trigeminal Neuralgia

Clinicians are commonly called upon to evaluate pain in the face. The first step is to localize the structures involved. A history of upper respiratory infections should raise consideration for sinusitis and direct attention to tenderness over the frontal and maxillary sinuses. Occasionally a dental abscess will present as diffuse unilateral facial pain. Malocclusion and bruxism are additional causes of dental pain. Temporal arteritis in the elderly presents as unilateral pain and tenderness of the temporal arteries in the temporal muscle. Muscle tension headache comes from bilateral sustained contraction of facial muscles (see below). In addition, since cranial nerve V supplies the inside of the cranial vault, pathological conditions there can be referred to the face. An MRI scan will identify these.

The condition of trigeminal neuralgia can usually be diagnosed from the characteristics of the facial pain alone. Excruciating paroxysms of lightning pain lasting from a few seconds to a minute occur at a single point on the face. It is one of the most severe pains known in clinical medicine. Usually the trigger zone is in the second (maxillary) or third (mandibular) division (or both) of cranial nerve V, often around the mouth (Figure 4–4). The first (ophthalmic) division is only rarely involved. The pain can occur spontaneously or be set off by touching the trigger zone, talking, eating, brushing the teeth, etc. Attacks can occur many times an hour when the condition is severe. Between attacks there is no pain, although patients live in dread of the next attack. Many lose weight because they avoid eating. Examination of the face does not reveal any abnormality in sensation.

In the majority of cases, the pain is thought to be due to irritation or compression of a division of the trigeminal nerve by the superior cerebellar artery where the nerve enters the pons. A tortuous bend in the artery or a small branch is usually the culprit. Displacing the vessel away from the nerve cures the pain. It is thought that local irritation of a small portion of fibers explains the small trigger zone on the face. Spontaneous ectopic impulses are induced here by a pulsating vessel or triggered when action potentials from stimuli in the periphery pass through this abnormal zone. A short, high-frequency barrage of impulses are then projected to the brain stem. An alternative hypothesis is that abnormal discharges induce a burst of action potentials within the trigeminal nucleus in the pons. A lesion there from multiple sclerosis can cause this type of pain. The paroxysmal discharge is much like an epileptic discharge, and anticonvulsants are used medically to try to control the pain. Carbamazepine or phenytoin is given in increasing doses until the pain is controlled or stopped. Surgery is offered to patients for whom this treatment is insufficient.

Headache

Headache is a common experience, affecting up to 80% of the population at least once a year. An estimated 30% will take an analgesic medicine, and 2% will consult a physician. Of these, approximately 15% will be referred for laboratory investigation or subspecialty consultation. Less than 1% of these will have a brain tumor, arteriovenous malformation, or another intracranial lesion.

The pain of headache is conveyed to the brain by nociceptive fibers of cranial nerve V and upper cervical roots of the spinal cord. The source of extracranial pain is changes in levels of extracellular peptides and chemicals in tense muscles, arterial walls, or subcutaneous tissue or pressure on nerves themselves. Infection of nasal sinuses and dental problems must be excluded.

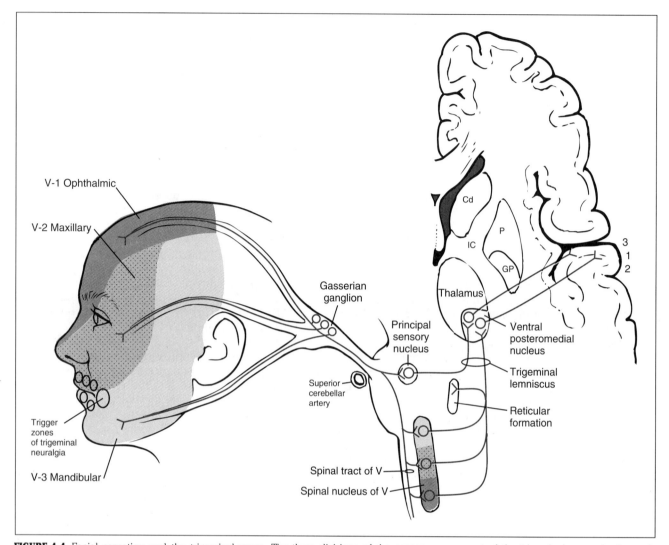

FIGURE 4–4. Facial sensation and the trigeminal nerve. The three divisions of the sensory component of the trigeminal nerve (motor and mesencephalic components not shown) have their cell bodies in the gasserian ganglion on the floor of the middle cranial fossa. This is the dorsal root ganglion for the face. The central axons of these neurons end in the principal sensory nucleus in the pons or descend in the spinal tract of V to synapse in the spinal nucleus. The principal sensory nucleus and the rostral part of the spinal nucleus receive heavily myelinated fibers and are concerned primarily with fine touch and pressure. Aδ and C fibers project into the spinal nucleus, which is essentially an extension of the substantia gelatinosa of the spinal cord, and convey pain and temperature sensations from the face. Second-order neurons cross the midline and project to the reticular formation and ventral basal thalamus. The pain of trigeminal neuralgia is caused by the superior cerebellar artery compressing the trigeminal nerve where it enters the pons. Cd, caudate; GP, globus pallidus; IC, internal capsule; P, putamen.

The source of intracranial pain is chemical irritation or stretching of meninges or the large vessels at the base of the brain that are innervated by cranial nerve V. Because the brain itself contains no nociceptive fibers, disease processes here do not cause pain until meninges or large vessels become secondarily involved.

The evaluation of patients with headache should focus on key points in the history and examination (Table 4–2). Once this information is gathered, it is often possible to classify the headache and initiate appropriate therapy. For many causes of headache, paying attention to simple common factors is often curative. Conversely, failure to pay attention to these factors impairs the effectiveness of analgesic therapy. These factors include removing potentially harmful items from the diet, especially caffeine, alcohol, chocolate, cheeses, and glutamate. Exercise and proper rest

are important. Avoiding prolonged uncomfortable postures is helpful for suboccipital headache and neck pain. Stretching exercises for stiff neck and shoulder muscles as well as massage, ice, or heat for face and neck muscles obviates the need for medicines in many cases. Finally, attention to psychological stress factors and the use of daily relaxation exercises are important for many patients with chronic headache.

Tension-type headache is the most common type of headache, affecting most people at some time in their life. It is a dull, aching pain usually localized bilaterally in the temporal, facial, or suboccipital muscles. It can last hours to days. Personal stress factors can often be identified, and patients may be anxious or depressed. There are no neurological abnormalities. In addition to the general measures given above, mild analgesics and muscle relaxants are helpful (Table 4–3).

TABLE 4-2. Evaluation of Headache

History

Typical attack: time of day, prodromal neurological symptoms, location, character, intensity, duration, activity during the attack, nausea or vomiting, sensitivity to light and sound
Recurrent attacks: age of onset; frequency; relationship to occupation, to activities, to stress, to menses; effect on employment, on recreation
Dietary factors: caffeine, alcohol, chocolate, spicy foods
Family history of headaches: clinical characteristics
Effects of medicines: previous drugs, doses, benefits, duration of use, side effects
Psychological factors: personal stress, anxiety, depression
Medical history: concurrent illness, hypertension, medications

Examination

Patient appearance during an attack, neck or facial muscle contraction, unilateral conjunctivitis, lacrimation, nasal discharge
Palpation of temporal arteries, suboccipital nerves, muscles, percussion over sinuses, teeth
Funduscopic examination: papilledema, hemorrhage
Cervical spine: mobility, tenderness, muscle spasm

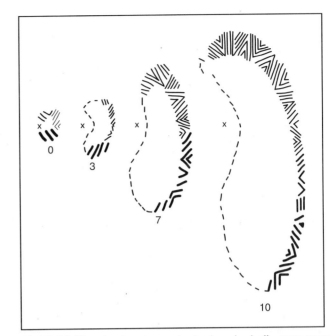

FIGURE 4-5. The visual scotoma of migraine classically starts near central vision (X) and migrates off to the periphery in one hemifield over 20 minutes. The fine details of the scotoma are short, bright line segments that pulsate in intensity and form an interdigitating pattern. These details are thought to reflect fluctuations in excitatory activity within orientation columns in primary visual cortex as a depolarizing wave of spreading depression spreads across it. Following the leading edge of these scintillating lights is an area where vision is temporarily lost (dashed lines). As the scotoma moves out of the visual field, vision is restored but the unilateral headache usually begins. (Reproduced, with permission, from K. S. Lashley. Patterns of cerebral integration indicated by the scotomas of migraine. Arch Neurol Psychiatry 46:331–339, 1941. Copyright 1941 American Medical Association.)

Migraine affects up to 10% of the population, beginning most often in young adult life and affecting women more than men. The headache may or may not be preceded by an aura. The aura may be a hemianopic scintillating scotoma, paresthesia, aphasia, or rarely weakness. Characteristically these symptoms last only 20–30 minutes and leave no deficit. There is usually a march of the abnormality, such as a scotoma that moves from central to peripheral vision and then disappears (Figure 4–5). The rate of movement of the scotoma, 1–3 mm/min, is the same as occurs during experimentally induced spreading cortical depression in animals. The mechanism of this abnormal phenomenon may be the contiguous release of potassium or glutamate from neurons or glia. PET studies of a patient taken during migraine showed a depression of cerebral blood flow beginning at the occipital poles and spreading bilaterally up to the central fissure.

The headache of migraine is usually unilateral, lasts 4–72 hours, and is associated with nausea and vomiting. There is sensitivity to light (**photophobia**) and sound (**phonophobia**), and activity of any kind, including mental work, seems to aggravate the syndrome. Patients often seek a quiet, dark room where they prefer to be left alone. Sleep often relieves the syndrome. Migraine headaches can recur several times in a month. The family history is often positive, and genetic studies are beginning to identify gene loci in some cases. Because the syndrome is characteristic, there is usually no need for laboratory testing unless features suggest transient ischemic attacks or intracranial bleeding (Chapter 15).

Acute migraine attacks usually require pharmacological treatment for relief of pain (Table 4–3). Mild cases will respond to simple analgesics (aspirin, acetaminophen, and other NSAIDs) and antiemetics (e.g., metoclopramide). More severe cases might require parenteral treatment to abort an attack (e.g., sumatriptan). Prophylactic treatment remains imperfect, as evidenced by the wide variety of pharmacological approaches: calcium channel blockers, β-blockers, serotonin reuptake inhibitors, and anticonvulsants. General measures should be instituted in all cases, and single medicines should be tried at full doses before switching to others.

TABLE 4-3. Treatment of Common Neurological Pain Syndromes

Drug	Daily Dose (mg)	Common Side Effects
Peripheral-acting analgesics for mild headache, neck pain, or low back pain		
Aspirin	650–1300	Dyspepsia, GI bleeding
Acetaminophen	500–2000	Dyspepsia
Naproxen sodium	750–2000	Dyspepsia, GI bleeding
Ibuprofen	200–800	Dyspepsia, GI bleeding
Muscle relaxants for muscle tension headache, neck pain, and low back pain		
Cyclobenzaprine	20–40	Drowsiness, dry mouth
Central-acting opioid analgesics for moderate to severe pain		
Oxycodone	5–20	Nausea, sedation
Central-acting tricyclic catecholamine reuptake inhibitors for chronic nerve pain		
Amitriptyline	25–100	Sedation, dry mouth
Anticonvulsants for trigeminal neuralgia and electric nerve pain		
Carbamazepine	400–1600	Dizzyness, sedation
Phenytoin	100–400	Confusion, ataxia
Central-acting serotonin agonists for aborting severe migraine headache		
Sumatriptan	6 subcutaneously	Flushing, chest heaviness
Dihydroergotamine mesylate	1–3 intramuscularly	Nausea, vomiting

Polypharmacy should be avoided, since combinations of different vasoactive drugs can sensitize vessels and aggravate headache.

Cluster headache is a type of vascular headache that occurs most commonly in middle-aged men. It is characterized by severe pain in or around the orbit, lasting up to 90 minutes, 1–3 times a day, for a 3- to 6-week period. Remissions between clusters are variable and can last from 6 months to many years. During an attack there is usually unilateral conjunctival injection, lacrimation, and nasal discharge. Treatment with a 2- to 3-week course of corticosteroids is often beneficial.

Certain types of headache should be investigated thoroughly. A sudden, severe "worst headache ever" should raise the suspicion of intracranial bleeding from an aneurysm or arteriovenous malformation (Chapter 15) or of meningitis if fever is present. The presence of neck pain and stiffness (meningismus) are additional signs of meningeal irritation from blood or infection. A CT scan should be performed emergently if bleeding is suspected, and a lumbar puncture when meningitis or encephalitis is being considered.

Patients above age 70 who present with unilateral temporal headache should raise concern for the possibility of giant cell arteritis, also called temporal arteritis. Women are affected more than men. Many patients have muscle aches of the neck and shoulders, low-grade fever, weight loss, and general malaise—symptoms that merge this condition with polymyalgia rheumatica. Upon palpation, the patient's temporal arteries will be found to be knotty and tender owing to inflammation from giant cells. This can be confirmed by biopsy. The erythrocyte sedimentation rate (ESR) will be elevated in 90% of cases and is an indication for starting high-dose corticosteroids. Treatment should be continued for 3–6 months, using the ESR to guide tapering and cessation of treatment.

Finally, a dull headache that increases over weeks to months should raise the suspicion of a brain tumor or chronic subdural hematoma. The headache is usually not severe. Occasionally there are changes in behavior with increased tiredness or mental dullness. Symptoms of mild depression may be present. This group of patients is challenging. Although most will have a poorly classifiable chronic headache syndrome, a few will have a meningioma, an early glioma that stretches blood vessels or meninges, or a chronic subdural hematoma. The only distinguishing feature on examination may be a slight weakness or sensory abnormality on one side of the body. CT or MRI scans are diagnostic.

Neck Pain

Pain in the neck is a common clinical complaint. It results from irritation of articular joints, ligaments, muscle tendons, and nerve roots. Trauma, arthritis, and chronic muscle strain are common causes. The goal of the initial clinical evaluation is to determine whether the nervous system is involved, imaging tests are required, and surgical consultation is needed. Mechanical signs are usually present when there is arthritis or disk disease. The examiner will find limitation of a particular movement of the head such as rotation, lateral bending, or extension because of pain. Palpation of the spine may reveal a tender disk interspace or muscle spasm due to nociceptive reflexes trying to hold the neck rigid. The Valsalva maneuver can be informative, since it raises intraspinal pressure and may add to irritation of a compressed root. Patients may report that coughing or even laughing causes neck or arm pain in this situation.

The presence of a cervical root syndrome (Table 4–4) indicates irritation or compression of a spinal ganglion or nerve as it exits the vertebral column due to arthritis, a bony spur, or protrusion of a disk. These syndromes are not uncommon in middle-aged people who have participated in physical sports and developed arthritic changes. Most will respond to conservative medical treatment with 2–7 weeks of analgesics, muscle relaxants, and physical therapy focusing on stretching exercises. Imaging tests and surgical consultation should be sought following acute trauma, in the presence of a severe root syndrome, when there are signs of spinal cord compression (e.g., weak spastic legs, Babinski's sign, loss of position sense in the toes), when there is suspicion of cancer, or when there is failure to respond to conservative medical treatment.

The Low Back Syndrome

Low back pain affects up to 80% of people at some time during their life and is often accompanied by muscle spasm, immobility, and radiation of pain into the buttock or leg. It is estimated that 2% of the population and 25% of working men seek medical attention each year for this condition. Age-related changes play a role, since autopsy series demonstrate changes of degenerative disk disease in 85% of adults by age 50. Weight-bearing activities, trauma, congenital abnormalities, and osteoarthritis are additive pathogenetic factors. The degenerative process leads to disk shrinkage, tears in the annulus fibrosus, and protrusion of disk material through the tear. In a minority of cases, the disk material may irritate or compress a ganglion or spinal nerve, causing a radicular syndrome (Table 4–5). Advanced disk space narrowing causes osteoarthropathy of the

TABLE 4–4. Cervical Root Syndromes

Root	Pain/Numbness	Weakness	Reflex Loss
C3/4	Shoulder	Diaphragm	None
C5*	Deltoid area	Deltoid Biceps	± Biceps
C6*	Dermatome into thumb	Biceps Brachioradialis	Biceps
C7*	Dermatome into second to fourth fingers	Triceps Fingers	Triceps
C8	Dermatome into fifth finger	Hand	± Triceps

*Common.

TABLE 4-5. Lumbar Root Syndromes

Root	Pain/Numbness	Weakness	Reflex Loss
L3	Lateral thigh	Quadriceps	± Knee
L4	Medial leg	Quadriceps Anterior tibial	Knee
L5*	Anterior/lateral leg Big toe	Toe extensor	None
S1*	Lateral/posterior leg Little toe	Foot evertor	Ankle

*Common.

facet joints, further adding to pain. The cause of pain in any particular case is difficult if not impossible to determine. In particular, there is little correlation between severity of symptoms and changes seen on an MRI scan. Conversely, 50% of normal adults will have degenerative changes seen on an MRI scan and 20% will have evidence of disk protrusion.

Mechanical signs are the hallmark of the low back syndrome. Patients discover that certain postures aggravate the pain, usually weight-bearing positions of sitting or prolonged standing. Lying in a position with flexion at the hips and knees usually relieves the pain. In the acute phase, patients will walk and move slowly and often require assistance for rolling over in the recumbent position and arising to the sitting position. These movements aggravate local inflammatory processes in joints, muscles, and nerve roots and cause reflex muscle spasms and more pain. During the examination, the patient will have limitation of movement at the waist for flexion, extension, and lateral bending. Palpation of the intervertebral spaces in the lumbar spine with the patient in the prone position usually reveals local tenderness. Paraspinal muscle spasm will be present. Raising the patient's leg while the patient lies in the recumbent position often causes or aggravates the back pain, and palpation of the sciatic nerve in the gluteal fold will reveal tenderness because this maneuver stretches an irritated nerve root.

The low back syndrome is usually self-limited, with 75% of patients able to return to full activities in 4–6 weeks. The initial approach to therapy is conservative medical management with a few days of bed rest, analgesics, muscle relaxants, and a program of physical therapy. Support girdles for the low back are useful in providing stability as the patient regains standing and walking postures. Imaging studies should be performed in the absence of improvement by 7 weeks, in the presence of a severe root syndrome, in the presence of bilateral root signs or bladder or bowel dysfunction, and with suspicion of cancer. Following recovery, avoidance of weight-bearing activities, correction of posture, and institution of a stretching and exercise program can help prevent recurrence.

VISUAL LOSS

Loss of vision is an alarming symptom when it affects central visual acuity and usually prompts patients to seek immediate evaluation from their physician. The causes of this condition affect structures between the cornea and the optic chiasm of one or both eyes (Table 4–6). In contrast, loss of peripheral vision does not necessarily alarm patients and may even go unnoticed until patients discover difficulty in reading or bump into unnoticed objects on one side. In this situation, lesions lie behind the optic chiasm, usually in the optic radiations in the temporal or occipital lobe, affecting the contralateral visual field (Figure 4–6). The difference between these two symptom complexes reflects the organization of the visual system. Central vision is organized to analyze *what* is being looked at. Peripheral vision is organized to detect *where* new visual stimuli are coming from.

The system for central vision begins in the macula of the retina, where there is the greatest density of color-sensitive cones. Cones are devoted to fine spatial resolution in the central 10 degrees of vision. The projection of this central vision from retina to geniculate body to calcarine cortex takes up almost as much anatomical space as does all the rest of the visual field (Figure 4–7). This principle of magnifying anatomy (number of circuits) to achieve fine discrimination is also found in the somatosensory system, where the

TABLE 4-6. Localization of Visual Loss

Site	Unilateral	Bilateral	Onset	Visual Acuity	Visual Field	Funduscopic Examination
Eye						
Cataract	Rare	Usual	Slow	↓	Normal	Cloudy lens
Glaucoma	Rare	Usual	Slow	Normal	Abnormal	Enlarged optic cup
Macular degeneration	Rare	Usual	Slow	↓	Normal	Mottled macula
Ischemia	Usual	Rare	Acute	↓ ↓	Abnormal	Pallor
Optic Nerve						
Optic neuritis	Usual	Rare	Acute	↓ ↓	Abnormal	Normal
Tumor	Usual	Rare	Slow	↓	Abnormal	Optic atrophy
Optic Chiasm						
Pituitary tumor	Occasional	Usual	Slow	Normal	Abnormal	Optic atrophy
Optic Radiations						
Stroke	Never	Always	Acute	Normal	Abnormal	Normal

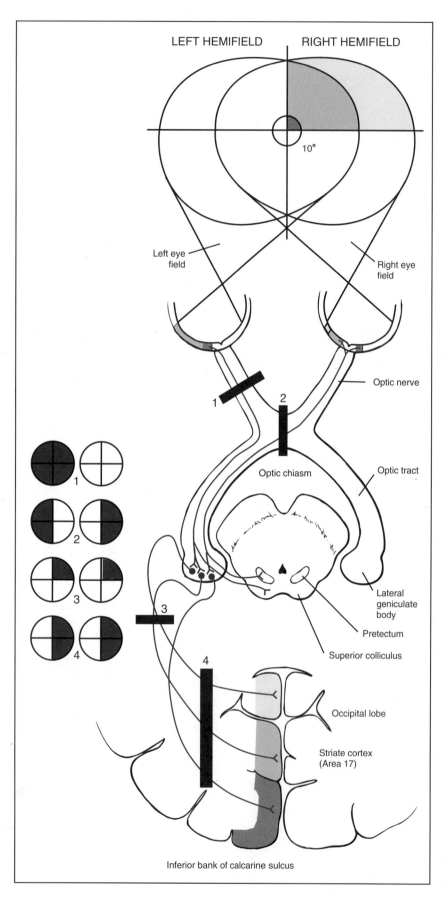

LEFT HEMIFIELD   RIGHT HEMIFIELD

10°

Left eye field

Right eye field

Optic nerve

Optic chiasm

Optic tract

Lateral geniculate body

Pretectum

Superior colliculus

Occipital lobe

Striate cortex (Area 17)

Inferior bank of calcarine sulcus

FIGURE 4–6. Visual pathways. Loss of central vision occurs with diseases in front of the optic chiasm (see Table 4–6) such as optic neuritis (1). Pituitary tumors can directly compress the chiasm from below and injure the crossing fibers from the nasal half of each retina. This causes bitemporal hemianopia (2). Behind the chiasm, the retinal fibers and optic radiation carry the contralateral visual field to the visual cortex. Lesions here can disrupt part of the hemifield ([3] right superior quadrantanopia from a temporal lobe lesion) or cause congruent hemianopia (4).

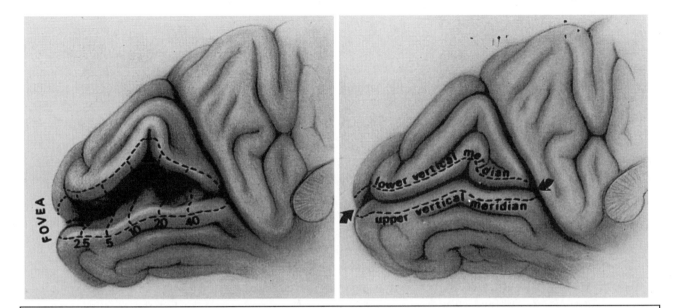

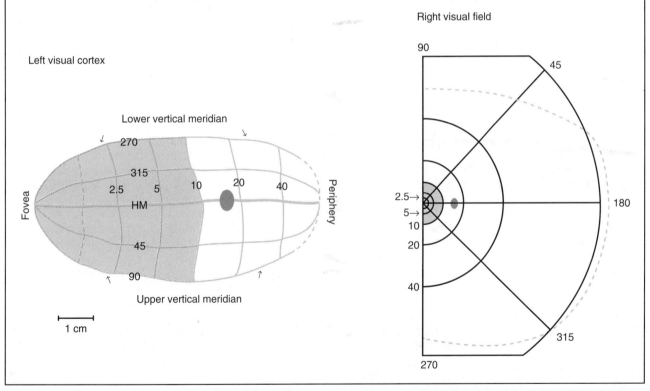

FIGURE 4–7. Summary figure of the right visual field in the left striate cortex. This representation was determined by defining the exact dimensions of visual field loss on a tangent screen test in patients with circumscribed lesions of the occipital cortex demonstrated by MRI. The calcarine fissure is opened to show the striate cortex. The horizontal meridian (HM) runs along the base of the fissure. The blind spot for the left eye (nasal retina) is located in the left visual cortex by the large dot. The dashed line on the cortex separates striate cortex on the inside (called V1) from extrastriate cortex on the outside (V2). The dashed line indicates the vertical meridian on the tangent screen. The vertical isocontour lines indicate the degrees of vision from the macula (occipital pole) to the periphery. Note that the first 10 degrees of vision occupy nearly half the representation of the visual field. Cortical circuits here are concerned with fine visual spatial resolution (see also Figure 4–2C). (Reproduced, with permission, from J. C. Horton and W. F. Hoyt. The representation of the visual field in human striate cortex: A revision of the classic Holmes map. Arch Ophthalmol 109:816–824, 1991. Copyright 1991 American Medical Association.)

cortical representation of the fingertips, lips, and toes is greater than that of the rest of the body surface (Figure 4–2C). When patients lose central vision, they discover they cannot determine what they are looking at.

The system for peripheral vision begins in the periphery of the retina, where the density of light-sensitive rods is greater than that of cones. Rods are sensitive to minute changes in light intensity across the visual spectrum. This part of the retina also projects upon the lateral geniculate body and then to the calcarine cortex to complete the visuotopic map of the external world. However, this system also has a great influence upon activity in the superior colliculus through retinotectal projections. The midbrain tectum, along with the parietal cortex with which it associates, orients the eyes and body toward new stimuli. When a person turns to see it, the new object falls upon the macula and the central visual system, where it will be inspected in detail. When patients lose peripheral vision, they simply are not alerted to new visual stimuli off to the side. They literally do not know what they are missing.

There are also two types of visual streams that project away from primary visual, striate cortex to extrastriate cortical areas for further analysis. Primates have more than 25 extrastriate visual areas. The *what* system is concerned with object recognition and projects inferiorly into the temporal lobe and limbic system. When bilateral lesions occur in this system, patients have difficulty with color discrimination (**achromatopsia**) and identification of faces (**prosopagnosia**). The *where* system is concerned with visuospatial perception and visuomotor performance. This functional stream projects superiorly into parietal cortex. Lesions here cause difficulty in depth perception, spatial localization, and motion perception. Patients may also have difficulty recognizing objects presented from an unconventional orientation, or in shifting their eyes to explore a static scene. Upon examining a picture, they will correctly report fine details but limit themselves to a small portion of the picture and miss the message of the entire picture altogether (**simultanagnosia**).

In evaluating a patient with visual loss, it is important to determine whether the symptom is acute, suggesting ischemia or demyelination, or chronically progressive, suggesting a degenerative etiology or compressive lesion (Table 4–6). Symmetric bilateral loss of central visual acuity suggests a degenerative disease such as cataract, glaucoma, or macular degeneration, diseases treated by ophthalmologists. Visual acuity is tested in each eye alone using an acuity card held at 14 inches. Patients should wear their glasses to correct for refractory errors. It is also best to test visual fields in each eye alone, having the patient count the examiner's fingers presented in each visual quadrant while the patient focuses on the examiner's eye. If a visual field defect is found, an MRI scan should be performed to localize and identify the lesion in the visual pathways.

HEARING LOSS

The causes of unilateral hearing loss affect structures between the external auditory canal and the coch-

lear nucleus in the brain stem (Table 4–7). Central auditory projections ascend bilaterally beyond the cochlear nucleus such that central lesions causing hearing loss would have to affect both sides of the brain and bilateral deafness would occur. This happens only rarely, as when a mass lesion compresses both inferior colliculi, or when bilateral strokes occur in the auditory cortex of the temporal lobes. In the latter situation, patients hear and orient toward sound but cannot identify it. In addition they cannot understand language although they speak perfectly well, a condition called pure word deafness. Bilateral deafness occurs most commonly in the elderly owing to end-organ disease. If it goes undetected, a patient may become paranoid or appear demented.

In examining patients for hearing loss, a 512-Hz tuning fork is used to test each ear individually. A simple method for the examiner is to ask the patient to indicate when the tuning fork goes silent and then determine by listening if it can still be heard. If a deficit is discovered, it is important to rule out canal obstruction with an otoscope, and middle ear disease with the Rinne test. In this test, the vibrating tuning fork is placed against the mastoid bone and the loudness is compared against hearing it in the air next to the ear. Normally, air conduction is better than bone conduction, since the ossicles of the middle ear magnify the air's vibration of the tympanic membrane. If middle ear disease affects the tympanic membrane (e.g., infection or trauma) or ossicles (e.g., otosclerosis), air conduction will be no better than bone conduction.

When sensorineural hearing loss is detected, a patient should have a pure tone audiometry test. More refined tests can be performed to identify inner ear disease of the cochlea (e.g., Meniere's disease) and lesions of cranial nerve VIII (e.g., acoustic neurofibroma). An MRI scan is important for diagnosing nerve and brain stem lesions. A lumbar puncture should be performed if infection or carcinomatous meningitis is under consideration.

Appropriate treatment is directed at the cause. Advances in hearing aid design have greatly helped overcome middle and inner ear damage.

Table 4–7. Localization of Hearing Loss

External ear
    Obstruction
    Trauma
Middle ear
    Otitis media
    Trauma to tympanic membrane
    Otosclerosis
Inner ear
    Advancing age—presbycusis
    Meniere's disease
    Acoustic trauma
Nerve lesion
    Acoustic neurofibroma
    Infection: syphilis, tuberculosis, sarcoidosis
    Carcinomatous meningitis
Lateral brain stem
    Multiple sclerosis
    Stroke

SUMMARY

Disorders of sensation can occur as isolated problems due to lesions of the central nervous system or as part of larger or more complex disease processes. Abnormalities of vision and hearing are treated by ophthalmologists and otolaryngologists when the eye and the ear are damaged peripherally. When the nerves and central pathways become involved, a neurologist and occasionally a neurosurgeon are best prepared to help the patient. Loss of sensation on the face or body is most often part of a peripheral nerve disorder, but central lesions can disrupt sensory function also. In the former situation, patients usually report their abnormal sensation as numbness, tingling, or pain. With central lesions, many patients are unaware of their deficit. Pain is the most common complaint in clinical medicine, and neurologists are often called upon to help patients with headache, neck, or low back pain. An anatomical approach to diagnosis and a neuropharmacological approach to therapy is the best clinical practice.

Selected Readings

Asbury, A.K., and H. L. Fields. Pain due to peripheral nerve damage: An hypothesis. Neurology 34:1587–1590, 1984.

Ellenberger, C., Jr. MR imaging of the low back syndrome. Neurology 44:594–600, 1994.

Felleman, D.J., and D. C. Van Essen. Distributed hierarchical processing in the cerebral cortex. Cereb Cortex 1:1–47, 1991.

Kozin, F. Reflex sympathetic dystrophy syndrome. Curr Opin Rheumatol 6:210–216, 1994.

Ochoa, J. L., and H. E. Torebjork. Paraesthesiae from ectopic impulse generation in human sensory nerves. Brain 103:835–853, 1980.

Solomon, S., and R. E. Lipton. Criteria for the diagnosis of migraine in clinical practice. Headache 31:384–387, 1991.

Vaina, L. M. Functional segregation of color and motion in the human visual cortex: Clinical evidence. Cereb Cortex 5:555–572, 1994.

Woods, R. P., M. Iacoboni, and J. C. Mazziotta. Bilateral spreading cerebral hypoperfusion during spontaneous migraine headache. N Engl J Med 331:1689–1692, 1995.

CHAPTER FIVE

DISORDERS

OF HOMEOSTASIS

INTRODUCTION 53

DIZZINESS AND VERTIGO 53

CONSCIOUSNESS AND COMA 55

DISORDERS OF SLEEP 59

DISORDERS OF AUTONOMIC FUNCTION 63

SUMMARY 64

INTRODUCTION

The brain plays a dominant role in maintaining necessary but unconscious functions essential for everyday life that include posture and balance, level of consciousness, sleep-wake cycles, and the control of blood pressure, bladder, and sexual performance. Disorders affecting the neurological systems that serve these functions cause unique clinical symptoms—dizziness, stupor, insomnia, hypotension, incontinence, and impotence. The diagnostic approach to patients who suffer such disorders of homeostasis is the same as for all neurological problems. The patient's symptoms must be translated into pathophysiological terms. The site of the lesion must be localized within neuroanatomical pathways. Etiological hypotheses must be generated to guide further evaluation and therapy.

DIZZINESS AND VERTIGO

Dizziness is a common but vague clinical complaint that by itself cannot lead to diagnosis or treatment. The first step is to help the patient translate the symptom into one of four possible conditions, each of which has several possible etiologies: syncope, unsteadiness, lightheadedness, or vertigo.

Syncope. Syncope, or fainting, is a common enough experience to be known by most adults. Dim vision, "gray out," or "spots in front of the eyes" is the first abnormality noticed when blood pressure drops and perfusion pressure to the brain falls below intraocular pressure. When retinal ischemia results, patches of electrical failure occur and quickly coalesce. A feeling of cold clamminess of the skin may be appreciated as the adrenal and sympathetic nervous systems respond, but usually weakness occurs rapidly and the patient falls down as consciousness is lost. In a simple faint, this fall results in an increased return of venous blood to the heart. Vasovagal bradycardia ceases, and cardiac output returns to normal, restoring brain perfusion and neurological function within 1–3 minutes. There are no neurological deficits following a simple faint. The cause of pathological syncope is usually related to cardiac disease (arrhythmia, valvular disease, ischemia) or orthostatic hypotension. Suspicion of heart disease necessitates a full cardiac evaluation. Orthostatic hypotension is the most common cause of syncope in clinical medicine and is diagnosed by finding a drop in blood pressure of 30/20 after a patient goes from the lying to the standing position. The use of diuretics and other medicines, dehydration from exercise, and the deconditioning that comes from prolonged bed rest are the usual culprits. Primary orthostatic hypotension (the Shy-Drager syndrome; Chapter 11) is a rare condition that occurs in patients with signs of parkinsonism. There is a failure of all autonomic function such that, in contrast to normal people, when there is a drop in blood pressure upon standing there is no compensatory increase in heart rate.

Unsteadiness. Unsteadiness is also a vague complaint that requires further analysis. Upon questioning, patients indicate that they do not feel steady on their feet, or their feet are disobedient, or they fear falling. If true vertigo (see below) is ruled out, there may be problems with vision, joint position sense, the joints themselves, or the motor system, particularly cerebellar pathways. In the elderly, cataracts and osteoarthritis are common nonneurological causes of unsteadiness. Neurologically, a decrease in joint position sense in the feet indicates abnormalities of large myelinated fibers in the peripheral nerves or dorsal columns, and appropriate evaluation must follow (Chapters 4 and 9). Similarly, if the examination discloses weakness or ataxia, the workup should focus upon the localization of abnormalities which may lie within muscle, nerve, or the central nervous system (Chapter 3).

Lightheadedness. Lightheadedness should be considered a diagnosis of exclusion in the evaluation of the dizzy patient. The symptoms are vague and cannot be translated into dysfunction of either cardiovascular or neurological systems. The examination will be normal. There may be underlying anxiety or depression in such patients, with or without a hyperventilation syndrome. The patient's medicines should be reviewed. Substance abuse should be considered.

Vertigo. Vertigo is defined as a conscious experience of spinning. Patients are aware of an abnormality in balance and find it extremely unpleasant. They may describe themselves or the environment as moving, spinning, or tilting. When it occurs suddenly, there may be nausea and vomiting and a patient can be thrown to the ground as in an earthquake. A sense of doom and dread is commonly evoked by such an experience. In history taking, attention should be paid to the onset and duration of the symptom, recurrent bouts, the effect of changing position on causing the symptom, the presence of tinnitus or hearing loss, and any past or concurrent brain stem symptoms. This information will usually lead quickly to a consideration of the location of the lesion and the common causes of vertigo (Table 5–1).

The neurological examination of a patient with vertigo focuses on determining whether the lesion is peripheral or central. Tests of hearing are required to determine whether the acoustic portion of cranial nerve VIII or the cochlea is involved as part of a peripheral cause of vertigo. This situation occurs in Meniere's dis-

---

TABLE 5–1. Localization of Vertigo

Peripheral Labyrinth or Nerve

Benign positional vertigo: crystals from otoliths in the posterior semicircular canal
Vestibular neuronitis: paralyzed labyrinth or nerve
Meniere's disease: endolymphatic hydrops
Infection: syphilis, herpes zoster
Vascular disease: ischemia of anterior inferior cerebellar artery
Tumor: acoustic neuroma
Toxin: aminoglycosides; salicylates; alcohol
Trauma

Central Vestibular Nuclei or Pathways in the Brain Stem or Cerebellum

Vascular disease: vertebrobasilar system ischemia and infarction
Migraine
Metabolic disorder: alcohol, thiamine deficiency
Multiple sclerosis
Tumor: in vestibulocerebellum or brain stem

ease and acoustic nerve tumors. Central causes of vertigo are most commonly a result of posterior (vertebrobasilar) ischemia (Chapter 15). The presence of a visual field defect (posterior cerebral artery), ataxia (superior cerebellar artery), dysarthria, diplopia, cranial nerve abnormalities, or crossed sensorimotor signs (basilar artery) are positive findings indicating that vertigo is the result of a central lesion of vestibular pathways.

Nystagmus (see below) is always present with true vertigo, reflecting imbalance within the vestibular projections upon the brain stem oculomotor system (Figure 5–1). In the normal situation, whenever the head moves the semicircular canals in the periphery send a signal to the oculomotor system that keeps the eyes focused on a target. Reflex fixation of eyes during head movement is called the vestibulo-ocular reflex (VOR). Patients who have had bilateral damage to their semicircular canals due to toxins (e.g., streptomycin, ethacrynic acid) have impaired or absent reflexes. Clinically, they have difficulties such as reading signs while riding in a moving car or on a bicycle. Their eyes cannot maintain fixation during sudden changes in head position. If the hair cells of the utricle and saccule are also destroyed, there is loss of detection of vertical acceleration and appreciation of gravity. Patients with

this problem have difficulty swimming underwater because they lose orientation for up and down.

Nystagmus is a rapid jerking of the eyes seen on examination. It is named for the direction of the fast, or jerk, component. In left nystagmus, the eyes jerk to the left. With vestibular system lesions, this movement is caused by a loss of tonic forces that keep the eyes from drifting off target to one side or the other, the drift being called the slow-phase component of nystagmus. With a lesion of the right horizontal semicircular canal, the eyes will drift to the right and the corrective fast component will jerk them back to the left. Horizontal or rotatory nystagmus can occur with either peripheral or central lesions of vestibular pathways although there are some distinguishing features (Table 5–2).

Benign positional vertigo is a common syndrome in the elderly. It is caused by carbonate crystals breaking off from the otoliths in the utricle and becoming clogged in a semicircular canal, most often the posterior canal. Some cases follow head trauma, but most are idiopathic and presumed degenerative. Patients experience vertigo and nausea with rapid changes in head posture such as rolling over in bed or turning a corner while walking. Seventy percent recover spontaneously in weeks to a few months, but the symp-

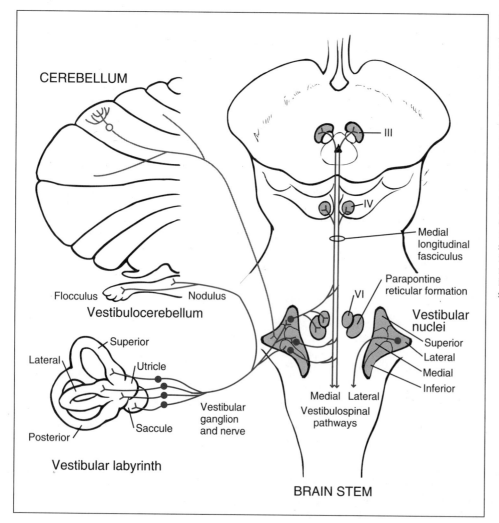

FIGURE 5–1. Vestibular pathways. The three semicircular canals originate from the utricle, where each ampulla with its hair cells and otoliths is innervated by a branch of the vestibular nerve. Changes in head position send impulses into the superior, medial, and inferior vestibular nuclei as well as directly into the vestibulocerebellum. The vestibular nuclei send fibers into the medial longitudinal fasciculus to reach the nuclei of cranial nerves III, IV, and VI for maintaining eye position during head movements (the vestibulo-ocular reflex). The lateral vestibular nucleus receives its principal input from the cerebellar cortex. Descending vestibulospinal pathways innervate proximal muscle motor neurons to maintain posture during changes in head and body position.

TABLE 5-2. Common Types of Nystagmus

Type	Features	Location	Etiology
Vestibular, peripheral	Rotary, unidirectional, inhibited with visual fixation	Labyrinth or cranial nerve VIII	Benign positional vertigo
Vestibular, central	Rotary, unidirectional, not inhibited with visual fixation	Vestibular nuclei or pathways	Stroke
Unilateral gaze paretic	In direction of one gaze	Lateral brain stem or cerebellum	Stroke
Symmetric gaze paretic	In all directions of gaze	Diffuse	Alcohol and drugs
Vertical, upgaze	Upon looking up, with diplopia, unreactive pupils, convergence spasm	Midbrain tectum	Pineal tumor
Vertical, downgaze	Upon looking down	Lower medulla—foramen magnum	Arnold-Chiari malformation
Dissociated	Abducting eye on lateral gaze	Medial longitudinal fasciculus	Multiple sclerosis

tom can be frightening and occasionally incapacitating. The diagnosis is made by an examination technique. The patient is supported by holding the head and then moved quickly from a sitting position to a recumbent head-hanging position so that one ear hangs below the examination table (Figure 5–2A). First one side then the other is tested. When the affected side is down, there will be a sense of vertigo and rotary nystagmus toward the affected ear. The nystagmus shows a delay in onset, is of short duration, returns in moving the patient to the sitting position, and fatigues with repeated maneuvers. These characteristics are diagnostic of benign positional vertigo. The condition can usually be cured by putting the patient through positional maneuvers that dislodge the debris from the canal and float it into the utricle (Figure 5–2B).

Vestibular neuronitis is a term used to describe the acute onset of vertigo, postural imbalance, nausea or vomiting, and persistent horizontal-rotary nystagmus. The nystagmus diminishes with visual fixation. Patients usually feel sick, remain immobilized in bed for 1–3 days, and gradually recover over 2–4 weeks. It is the second most common cause of vertigo affecting people from 30 to 60 years of age. A viral etiology affecting the nerve or labyrinth is presumed but not proved. Caloric testing is diagnostic. Irrigation of the external ear canal with cold (30°C) or warm (44°C) water in a normal person induces convection currents in the semicircular canals that cause nystagmus away from or toward the side of irrigation, respectively. In vestibular neuronitis, the caloric response is reduced or absent. Hearing, however, is normal.

Meniere's disease is the third most common cause of vertigo and is characterized by tinnitus, fluctuating hearing loss, and attacks of vertigo and nystagmus lasting for hours. The attacks are often preceded by a sense of fullness in the ear. Symptoms are thought to be caused by expansion of endolymph (endolymphatic hydrops) with rupture of membranes and spillage of high-potassium fluid into the perilymph, blocking vestibular and auditory function. The illness begins on one side generally between ages 30 and 50. Only 20% of cases become bilateral, usually after 10–20 years. The vertigo disappears between attacks, but the hearing loss is progressive. Remissions between attacks can last years. The diagnosis rests upon finding fluctuations of hearing loss using pure tone audiometry and on the phenomenon of recruitment using impedance audiometry. Recruitment can sometimes cause symptoms. Patients with cochlear damage report increased difficulty hearing voices distinctly when more than one person is talking, euphemistically called the "cocktail party" phenomenon. The cause of Meniere's disease is unknown. Autoimmunity may play a role. Since there are many familial cases, genetic factors are being sought.

The treatment of vertigo in patients with vestibular neuronitis or Meniere's disease is symptomatic. Anticholinergic medicines are helpful, e.g., meclizine (25–100 mg/d) or a scopolamine patch. Bed rest during the acute phase of the attack is recommended, but then patients should return to full activity. Head and neck movement exercises induce mild vertigo, but they stimulate healthy labyrinthine functions to compensate and correct imbalance of activity in vestibulo-ocular pathways. Thus, the exercises hasten recovery of vestibulo-ocular reflexes and cessation of vertigo and nystagmus. There is some evidence that a low-sodium diet and the use of diuretics are also beneficial in Meniere's disease.

CONSCIOUSNESS AND COMA

Consciousness is defined medically as continuous awareness of environment and self. There are two neurophysiological components. First, there is the state of arousal—the degree to which a patient may open eyes, move the body, and direct attention to stimuli, however briefly. Second, there is the content of consciousness—the degree to which a patient's attention to stimuli is appropriate and meaningful. For example, a patient who has taken an overdose of barbiturate will be difficult to arouse but for brief moments may give accurate verbal responses to questioning. In contrast, patients who "awake" following widespread ischemic damage to the brain from cardiac arrest may be easily arousable but exhibit no meaningful evidence of awareness of self or environment. Both patients have abnormalities of consciousness.

A variety of terms are used to describe altered states of consciousness ranging from mild states of confusion to brain death. Definitions are given in Box 5–1, and usages vary somewhat among physicians from different institutions. Practically, it is useful to think of these terms in relationship to two simple mechanisms that underlie consciousness: the brain stem reticular

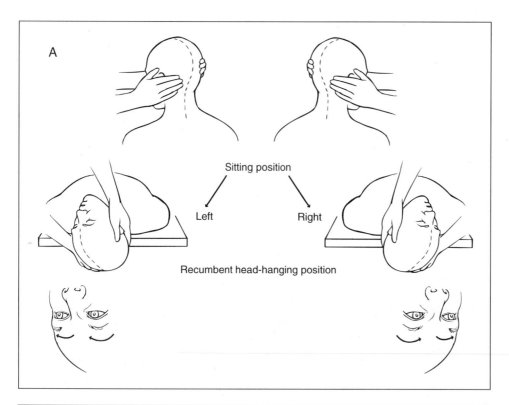

Sitting position

Left   Right

Recumbent head-hanging position

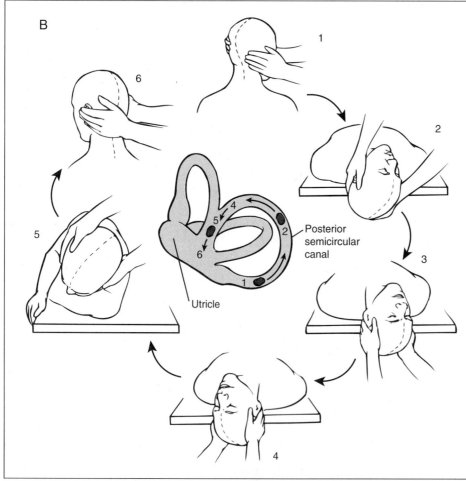

6

Posterior
semicircular
canal

5

Utricle

4

1

2

3

FIGURE 5-2. Positional maneuvers to test and treat benign positional vertigo. *A,* To diagnose benign positional vertigo, the patient is moved rapidly from a sitting to a recumbent, lateral head-hanging position on the right or left. This induces vertigo and rotary nystagmus toward the affected ear when it is down. *B,* To cure this syndrome, the patient is put through positions to dislodge and clear obstructive debris in the posterior canal. After the nystagmus has stopped (approximately 30 seconds in position 3), rotating the patient quickly to the other side will dislodge and begin to float the crystals toward the utricle. After 30 seconds at step 4, the patient is fully rotated into the face-down position for 30 seconds and then brought into the upright position facing the other way. The crystals should now be in the utricle and no longer obstructing fluid movement in the semicircular canal. The procedure can be repeated until vertigo and nystagmus completely disappear. (Slightly modified and reproduced, with permission, from C. A. Foster and R. W. Baloh. Episodic vertigo. *In* R. E. Rakel [ed.]. *Conn's Current Therapy.* Philadelphia, W.B. Saunders Co., 1995, pp. 837–841.)

BOX 5-1   Altered States of Consciousness

Delirium: An acute state characterized by lack of attention, disorientation, misperceptions, agitation, and visual hallucinations. Medicines (e.g., morphine), illicit drugs, alcohol withdrawal, infections, and diffuse cerebral hypoxia are common causes.

Obtundation: A depressed level of consciousness with diminished spontaneous activity and a slow and blunted response to environmental stimuli. Patients may appear to be sleeping excessively, since they can be alerted by vigorous physical or noxious stimuli. If sedative drugs are not being used, the patient requires emergent evaluation for other causes. **Stupor** is a synonym.

Concussion: A brief, 1- to 3-minute loss of consciousness following head trauma commonly due to sports activities (e.g., boxing, football), automobile accidents, or violence. Pathologically there is direct trauma to the brain stem with or without diffuse shearing injuries in white matter pathways.

Coma: A condition in which a person is unresponsive to stimuli and totally unaware of the environment. The patient usually lies motionless with eyes closed. In response to strong noxious stimuli, there may be inappropriate movement or postures, brief facial grimacing, or eye opening. These signs signify spinal cord and brain stem nociceptive reflex function only. Ventilation may or may not be depressed depending on the location of the process and the underlying cause.

Persistent Vegetative State: A permanent state characterized by normal sleep-wake cycles, preserved brain stem control of breathing and autonomic functions, but absence of all meaningful cortical activity. Patients may appear awake in this condition, but there is no evidence of sentient awareness of self or the environment. Patients lapse into this state following coma caused by diffuse, severe hypoxia/ischemia due to cardiac arrest or drug overdose. The term is applied only after there is failure to improve for one month following the onset of coma. Pathologically there is diffuse destruction of the cerebral cortex and hippocampus. Rarely, destruction of the frontal basal part of the forebrain by a ruptured aneurysm or a third ventricular tumor can cause this syndrome. **Coma vigil** and **akinetic mutism** are synonyms.

Locked-in Syndrome: A state in which the patient is conscious but unable to move anything but the eyes or eyelids. The cause is a severe infarction of the pons, disconnecting the hemispheres from volitional control of lower bulbar and all spinal muscles. Brain stem control of breathing and autonomic functions located below the lesion remain normal. Once discovered, it is occasionally possible to instruct such patients to communicate through a code of vertical eye movements or blinking. Patients in this tragic state either recover some additional movements or die.

Brain Death: Complete and irreversible cessation of cortical and brain stem function. There is no spontaneous or reflex pupillary, doll's eye, corneal, caloric, gag, or ventilatory function. The term has come to be defined in the bylaws of most hospitals in order to aid in decisions regarding patients in intensive care units when mechanical ventilation is required to maintain continued oxygenation of the heart and other organs after the brain stem has been irreversibly damaged. In practice, two physicians familiar with the neurological condition are required to document brain death. Reversible conditions due to sedative drugs, muscle paralyzing agents, metabolic abnormalities, and hypothermia must be ruled out. Laboratory tests such as EEG are not required.

Other Conditions: Technically, **dementia** is an altered state of consciousness, since the diffuse disruption of cortical processes results in an abnormal content of consciousness and permanent degradation of cognitive skills. The end result of dementia is no different from the persistent vegetative state in its destruction of the human quality of life. Similarly, **depression** might be viewed as altered consciousness, since patients exhibit a decreased capacity for arousal to environmental and internal stimuli. However, both terms are clinical entities encompassing a wide variety of phenomenology in addition to alterations in consciousness. For this reason they are not usually grouped with the other disorders of consciousness

---

activating system and the diffusely interconnecting cerebral cortical systems. Physiological activity in the reticular nuclei that run from the midpontine level to the interlaminar, midline, and periventricular thalamic and hypothalamic nuclei is integral for maintaining consciousness. Depression of this reticular activating system by drugs is similar to turning out the lights with a rheostat, whereas sudden destruction of this system as from a hemorrhage is like turning off a light switch. By way of contrast, damage to the cerebral cortex is like removing light bulbs one by one. Loss of consciousness is proportionate to the amount of damage done to the cerebral hemispheres by diffuse or multifocal processes. Encephalitis and meningitis are examples. Metabolic diseases and toxins are conditions that can affect both the reticular activating and diffuse cortical systems at the same time.

Despite a potentially confusing array of descriptive terms, operationally a clinical scale is commonly used in emergency rooms and intensive care units to numerically grade a patient's level of consciousness and follow progress over time. The Glasgow Coma Scale (Table 5–3) is easily used by nurses and physicians and allows for direct communication of changes in a patient's status. In addition, once the cause of coma is determined, the scale can be used to guide therapy as well as to estimate prognosis. For example, a patient with a brain stem hemorrhage with a persistent score of 6 for 3 days has a poor likelihood of recovering meaningful function. The same situation due to a drug overdose does not imply a bad outcome, since neuronal function is depressed but not destroyed. With proper care, complete recovery is the expectation.

Alterations of consciousness are a medical emergency. Failure to institute timely and appropriate treatment allows pathophysiological mechanisms to damage the brain irreversibly or lead to depression of brain stem functions and cessation of breathing. When a

TABLE 5–3. Glascow Coma Scale*

Eye opening	
Spontaneous	4
To speech	3
To pain	2
None	1
Best verbal response	
Oriented	5
Confused	4
Inappropriate	3
Incomprehensible	2
None	1
Best motor response	
Obeys commands	6
Localizes stimulus by appropriate movement	5
Demonstrates weak flexion	4
Demonstrates abnormal flexion	3
Demonstrates abnormal extension	2
None	1

*The patient's best performance is scored on sequential examinations.

physician encounters an obtunded or comatose patient, the first steps are the ''ABCs'' of emergency treatment: establish a clear *a*irway, assure normal *b*reathing, and support *c*ardiovascular function. These steps, together with starting intravenous glucose, assure that the brain will be supplied with normal levels of oxygen and glucose. A careful history and examination can then be performed to localize the abnormality and determine the underlying cause.

The differential diagnosis for causes of coma is long, but if a few points of history can be obtained, the list can be shortened (Table 5–4). A history of trauma, alcohol or drug abuse, epilepsy, or the presence of a systemic disease provides a leading hypothesis. A description of events from the prior 2 weeks may reveal the subacute course of an expanding mass lesion with progressive weakness and somnolence. A history of rapidly deteriorating neurological function in the preceding hours may indicate a brain stem, cerebellar, or subarachnoid hemorrhage. Prior headache and the presence of fever point to a severe CNS infection.

The examination of a comatose patient is focused on localizing a lesion in the reticular activating system, the cerebral cortex diffusely, or both. The examination is recorded in detail to provide a point in time against which serial examinations will judge the evolution of the patient and the effect of treatment. First, simple observations and tests will allow quick scoring on the Glasgow Coma Scale (Table 5–3). Second, observations of movements of the face, eyes, and body spontaneously or in response to noxious stimuli will reveal whether a focal, asymmetric process is involved or whether a metabolic process is depressing brain function diffusely. Third, particular attention is paid to brain stem reflex function.

Examination of the pupils provides important information in comatose patients and can be performed quickly (Figure 5–3). The diameter of the patient's pupils if normal should be within the range of diameters of other people in the same room under the same lighting conditions. Very small pupils indicate either excessive parasympathetic pupilloconstriction, as with

opioid administration, or block of sympathetic pupillodilation, as from the interruption of descending sympathetic pathways in the brain stem due to a pontine hemorrhage. Very large pupils on both sides indicate interruption of parasympathetic pupilloconstriction in the midbrain and suggest a metabolic cause of coma. Dilation of pupils occurs quickly following cardiac arrest as an early sign of cerebral ischemia.

Shining a bright light into one eye produces prompt, brisk constriction of both pupils in the normal condition. The response of both pupils upon illuminating each eye independently should be carefully observed and recorded. An asymmetric or absent efferent pupillary response on one side is strong evidence for compression of the pupilloconstrictor fibers in the ipsilateral third nerve. This occurs most commonly from an aneurysm on the posterior communicating artery or from the medial aspect of the temporal lobe when it becomes pushed over the edge of the tentorium by a mass lesion in a process called transtentorial herniation (Figure 5–4).

Inspection of the position of the eyes at rest in a normal sleeping person will reveal they are very slightly

TABLE 5–4. Common Causes of Coma

Metabolic Brain Disease

The neurological examination does not show any focal or asymmetric abnormalities. As coma deepens, there is progressive loss of the pupillary light reflex, vestibulo-ocular reflex, and ventilation. These functions are the first to return with recovery.
- Drugs and toxins: alcohol, barbiturates, opioids
- Cardiovascular disease: hypotension from arrhythmias, hemorrhage, cardiac arrest
- Diabetes mellitus: ketoacidosis, nonketotic hyperosmolarity
- Hypoglycemia: spontaneous, insulin overdose
- Infection: encephalitis, meningitis
- Pulmonary disease: hypoxemia, CO_2 narcosis
- Hepatic encephalopathy
- Uremia

Supratentorial Mass Lesions

There is usually a history of focal abnormalities leading progressively to obtundation over hours (hemorrhage), days (abscess), or weeks (tumor). The examination shows asymmetric or focal signs of weakness, pupillary response, and eye movements. The development of a third nerve palsy with a dilated fixed pupil is the classic sign of an expanding mass lesion in a hemisphere causing transtentorial herniation with compression of the midbrain reticular formation (Figure 5–4).
- Intracerebral hemorrhage
- Subdural hematoma
- Massive infarction
- Tumor
- Abscess

Posterior Fossa Lesions

These conditions can cause coma within minutes to hours after onset, since they can destroy or compress the reticular activating system. Mass lesions in the cerebellum can cause herniation of the tonsil through the foramen magnum (Figure 5–4). Death can occur quickly when ventilation is depressed. Acute headache accompanied by ataxia, dysarthria, and diplopia is an early warning symptom. Asymmetric brain stem signs are found on examination.
- Brain stem infarction
- Pontine hemorrhage
- Cerebellar mass lesion: hemorrhage, tumor, abscess

divergent. Finding this position in a comatose patient suggests that no focal lesions are causing asymmetric positioning of the eyes. For example, if the eyes are tonically deviated to one side, there could be a lesion of the ipsilateral frontal lobe eye fields, since the adversative action of the contralateral frontal lobe would be unopposed. In this situation, there often is weakness of the arm and leg on the side opposite to the deviation of the eyes. Conversely, there could be a lesion of the contralateral brain stem, leaving the ipsilateral gaze center's influence on cranial nerve VI and opposite nerve III unopposed, yoking the eyes away from the side of the lesion. In this situation, there is weakness on the same side as the deviation of the eyes. Since these conditions can be confusing, it is important to test the movement of the eyes by stimulating the vestibulo-ocular reflex.

In the "doll's eye maneuver," the VOR is tested by turning the patient's head quickly to one side and then the other and watching the movements of the eyes. In a normal awake person, the eyes either maintain their state of visual fixation or go where the person directs them. There is no reproducible reflex pattern. When this is done to a doll, the weights at the back of the eyes keep the gaze directed forward as the head is turned. When this is done to a comatose patient with a depressed cortex but intact brain stem, the VOR keeps the eyes directed forward (a positive "doll's eye reflex"). When the brain stem is depressed in addition to the cortex, the eyes will remain in a fixed position and turn with the head. A cold-water caloric test can be used to confirm abnormalities of the VOR. Irrigating the ear canal with ice water is the most potent stimulus for this reflex and is used to identify unilateral or bilateral brain stem dysfunction (Figure 5–5).

Upon completion of the history and the neurological examination, together with observations of ongoing changes in the state of the patient, the examiner should be able to conclude whether coma is caused by a diffuse metabolic process or a focal structural lesion above or below the tentorium (Table 5–4). This conclusion will lead to decisions regarding the need for blood tests to explore toxic and metabolic causes, for lumbar puncture to rule out infection, or for imaging studies to evaluate structural lesions. A CT scan is done emergently because it is faster than an MRI scan and has a high sensitivity for blood, since the majority of coma-producing mass lesions are hemorrhagic.

The specific treatment of the comatose patient depends on the diagnosis, but all patients are best managed in an intensive care unit until consciousness is recovered. Patients who have suffered head trauma or intracranial bleeding or who have required craniotomy for a mass lesion are prone to develop episodes of raised intracranial pressure. When high-pressure waves exceed arteriolar perfusion pressure, they can secondarily damage brain. In these patients, an intracranial pressure gauge is used to follow changes and direct therapy that lowers intracranial pressure. Hyperventilation is used to lower arterial pCO_2, which will constrict intracranial vessels. Osmotic diuretics (e.g., intravenous mannitol) will lower pressure by drawing water out of

normal areas of the brain where the blood-brain barrier is intact. However, such agents will increase edema and pressure where the blood-brain barrier is damaged such as around tumors and areas of hemorrhage. These treatments are used to buy time until the primary pathological process abates or surgical intervention is pursued. Continuous electroencephalographic monitoring, intracranial Doppler sonography, and xenon CT blood flow measurements are techniques that have been brought to the bedside to improve the care of comatose patients.

DISORDERS OF SLEEP

The natural circadian rhythm of animals includes sleep. In humans, the diurnal pattern becomes established by age 5, and the nightly amount of sleep for an individual remains relatively constant after age 20, declining slightly in the elderly. During the night, electroencephalographic recordings indicate that sleep passes between cycles of slow-wave sleep and rapid eye movement (REM) sleep. Slow-wave sleep has four stages, in which the dominant frequency of the electroencephalogram becomes slower and the amplitude higher as the sleep becomes deeper. The first REM phase usually begins after 90 minutes and is characterized by a low voltage and fast desynchronized electroencephalogram. There is complete inhibition of body tone during REM sleep except for the muscles to the eyes and ear ossicles. The eyes can be seen to move under the eyelids during REM sleep. There are four to six sleep cycles per night with the REM phase becoming longer toward morning. Greater than 75% of people report vivid dreams when awakened from REM sleep.

The cause of sleep is unknown. Experiments in animals indicate that the dorsal pontine reticular formation plays an important role. During REM sleep, EEG records spikes in the visual cortex that are known to originate in the pons and are relayed through the geniculate nucleus. These are called PGO spikes. This activity may be responsible for dreaming. The injection of carbachol, a cholinergic agonist, into the dorsal pons can induce REM sleep in cats. The injection of serotonin can induce slow-wave sleep. Blocking serotonin synthesis temporarily causes insomnia. The balance between neuronal activity and specific neurotransmitters in the dorsal pons during sleep is under active investigation.

Disorders of sleep are called **parasomnias** and occur mostly during slow-wave sleep in children. These include enuresis (bedwetting), sleepwalking, and night terrors. These benign problems often run in families. Children outgrow them. If they are disturbing, imipramine can be given to help control enuresis, and briefly waking the child after one hour of sleep may prevent night terrors. Some adults will have one or a few myoclonic jerks of muscles upon falling asleep. These are not pathological. Additionally, some people, as well as patients with peripheral neuropathy, report having "restless legs" upon retiring that prevents falling asleep. There is also a rare parasomnia in adults called REM behavioral disorder. When such patients enter REM sleep, they become behaviorally activated and can be

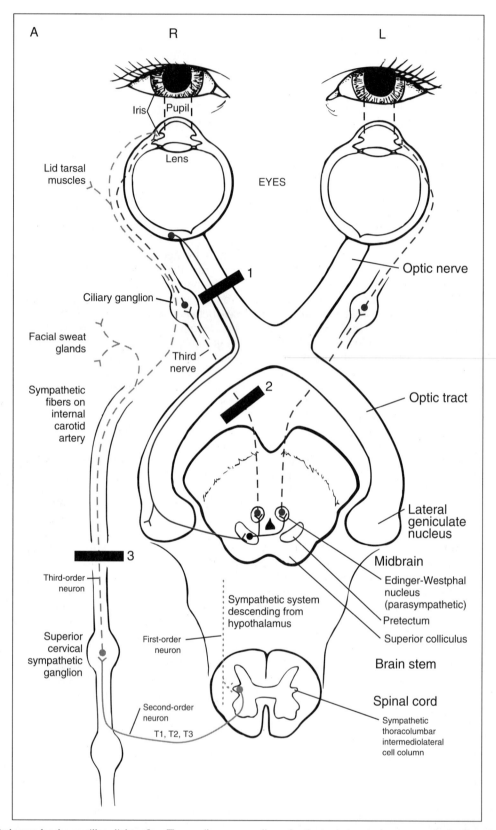

A, R, L

Iris | Pupil

Lens

Lid tarsal muscles

EYES

Optic nerve

1

Ciliary ganglion

Facial sweat glands

Third nerve

Sympathetic fibers on internal carotid artery

2

Optic tract

Lateral geniculate nucleus

Midbrain

Edinger-Westphal nucleus (parasympathetic)

Pretectum

Superior colliculus

3

Third-order neuron

Sympathetic system descending from hypothalamus

Brain stem

First-order neuron

Superior cervical sympathetic ganglion

Spinal cord

Sympathetic thoracolumbar intermediolateral cell column

Second-order neuron T1, T2, T3

FIGURE 5–3. *A,* Pathways for the pupillary light reflex. The pupils are normally under the tonic input of parasympathetic fibers from the Edinger-Westphal nucleus in the midbrain. With a decrease in ambient light, the tonic activity decreases and the pupils dilate. With any increase in light to either eye, both pupils constrict. The sympathetic input dilates the eye and can override parasympathetic influence in conditions of fright.

Legend continued on opposite page

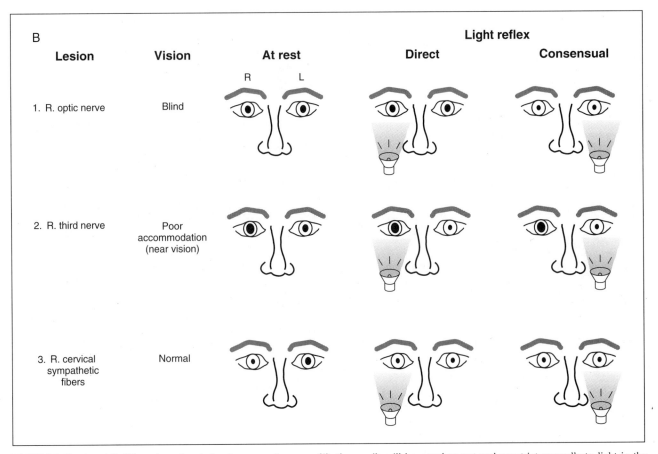

FIGURE 5-3 *Continued B*, When there is a lesion in one optic nerve (1), the pupils will be equal at rest and constrict normally to light in the opposite eye but constrict poorly to light in the affected eye. When the parasympathetic system is damaged (2), there is full dilatation of the eye. Conversely, when the sympathetic system is damaged (3), there is pupilloconstriction, often accompanied by ptosis and anhidrosis (Horner's syndrome; see text).

quite violent, injuring themselves or their partner. Clonazepam is useful for the restless leg syndrome as well as the REM behavioral disorder.

Insomnia is a common complaint in clinical medicine and has many causes. Most often there is an underlying emotional problem causing either anxiety with difficulty falling asleep, or depression with early morning awakening. Therapy should be directed at treating the underlying problem rather than prescribing hypnotic or sedative medicines. Chronic use of such medicines can cause abnormal sleep architecture. Most depress REM sleep, with a resultant rebound of REM sleep once they are stopped. Additionally, these medicines can be addictive (e.g., barbiturates) or habit forming (e.g., benzodiazepines) and should be used only for short periods of time to avoid developing dependence and withdrawal symptoms.

Excessive daytime sleepiness usually is the result of insufficient nighttime sleep. The brain will extract a fixed total amount of sleep over time. Occasionally, poor nocturnal sleep is due to **sleep apnea**. This condition occurs most often in overweight people with wide necks. During sleep, the uvula and posterior pharynx relax and block the airway. Snoring occurs on inspiration and leads to choking, which awakens the

patient and disrupts the amount and quality of sleep. Polysomnography is the clinical neurophysiological test for recording a patient's electroencephalogram, breathing pattern, arterial oxygen, and other variables during sleep. During obstructive sleep apnea, this test shows a fall in arterial oxygen saturation. The first line of treatment is weight reduction. Use of a tight-fitting mask and controlled positive airway pressure is helpful in keeping the posterior pharynx open. Rarely patients will require surgical removal of obstructive adenoids or posterior pharyngeal tissue.

Narcolepsy is another cause of daytime sleepiness. This condition is characterized by an intense and irresistible desire to sleep. Patients have short, 5- to 30-minute attacks of sleep, occasionally in awkward social circumstances or even while driving a car. When asked to try to go to sleep during the daytime, patients exhibit a rapid onset of REM sleep. This behavior is diagnostic of the disorder. Approximately 25% of patients will also have **cataplexy**, which is the sudden loss of motor tone brought on by excitement. One patient with narcolepsy, an opera singer, would become weak in the knees and occasionally fall down during particularly emotional arias. Other minor symptoms associated with this condition include hallucinations upon falling

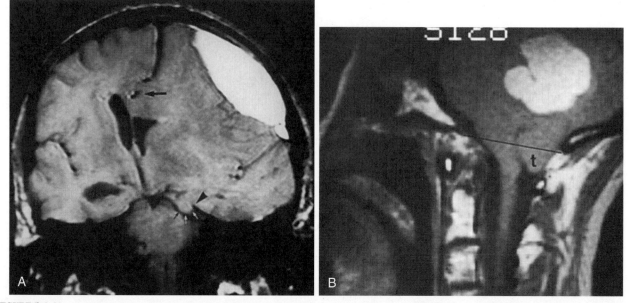

FIGURE 5–4. Herniation and coma. *A,* A subdural hematoma from head trauma has caused swelling of the left hemisphere and transtentorial herniation of the uncus of the temporal lobe (small arrows) through the incisural notch (arrowhead) to compress the midbrain. There is also herniation of the cingulate gyrus under the falx with lateral displacement of the anterior cerebral arteries (large arrow). The patient is comatose and has a left third nerve palsy, fixed dilated left pupil, and right hemiparesis. *B,* A large metastatic lesion in the cerebellum has pushed the tonsil of the cerebellum (t) through the foramen magnum (solid line). Tonsillar herniation can compress the medullary respiratory centers and lead quickly to cessation of breathing and death. (*A* and *B* are reproduced, with permission, from S. J. Willing. *Atlas of Neuroradiology.* Philadelphia, W.B. Saunders Co., 1995.)

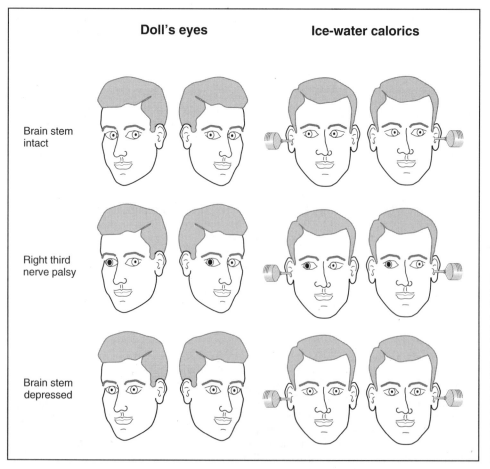

FIGURE 5–5. Vestibulo-ocular reflexes in comatose patients. When the brain stem VOR is intact, the doll's eye phenomenon will be present upon turning the head quickly from one side to the other, and cold calorics will tonically yoke the eyes to the side of irrigation. With a third nerve lesion, the affected eye fails to move with either the doll's eye maneuver or cold calorics. When there is deep depression of brain stem function, the doll's eye phenomenon is absent and cold caloric testing has no effect.

asleep and sleep paralysis. Rarely these symptoms can occur in isolation in otherwise healthy people. Usually they are transient phenomena.

The cause of narcolepsy is unknown. There is a strong familial occurrence, with most patients being positive for the Dw2 haplotype at the MHC gene locus on chromosome 6. This haplotype is also prominent in multiple sclerosis (Chapter 14), but there is no overlap between the two disorders. The Dw2 locus in narcolepsy may be a marker for an adjacent gene. Drugs that help alleviate narcolepsy (amphetamine and methylphenidate) cause release of catecholamines. Methylphenidate is used therapeutically. Additionally, tricyclic antidepressants, particularly clomipramine, are effective in abolishing cataplexy. Taken together, these facts suggest that the symptoms of narcolepsy are related to a genetic disorder of catecholamine pathways in the sleep centers in the brain stem.

DISORDERS OF AUTONOMIC FUNCTION

The sympathetic and parasympathetic nervous systems innervate the smooth muscle and secretory glands of the body. The sympathetic nerves leave the intermediolateral cell column in the thoracic and lumbar cord to synapse in the sympathetic chain ganglia adjacent to the spinal column. Postganglionic cells leave the ganglion to innervate their targets, where they release norepinephrine to act upon different classes of α- and β-receptors. The two exceptions to this plan are the sympathetic innervation of sweat glands, which release acetylcholine, and the preganglionic fibers to the adrenal medulla, which use acetylcholine to stimulate the release of epinephrine into the general circulation. Acting in unison, the sympathetic nervous system and the adrenal gland cause the emergency "fight or flight" reaction; signs include pupil dilatation, increase in heart rate and blood pressure, bronchodilatation, piloerection and sweating, and an increase in blood glucose and lipid levels. The hypothalamus and pituitary participate in this reaction by secreting corticotropin-releasing factor (CRF) and ACTH, which increase adrenal cortical secretion of glucocorticoids.

The parasympathetic nervous system travels with cranial nerves and pelvic nerves (S2, 3, and 4) to synapse upon postganglionic cells in the target organ. Postganglionic neurons release acetylcholine upon muscarinic receptors. Activity in this system is generally thought to control vegetative behaviors by slowing the heart rate, increasing secretion of salivary and digestive glands, and increasing gastrointestinal motility. The sympathetic and parasympathetic nervous systems often have opposing effects such as raising and lowering heart rate or pupillary dilatation or constriction. However, the two systems work together in controlling bladder and male sexual functions.

The integration and control of autonomic functions occur in the hypothalamus, which receives strong input from the limbic system—the amygdala, hippocampus, and olfactory cortex. In addition to orchestrating the emergency "fight or flight" reaction, a relatively rare event, the hypothalamus controls eating behavior, sex-

ual function, and body temperature. Through its direct influence on the pituitary and endocrine glands, it controls reproduction, lactation, and the body's use of fuels (glucocorticoids from the adrenal gland) and rate of metabolism (thyroxine from the thyroid gland). Small tumors of the hypothalamus or pituitary can disrupt these homeostatic functions. Craniopharyngiomas in children and prolactinomas and chromophobe adenomas in adults are examples. These are discussed in detail in textbooks of endocrinology. When these tumors enlarge, they compress the optic chiasm and cause visual field defects (Chapter 4).

There are several common syndromes of autonomic failure in clinical medicine. In evaluating each one it is best to try to locate the lesion either peripherally or centrally. The common peripheral causes of autonomic neuropathy include diabetic and amyloid neuropathy and the Guillain-Barré syndrome (Chapter 9). The central causes include multiple system atrophy (Shy-Drager syndrome; Chapter 11) and lesions that disrupt descending influences on spinal autonomic centers.

Horner's syndrome is the triad of unilateral ptosis, meiosis, and facial anhidrosis. It is caused by an interruption of the sympathetic innervation of the face due to a lesion that affects the first-order neuron (hypothalamus to thoracic cord), second-order neuron (thoracic cord to sympathetic chain), or third-order neuron (sympathetic ganglion to lid elevator muscle, iris, and face sweat glands; Figure 5–3). In practice, the presence of this syndrome in a patient should raise the possibility of a tumor affecting the second- or third-order neurons in the sympathetic chain, and search for a lesion in the lung or mediastinum should be undertaken.

Orthostatic hypotension is a leading symptom of diffuse autonomic failure once other causes are ruled out as discussed above. The presence of orthostatic hypotension in an elderly patient may signal an autonomic neuropathy. The presence of bradykinesia and rigidity indicates multiple system atrophy.

Urinary incontinence is usually evaluated by gynecologists (stress incontinence in women) and urologists (benign prostatic hypertrophy in men). There are three common neurological causes of incontinence. Peripheral autonomic neuropathy or compression of the S2–4 nerve roots in the spinal canal can disrupt both the afferent and efferent reflex pathways to the bladder. This leads to a distended, poorly contracting bladder and overflow incontinence. Urination is difficult and incomplete. Treatment with cholinergic stimulants that increase reflex contraction of the bladder (e.g., bethanechol chloride, 10–25 mg every 8 hours) or an α-adrenergic antagonist to relax the internal sphincter (e.g., phenoxybenzamine, 20–40 mg three times a day) can be useful.

Second, lesions above the sacral spinal cord that affect bilateral descending autonomic pathways will cause a spastic bladder. These pathways lie just medial to the corticospinal pathways so that patients commonly have spastic weakness of the legs in addition. An upper motor neuron lesion to the bladder results in a hyperactive bladder reflex. Distention from small volumes of urine (<200 mL) induces a strong reflex contraction and symptoms of urgency and frequency. Multiple sclerosis is a common cause. Occasionally a spinal cord tumor will present in this fashion. The use of anticholinergic medicines will help inhibit the hyperactive reflex (e.g., propantheline bromide, 15 mg four times a day). Limiting fluid intake and caffeine, setting regular times for urination, and intermittent catheterization are useful techniques that patients can learn to perform.

The third neurological cause of incontinence is damage to the frontal lobes and their fibers in the superior frontal gyrus and cingulum. Rarely, a meningioma of the falx will affect these areas bilaterally. The syndrome of normal-pressure hydrocephalus is a more common cause. This is a poorly understood condition that is characterized by a "glue footed," festinating gait, mild mental changes, and urinary incontinence. The loss of urine occurs without warning in a setting of otherwise normal bladder function. It surprises and embarrasses the patient. It is believed that the symptoms are caused by enlargement of the anterior horns of the lateral ventricles with stretching of descending fibers from the cortical representation for the bladder and the lower extremities. Surgical treatment of the hydrocephalus with ventricular shunting can be helpful for many patients.

Male impotence, defined as loss of erections, can be a sign of autonomic failure. If loss of libido, or sexual drive, is also present then depression, anxiety, or another psychological cause is usually involved. In this situation, nocturnal or early morning erections are usually preserved. These occur during REM sleep. Many commonly used drugs can interfere with libido, sexual performance, and orgasm in men and women, including antihypertensives, antidepressants, and antianxiety drugs. Alcohol is the most common offending agent. Loss of all erections with preserved libido can occur with peripheral autonomic neuropathy, destruction of the S2–4 spinal cord parasympathetic center, or central degenerative diseases. Spinal cord lesions above the lumbosacral cord leave autonomic reflexes intact, and

erections and ejaculation can occur. The use of testosterone, local intrapenile injection of vasoactive drugs (e.g., papaverine, prostaglandin E1), and mechanical devices can be helpful in restoring male potency.

SUMMARY

Neurological systems that control balance, sleep-wake cycles, consciousness, and internal homeostasis are vulnerable to the same disease processes that affect the rest of the nervous system. Disruption of these systems causes symptoms and signs that are usually specific for the site of the lesion peripherally or centrally. Neurological examination and laboratory procedures can localize and determine the pathological process in most cases. Disorders of labyrinthine function are profoundly disturbing to patients but often are self-limited and benign. Depression of consciousness is a medical emergency that should lead to rapid diagnosis and treatment to prevent irreversible brain damage due to a variety of causes. Evaluation of disorders of sleep and autonomic function can proceed in an orderly fashion and will likely reveal different treatable causes.

Selected Readings

Aldrich, M. S. Narcolepsy. N Engl J Med 323:389–394, 1990.
Baloh, R. W., and V. Honorubia. *Clinical Neurophysiology of the Vestibular System.* Philadelphia, F. A. Davis Co., 1979.
Brandt, T. *Vertigo, Its Multisensory Syndromes.* London, Springer-Verlag, 1991.
Epley, J. M. The canalith repositioning procedure for treatment of benign positional vertigo. Otolaryngol Head Neck Surg 107:399–404, 1992.
Levey, D. E., et al. Predicting outcome from hypoxic-ischemic coma. JAMA 253:1420–1426, 1985.
Plum, F., and J. B. Posner. *The Diagnosis of Stupor and Coma,* 3rd ed. Philadelphia, F. A. Davis, 1980.
Prinz, P. N., et al. Current concepts in geriatrics: Sleep disorders and aging. N Engl J Med 323:520–526, 1990.
Quality Standards Subcommittee of the American Academy of Neurology. Practice parameters: Assessment and management of patients in the persistent vegetative state (summary statement). Neurology 45:1015–1018, 1995.
Quality Standards Subcommittee of the American Academy of Neurology. Practice parameters for determining brain death in adults (summary statement). Neurology 45:1012–1014, 1995

CHAPTER SIX

DISORDERS

OF HIGHER

FUNCTIONS

INTRODUCTION **66**

NEUROBIOLOGY OF HUMAN BEHAVIOR **69**

   The Cerebral Cortex **69**

   The Prefrontal-Limbic System **70**

   The Temporal-Limbic System **70**

LANGUAGE FUNCTIONS **71**

   Aphasia **71**

   Alexia **73**

   Apraxia **73**

ATTENTIONAL SYSTEMS **74**

   The Parietal Lobe Syndrome **74**

FRONTAL LOBE FUNCTIONS **75**

   Circuit-Specific Behaviors **75**

LEARNING AND MEMORY **75**

   Amnesia Syndromes **77**

MOOD AND EMOTION **79**

   Depression **79**

   Obsessive-Compulsive Disorder **80**

   Schizophrenia **81**

SUMMARY **81**

INTRODUCTION

Human behavior is uniquely characterized by *capacities* to willfully direct and sustain attention, to create and communicate representational symbols, to search internally for past memories, and to make plans that guide future behavior. Humans alone create internal mental states, abstract or emotionally charged, through which they explore the world and analyze the self. These higher functions are largely the property of the cerebral cortex and the limbic system, areas that have expanded as much as tenfold in the evolution of

the human brain compared with the closest primate (Figure 6–1).

Focal disease processes that affect the cerebral cortex or the limbic system can disrupt individual components of integrated human behavior and cause difficulty with language, spatial orientation, and memory. Determining the site of lesions causing behavioral dysfunction has allowed mapping of the brain for normal higher brain functions. The science of functional localization began in the 19th century when the French physician Pierre Paul Broca first described a lesion in the left inferior frontal gyrus as a cause of aphasia (Box

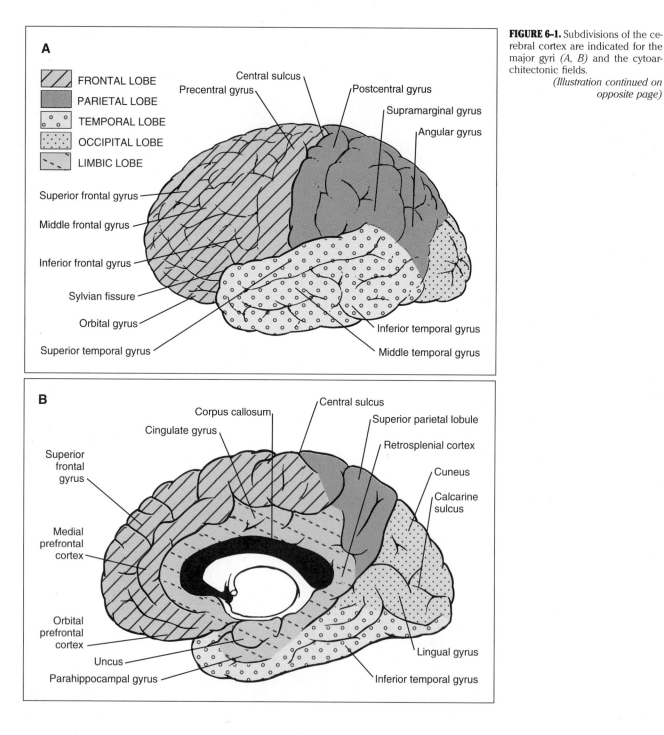

A

- FRONTAL LOBE
- PARIETAL LOBE
- TEMPORAL LOBE
- OCCIPITAL LOBE
- LIMBIC LOBE

Superior frontal gyrus
Middle frontal gyrus
Inferior frontal gyrus
Sylvian fissure
Orbital gyrus
Superior temporal gyrus

Central sulcus
Precentral gyrus
Postcentral gyrus
Supramarginal gyrus
Angular gyrus
Inferior temporal gyrus
Middle temporal gyrus

B

Corpus callosum
Cingulate gyrus
Central sulcus
Superior parietal lobule
Retrosplenial cortex
Cuneus
Calcarine sulcus
Superior frontal gyrus
Medial prefrontal cortex
Orbital prefrontal cortex
Uncus
Parahippocampal gyrus
Lingual gyrus
Inferior temporal gyrus

FIGURE 6–1. Subdivisions of the cerebral cortex are indicated for the major gyri *(A, B)* and the cytoarchitectonic fields.
(Illustration continued on opposite page)

6–1). Today functional imaging techniques are being used to corroborate and extend observations of patients with focal neurological lesions. Positron emission tomography (PET scanning) and functionally activated magnetic resonance imaging (fMRI) are two potent methods for localizing higher brain functions in healthy people. These noninvasive techniques can be performed many times over in the same subject. These features allow using the subject as his or her own control such that a brain image taken while resting can be subtracted from an image obtained during the performance of a higher brain function. Subtraction images have been used to localize cortical sites for color vision, individual steps in language processing,

attentional systems, motor learning, working memory, and aspects of emotion.

One goal of neuroscience is the explicit description of brain functions unique to humans. Different models have been proposed to help guide experiments. Development of the first model is credited to the British neurologist Hughlings Jackson for his analysis of patients around the turn of the century. It is called the **hierarchical model**. Jackson observed that lesions of lower brain centers disrupted simple automatic functions, whereas lesions of prefrontal cortex disrupted purposeful movement—the "least automatic," or higher, brain functions. The higher centers were evolutionary elaborations of the lower centers and arose as

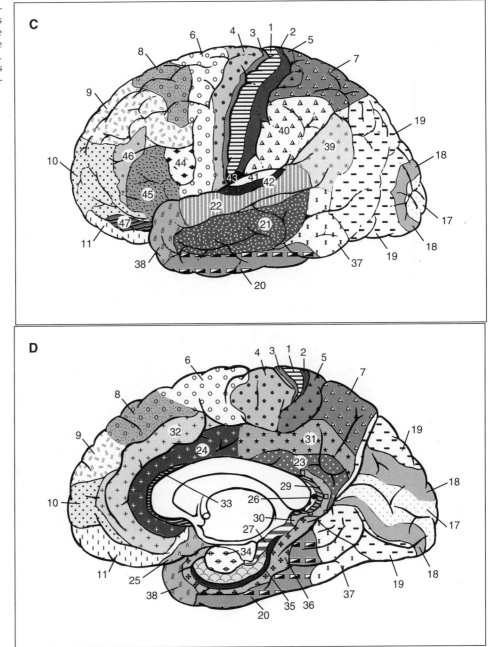

FIGURE 6–1 *Continued.* (*C, D;* numbered according to Brodmann's 1907 map). These illustrations are stylized, and there is considerable variability among human brains. Note that cytoarchitectonic fields do not coincide with gyral patterns.

BOX 6-1   Broca's Aphasia

Pierre Paul Broca (1824–1880), French surgeon and anthropologist, is credited with the first demonstration of a focal lesion of the left hemisphere associated with loss of language. In his seminal report of 1861 he called the deficit *aphemia*, and it came to be called aphasia by others. At autopsy of the patient in question, a large cyst emanating from the sylvian fissure was compressing the inferior frontal convolutions, the insula, and the underlying striatum. Since the greatest area of destruction was the posterior extent of the third (inferior) convolution and the longest standing symptom was total lack of verbal expression but for a single syllable, he assigned localiza-

tion for articulation of speech to this gyrus, naming it the *circonvolution du langage*. Others later named it Broca's convolution. The report was controversial from the start—and modern studies have found that infarction of Broca's convolution does not always cause Broca's aphasia—but the principles and practice of localization of higher functions were established. The notion of Broca's *area* survives today when considering the localization of nonfluent or expressive aphasia (Figure 6–4), but assignment of articulation of language to a portion of one specific gyrus is not possible.

AN OBSERVATION OF APHEMIA *

On April 11, 1861, a fifty-one-year-old man named Leborgne suffering from a diffuse gangrenous inflammation of the entire right lower limb . . . was admitted as a surgical patient to the general infirmary of the Bicêtre. When I questioned him the next day about the onset of his illness his only response was the monosyllable "tan," repeated twice in succession and accompanied by a movement of the left hand.

Leborgne had been subject to epileptic fits since his youth, but he worked as a lastmaker until the age of thirty, when he lost his speech and was admitted to the hospice of the Bicêtre as an invalid.

He was intelligent and in excellent general health, suffering only from loss of articulate speech. He came and went in the hospice where he was known by the name of Tan. He understood everything that was said to him . . . but regardless of the question put to him, he always answered "tan, tan."

Ten years after he lost the ability to speak, a new symptom appeared: the muscles of his right arm gradually weakened and eventually became completely paralyzed. Tan continued to ambulate without difficulty, but the paralysis slowly spread to involve the right lower extremity. Tan had been confined to bed for almost seven years when he was transferred to the Bicêtre infirmary.

Tan's right arm and leg were completely paralyzed. His

face was symmetrical at rest; however, when he inflated his cheeks the left cheek ballooned out slightly more than the right. The tongue moved freely and did not deviate; the patient was able to protrude it and move it in all directions.

It was not possible to reach any firm conclusions about Tan's intellect. . . . He fared best with numerical answers, which he communicated with his fingers . . . I showed him my watch on two successive days. The second hand was not working, and, consequently, he could only distinguish the three hands by their shape and length. Nevertheless, after examining the watch for a few moments he was able to indicate the correct time on each occasion. There can be no doubt, therefore, that this man was intelligent, that he was able to think, and that he had retained in some measure his memory for past events.

It was obvious from the history and from the results of my examination that this was a progressive cerebral lesion, which at the outset and during the first ten years of Tan's illness had remained limited to a rather circumscribed region, sparing the motor and sensory organs [sic] and that after ten years the lesion spread to involve one or more motor organs. Since Tan's right side was completely paralyzed and since sensation in his right limbs was slightly impaired, the principal cerebral lesion must have been in the left hemisphere.

The patient died at 11 AM on April 17.

*P. Broca. Remarques sur le siège de la faculté du langage articulé d'une observation d'aphemie (perte de la parole). Bull Soc Anat Paris, 2e série 6:332–333, 343–357, 1861. Excerpted from a translation by C. Westerlain and D. A. Rottenberg. Remarks on the seat of the faculty of articulate speech, followed by the report of a case of aphemia (loss of speech). Excerpted, with permission of Simon & Schuster, from D. A. Rottenberg and F. H. Hochberg (eds.). *Neurological Classics in Modern Translation*. Copyright 1977 by Hafner Press, pp. 136–145.

---

a process to control them. This model remains current, albeit modified, in studies of perceptual systems in experimental primates. For example, neurons in primary visual cortex become active in response to simple orientations of lines, whereas neurons located in visual centers farther downstream in temporal cortex become active only in response to complex shapes such as faces. This model proposes that perceptions of the external world are built up hierarchically as neuronal activity is relayed from primary sensory cortex to association cortex and onward.

Two additional models guide current thinking of higher brain function. The model of **parallel processing** takes note of the redundancy of pathways available to analyze sensation and support behavior. A

simple example is given by the two pathways that carry touch sensations from the periphery up the spinal cord and into the cortex (Chapter 4). Individual modalities are partially separated in the two somatosensory systems such that information is processed in parallel. In animals the information in each pathway is linked to behavior, but in humans the pathways must become merged in the cortex before a felt sensation can be fully appreciated and identified mentally.

The third model is called the **distributed system**. This model notes that the performance of complex functions is the expression of concurrent activity within widely distributed but localizable modules of cortex and their subcortical targets of projection. Functional imaging is one technique that is useful in identifying these different sites in humans. For example, PET scans have shown that as many as seven different cortical sites become active during the reading of simple words. However, owing to the spatial and temporal limits of resolution of such technologies, the functional activation map of humans is still relatively crude. Ideally, one would like to record directly any changes in neuronal firing throughout the brain in association with a particular behavior in order to explore this model fully.

A second goal of human neuroscience is to discover the neurobiological substrates that make each human unique. Why can some people process information more rapidly and accurately than others? Why do others have larger capacities for working memory, or special skills in mathematics, music, or dance? To what degree are these attributes inherited or learned? How does this learning take place? How can it be facilitated? The answers to these questions lie largely in studies of the structure and function of the cerebral cortex.

NEUROBIOLOGY OF HUMAN BEHAVIOR

Higher brain functions in humans are defined simply as those requiring the integration of perception, thought, and emotion with movement. Anatomically the key components of these functions lie in the association areas of the cerebral cortex and the limbic system. They are also greatly influenced by four neuropharmacological systems that project from subcortical sites upon the cortex. The acetylcholine system projects from the basal forebrain into the dentate gyrus of the hippocampus and diffusely upon the cortex. The dopamine system in the ventral tegmentum projects heavily upon the prefrontal cortex. The norepinephrine system ascends from the locus caeruleus, and the serotonin system from the raphe nuclei, to project diffusely upon cortex. Abnormalities in these four systems can have a profound influence on attention, memory, mood, and cognitive processing.

The Cerebral Cortex

The *neo*cortex of mammals is the six-layered sheet of neurons covering the cerebral hemispheres. This structure has many common features among different species. Layer IV contains a high density of granule cells in the zones of termination for the specific afferents from the thalamus. This "granular cortex" histologically characterizes the primary receptive cortices for vision, hearing, and somatosensory sensation, as well as the prefrontal cortex, which receives primary afferents from the dorsomedial thalamic nucleus. Other cortical areas have far fewer layer IV granule cells. Layers V and VI contain neurons that primarily project out of cortex. Motor cortex is distinguished by giant pyramidal neurons in these deep layers whose axons make the greatest contribution to the corticospinal pathway. Layers II and III neurons contribute to short and long corticocortical and callosal pathways, connecting one zone to another.

Variations in the density of neurons in the different layers were used by scientists at the turn of the century to produce cytoarchitectonic maps of the human brain. The Brodmann map of 1907 (Figure 6–1C and D) is still used to assign locations of cerebral functions, although the exact boundaries between areas are highly variable among individuals. In monkeys, different cytoarchitectonic zones can be further subdivided by input and output connections. Taken altogether, each point on the cortical sheet can be characterized by cytoarchitectonics, thalamic input, local and long cortical connections, subcortical projections, and the receptive field properties of the area's neurons. The last term denotes the types of sensation, movement, emotion, and conditional stimulus attributes that cause the neuron to change its rate of firing.

Through evolution the cortical sheet has become up to tenfold larger in surface area from monkeys (200 cm^2) to humans (1900 cm^2) but only two- to threefold thicker. The vertical histological organization of cortex has remained constant in evolution. This finding reflects the common pattern of development of cortex during embryogenesis among mammals. In the earliest stages of brain formation, primordial neurons divide in the germinal matrix around the ventricle and daughter neurons migrate radially outward along glial "guide wires" to their position in the cortex. The final number of neurons in any one column of cortex running from the white matter to the surface is constant from area to area, except for the visual cortex, where the number is doubled. The number is also constant from species to species. Thus, evolution has advanced by increasing the number of cell divisions in the germinal matrix and simply adding on more cortical columns over time rather than by creating an entirely new architectural design. The expanding thickness of cortex in primates has been caused by an elaboration of local circuitry within each column. The greater thickness of human cortex is an expression of the greater complexity of wiring. There has also been some expansion of older, three-layered cortex in the hippocampus (*archaeo*cortex), as well as in transitional zones between archaeocortex and neocortex, e.g., the entorhinal cortex in the parahippocampal gyrus (*palaeo*cortex).

The greatest areal expansion within *neo*cortex has occurred in association areas, particularly the prefrontal cortex. The primary sensory areas of cortex subserving somatic sensation (areas 3, 1, and 2), vision (area 17), and hearing (areas 41 and 42) occupy less than 10% of the cortical surface area (Figure 6–1C and D). Studies in monkeys show that each of these primary zones projects into immediately adjacent association cortex for further processing of these sensations. These primary association zones subsequently project upon four common targets: the parietal cortex, prefrontal cortex, cingulate gyrus medially, and parahippocampal gyrus inferiorly. Studies of neurons in these zones in monkeys indicate highly complex receptive field properties. Rather than firing in response to a single type of sensation, their activation is conditional upon the timing and place of the stimulus, the presence or absence of other sensory stimuli, the emotional state of the monkey, and the intended use of the sensation for subsequent movement. Functional images of these zones in humans indicate that they are never activated in isolation but rather within a network of sensory and motor areas. This networking occurs during a single sensation as well as during the imagination of sensation. It also occurs during movement as well as in anticipation of movement. In addition, these areas become functionally stimulated by many different types of behaviors, indicating a convergent activation of common behavioral attributes elaborated within the areas, such as attention to novelty (cingulate cortex) or working memory (dorsolateral prefrontal cortex).

The size of any cortical area is influenced by its use. For example, when a nerve to a finger is cut, the cortical representation of adjacent fingers expands. If one eye is removed in a young animal, the ocular dominance columns of the other eye enlarge in the visual cortex. The association areas are particularly malleable during development. Damage to the left, or dominant, hemisphere of an infant shifts language functions to the right hemisphere. In addition, the field of activation of a cortical area is influenced by experience. For example, when a human first attempts a novel motor task, a large area of the motor cortex becomes functionally activated. With practice and improvement in performance, the area of activation becomes more discrete, reflecting attainment of a "functional efficiency." These findings indicate that the cerebral cortex is much more plastic than was once thought.

The Prefrontal-Limbic System

The frontal lobe, defined as the cortical area anterior to the central gyrus, is divided into motor cortex (area 4), premotor cortex (areas 6 and 8), and prefrontal cortex (areas 9, 10, 11, 44, 45, 46, and 47) (Figure 6–1C and D). The prefrontal cortex is characterized histologically as granular cortex owing to its strong afferent input to layer IV from the dorsomedial thalamic nucleus. Prefrontal cortex is divided into three areas (Figure 6–2). The dorsolateral area receives input from the lateral (parvicellular) part of the dorsomedial nucleus, which also projects to the cingulate, retrosplenial, and parahippocampal gyri as well, thus linking prefrontal *neo*cortex with limbic *palaeo*cortex (Figure 6–2). Similarly, the orbitofrontal and mediofrontal divisions of the prefrontal cortex are reciprocally connected to the medial (magnicellular) part of the dorsomedial nucleus as well as the amygdala, thus forming another neocortical-limbic unit. These latter two areas of frontal cortex and the amygdala project down upon the medial and ventral aspects of the striatum, called the *limbic striatum*. Through its projections to globus pallidus and substantia nigra and hence to thalamus, the limbic striatum forms a loop circuit back to cortex. Similar to the neocortical-striatal-thalamic loop circuits subserving motor functions (Chapter 3), these loop circuits serve cognitive and emotional functions. Disorders affecting these pathways cause abnormalities in emotions, motivation, and decision making while leaving sensation and movement unaffected (see below).

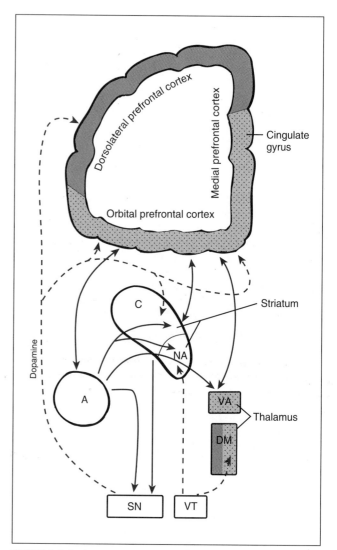

FIGURE 6–2. Prefrontal-limbic systems. Prefrontal granular cortex is defined by its input from the dorsomedial nucleus. The lateral part of the dorsomedial thalamic nucleus (DM) has reciprocal connections with the dorsolateral cortex, and the medial part with the orbital prefrontal and medial prefrontal areas, as indicated by the shading. In addition, the ventral anterior nucleus (VA) projects to the cingulate cortex. There are strong interconnections of the prefrontal cortex with the amygdala (A) and the medial and ventral striatum. Dopamine input to these areas comes from the substantia nigra (SN) and ventral tegmentum (VT). C, caudate; NA, nucleus accumbens.

The Temporal-Limbic System

The hippocampus, lying within the medial folds of the temporal lobe, is the cortical structure uniquely required for the formation of memory in animals including humans. In lower species, the hippocampus is primarily concerned with spatial memory, particularly in recollecting the location of odors linked to food, sexual mating, and the territory of predators. The olfactory system forms a major input to the hippocampus in these species. In humans, the major input to the hippocampal formation comes from the temporal and parietal association cortices via the parahippocampal gyrus. Activity in frontal cortex gains access to the hippocampal formation via projections upon the cingulate and retrosplenial cortex and reaches the amygdala via the uncinate fasciculus (Figure 6–3).

Projections into the hippocampus from the parahippocampal gyrus go through a loop circuit made up of the dentate gyrus and hippocampal pyramidal cell layers, which project back upon the subicular cortex. The subicular cortex projects down through the fornices into the septal nuclei of the basal forebrain and the mamillary bodies of the hypothalamus. In addition, the subicular cortex is strongly linked with the amygdala, lying anterior to the hippocampal formation. These circuits thus link highly processed neocortical information about the external world with systems concerned with internal homeostasis (hypothalamus) and emotion (amygdala).

Bilateral damage within temporal-limbic circuits can irreversibly destroy memory and emotional aspects of higher brain functions in humans. For example, patients with lesions within the hippocampal loop circuit cannot learn to recognize the identity of a new face. Nevertheless, they may show an emotional or covert autonomic nervous system reaction to the face, such as a change in galvanic skin response. By contrast, patients with bilateral damage to the amygdala will recognize the identity of a face but neither feel nor express any emotional reaction. Such patients with symmetric bilateral lesions are uncommon in clinical medicine, but studies of their behavior have revealed the distributed modular organization of individual components of complex human behavior.

LANGUAGE FUNCTIONS

Communication through spoken language is unique to humans. This capacity is highly localized to the left hemisphere and correlates with anatomic asymmetries in the temporal and frontal lobe cortex (Figure 6–4). In the temporal lobe the cortex associated with Wernicke's area (planum temporale), and in the frontal lobe the cortex associated with Broca's area (posterior third of the inferior frontal convolution), are larger in the left hemisphere compared with the right in the great majority of cases studied. There are no such asymmetries in subhuman primates. Those species and many others communicate vocally with sounds that signify emotional content largely related to eating, mating, and defense behaviors. The neuroanatomy subserving this type of vocalization is located bilaterally in limbic structures (cingulate gyrus, amygdala, preoptic area, hypothalamus, and midbrain reticular formation). Lesions in these areas in humans can result in muteness, indicating an important relationship between older vocalization systems and newer-dominant hemisphere language systems.

Aphasia

Aphasia is a common symptom in clinical neurology and largely reflects strokes due to occlusion of the left middle cerebral artery or its branches within the zone of language (Figure 6–4). Tumors, infections, and epileptic and degenerative conditions affecting this cortical area are additional causes. As with all lesions of the cortex, the speed of onset, severity, and accompanying symptoms and signs provide clinical clues about the etiology. Neurologists classify the phenomenology of aphasia symptoms into different syndrome types reflecting damage to different areas (Box 6–2).

Broca's aphasia (Box 6–1) is characterized by great difficulty in speaking. By contrast, understanding language is relatively well preserved. This syndrome is also called nonfluent, expressive, or motor aphasia. For example, a patient will be able to obey multiple-step commands (e.g., "put your left thumb over your right eye and stamp your foot twice") but be unable to say even a simple word (e.g., "thumb"). Patients can read

FIGURE 6–3. Temporal-limbic systems. The limbic lobe lies on the medial aspect of the hemisphere and includes the cingulate gyrus, parahippocampal gyrus (entorhinal cortex), amygdala, and their connections. The input to the temporal-limbic system through the parahippocampal gyrus comes from association areas of neocortex that receive reciprocal connections from the amygdala and subiculum (not shown). The parahippocampal gyrus sends information through the circuits of the hippocampal formation, where registration and consolidation of declarative memory occurs. Projections leave the hippocampus via the subiculum, which projects down through the fornix to the septal area and the hypothalamus (Box 6–5).

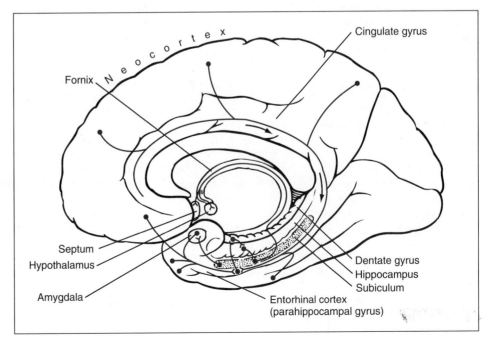

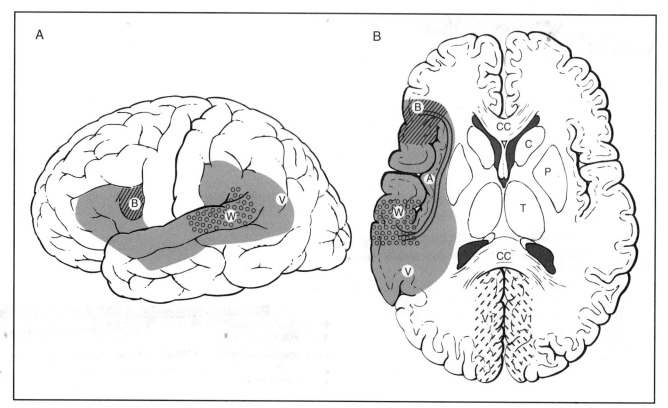

FIGURE 6–4. The zone of language. The concept of a "zone of language" was first proposed by Dejerine in 1914 to illustrate localization of the components of language as discovered by focal lesions of the left hemisphere in patients. Broca's area (B) is localized to the posterior (opercular) part of the inferior frontal gyrus. Wernicke's area (W) lies behind Heschl's gyrus (not labeled) and occupies the planum temporale. The arcuate fasciculus (A) connects the posterior parts of the zone to the anterior parts. Dejerine also proposed an area for the visual images of words (V). Patients who suffer a stroke within the distribution of the superior branch of the left middle cerebral artery have a Broca type aphasia, whereas infarcts from occlusion of the inferior temporal division or its branches cause a Wernicke type aphasia. C, caudate; CC, corpus callosum; P, putamen; T, thalamus; V1, primary visual cortex.

normally silently, but writing is impaired (**agraphia**). Thus, the dysfunction lies within language systems rather than in cortical motor systems *per se*. However, since Broca's area lies close to the motor strip, patients with Broca's aphasia due to stroke commonly also have weakness of the right side of the face and right hand. Patients are aware of their deficit and frustrated by their loss of communication. However, the prognosis for recovery of some spoken language is usually good, although it requires many months and usually leaves the patient with a shortened, telegraphic type of speech composed mostly of nouns and verbs.

Wernicke's aphasia is characterized by difficulty in understanding language. In addition, speech is fluent but often devoid of nouns and conveys little meaning. This syndrome is also called fluent, receptive, or sensory aphasia. For example, patients have difficulty understanding and thus obeying multiple-step commands. In the example given above, a patient might hold up a hand and ask quizzically, "you mean put the thing over this up here?" In contrast to patients with Broca's aphasia, they initiate speech spontaneously, although it is predominantly composed of prepositional phrases and is circumlocutious, leading farther and farther from the point as it continues. There may be paraphasias, with one word replacing another, such as calling a spoon a fork (literal paraphasia), or one sound

replacing another, such as calling a spoon a sploom (verbal paraphasia). Lesions in the posterior aspects of the zone of language cause no weakness or sensory loss. Relatives or friends who hear the patient speak often conclude that there is a psychiatric problem rather than a focal brain abnormality. Patients themselves are unaware of their deficit. The prognosis for recovery of full language comprehension in these patients is poor.

Global aphasia is the loss of all language skills: comprehension, speaking, reading and writing. The usual cause is a complete infarct within the territory of the left middle cerebral artery. Patients with this syndrome usually suffer a dense right hemiparesis in addition. Such a stroke leaves the patient essentially demented. The prognosis for recovery is poor. Two exceptions are noteworthy. Compression of the lateral convexity of the left hemisphere by a subdural hematoma following head trauma can cause global aphasia. Surgical drainage will restore language in most cases. Second, epileptic discharges within the zone of language can cause temporary, but recurring, aphasia. Anticonvulsant medications can prevent this type of aphasia.

Conduction aphasia is an uncommon but informative abnormality for students of language. Both comprehension and spontaneous fluent speech are rel-

CHAPTER 6   DISORDERS OF HIGHER FUNCTIONS   **73**

BOX 6-2 Glossary of Common Terms for Abnormalities of Higher Functions

Acalculia: loss of the ability to calculate, or perform simple arithmetic.

Agraphia: loss of the ability to write, a common symptom of aphasia.

Agnosia: loss of the ability to recognize objects within one sensory domain but not other domains. Recognition of objects by another sensory system indicates normal memory and naming functions.

> **Tactile agnosia:** inability to recognize objects by feeling them in the hand; also called astereognosis.

> **Visual agnosia:** inability to recognize objects by sight; also called cortical blindness.

> **Prosopagnosia:** inability to recognize familiar faces.

> **Anosognosia:** denial of deficit.

Alexia: loss of the ability to read.

Aphasia: Loss of the capacity and skills for spoken and written language.

> **Broca's aphasia:** difficulty in speaking. Comprehension is preserved. Also called nonfluent, expressive, or motor aphasia.

> **Wernicke's aphasia:** impaired comprehension. Speaking is relatively well preserved. Also called fluent, receptive, or sensory aphasia.

> **Conduction aphasia:** relatively preserved comprehension and spontaneous fluent speech but with inability to repeat words correctly.

> **Global aphasia:** difficulty with comprehension, repetition, and speaking.

Apraxia: loss of the ability to perform learned motor skills with the hands. Sensation, strength, and coordination are relatively well preserved.

---

atively well preserved. In contrast, patients have great difficulty repeating even simple phrases. A focal lesion affects the arcuate fasciculus, the pathway that connects Wernicke's area to Broca's area (Figure 6–4). Patients are recognized by the occurrence of paraphasic abnormalities in speech. In addition, as with all aphasic syndromes, patients are unable to write. This condition is cited as an example of a "disconnection syndrome," in which the deficit reflects an inability to send information from one cortical area to another while the cortical areas themselves remain relatively unaffected. Language that is heard and understood in temporal cortex cannot be relayed to the anterior frontal speech areas for repetition.

Alexia

The ability to read requires the integration of visual information from either of the two occipital lobes with word processing functions within the zone of language. Alexia, the inability to read, is often part of the Wernicke aphasia syndrome, reflecting damage to the posterior temporo-occipital cortex. There may be a total loss of reading ability, or patients may be able to read a few words, or spell out the words, but have difficulty in identifying the meaning of the words. Studies of such

patients suggest that separate cortical areas deal with the graphic, syntactic, and semantic aspects of language.

Alexia without agraphia is a second type of disconnection syndrome. In this situation, patients are unable to read but they can write, and the other language skills of comprehension, repetition, and fluency are normal. Writing is the most fragile language skill, and its preservation in this syndrome indicates that the loss of reading is a relatively isolated symptom. Indeed, patients cannot even read what they themselves write. Curiously, most patients also have difficulty naming colors. Although they cannot name a color to which the examiner points, they can correctly point to a color the examiner names. Thus, they have a deficit in the naming as opposed to the perception of color. Finally, most patients also have a right homonymous hemianopia. The cause of this syndrome is a stroke of the left posterior cerebral artery in its proximal portion. The stroke causes infarction of the posterior third of the corpus callosum as well as the left occipital cortex. The latter lesion causes the contralateral hemianopia. The infarct of the corpus callosum blocks communication from the uninvolved right visual cortex to the zone of language in the left hemisphere (Figure 6–4). The two areas are disconnected. If the corpus callosum were not infarcted, a patient's normal left visual field would see text and colors and convey the information normally to the left hemisphere for reading and color naming. The normal function of the right visual cortex is illustrated by a patient's capacity to identify colors by pointing.

On occasion, when the left angular gyrus in the temporoparietal cortex is included in the lesion or is the sole site of the lesion, a constellation of other symptoms occurs including right-left confusion, finger agnosia, and acalculia. This cluster of symptoms is called the Gerstmann syndrome after its discoverer. It is proposed that the clustering of these symptoms reflects how children are taught to count, add, and subtract as they learn to name their fingers. Thus, arithmetic, finger identification, and right-versus-left orientation would be functionally and anatomically linked in this cortical area.

Apraxia

The loss of the ability to execute learned motor skills upon command is called apraxia. Apraxia occurs most commonly with lesions of the dominant parietal lobe. For example, when a patient is asked to show how he would comb his hair using his hand he would have difficulty doing this correctly despite understanding the command and having no sensory, motor, or coordination deficits. Apraxia reflects a failure of language to invoke a well-learned motor program. The motor program itself is often preserved. In this example, the patient would probably show no deficit in combing his hair within the normal context of dressing in front of a mirror. With unilateral damage to the parietal cortex, the abnormalities of apraxia are usually manifested only within the artificial context of the examination. When there is bilateral damage, the apraxia disrupts ordinary daily behaviors such as dressing, bathing, and preparing and eating meals. This situation occurs in Alzheimer's disease.

ATTENTIONAL SYSTEMS

The capacity for focusing attention upon an external stimulus, an internal thought, or a behavioral task underlies all other cognitive functions. In clinical neurology, it is important to ensure that a patient has this capacity before testing memory, language, and cognition. Often this can be accomplished by noting a patient's ability to participate fully in a conversation, responding appropriately and correctly at the right time. A patient who exhibits distractibility or confusion should be tested directly for skills of attention. The examiner should ask such a patient to repeat a series of numbers forward, or give them backward, or raise a hand whenever the examiner says the letter "a" in a series of letters. Difficulty in performing these simple tests is common in diffuse metabolic and toxic abnormalities of brain as well as in dementia.

The Parietal Lobe Syndrome

Abnormalities of attention can occur with focal lesions of the cortex, being most prominent following damage to the inferior parietal lobule of the nondominant hemisphere. This area receives highly processed visual and somatosensory information and integrates it for the orientation of the eyes and movement of the body into contralateral space. It sends this information anteriorly to the frontal eye fields and premotor cortex for execution of movement and receives modifying influences in return. The receptive field properties of neurons in this parietal cortex are tuned to the visuospatial information of the stimulus as well as somatosensory information for the position of the head, eyes, and arm. In addition, parietal neurons become conditioned to past experience with the stimulus and its potential relationship with intended movements or rewards.

Patients with damage to the right parietal lobe do not take notice of objects in the left visual world despite having full visual fields on direct testing. The most subtle abnormality is neglect of left visual stimuli when bilateral stimuli are presented. This can be revealed by testing the visual fields of both eyes and both fields simultaneously, or simply by asking a patient to bisect a horizontal line. The patient will designate a center point to the right of true center, neglecting much of the left side of the line (Figure 6–5A). In addition, patients will have difficulty directing their eyes to the left and reaching for objects in left space. They may even fail to dress the left side of their body, or eat food off the left side of their plate. When asked to draw a clock, face, or a house from memory they will neglect many details on the left side (Figure 6–5B). In addition, they will have difficulty in copying drawings of two- or three-dimensional objects, an abnormality called constructional apraxia (Figure 6–5C). Curiously, patients will be largely unaware of their deficit in attention.

In addition to deficits in visuospatial attention and orientation due to parietal lesions, patients will have abnormalities of somatosensory function. These may be

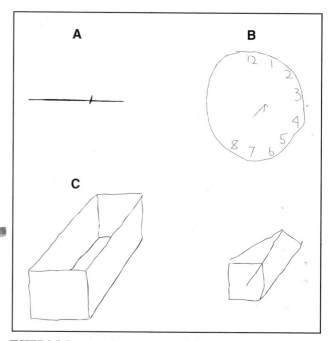

FIGURE 6-5. Drawings from patients with lesions of the right parietal lobe, retouched for purposes of illustration. *A,* The patient has attempted to bisect the line in the middle. Much of the left side is neglected. *B,* A patient's attempt to draw the face of a clock at 9:20 from memory. The left side is largely ignored. *C,* A patient's attempt (at right) to copy the examiner's drawing of a cube.

subtle, such as neglect of stimuli delivered to the left hand when both hands are stimulated simultaneously. However, most patients also exhibit **astereognosis**, or tactile agnosia. When a common object that the patient easily identifies by sight alone, such as a key, is placed in the patient's left hand, the patient will be unable to identify it with the eyes closed. In addition, the patient will not manipulate the object placed in the hand with normal manual dexterity, palming the object rather than passing it rapidly among the fingers. Occasionally, a patient will not even feel the object in the hand or may even fail to appreciate noxious stimuli to the left side of the body. If a left hemiparesis is present, some patients will not recognize their paralyzed limbs and even deny their deficit, a condition called **anosognosia**.

These deficits in attention due to damage to the right parietal lobe have been interpreted in a variety of ways. Some propose simply that there is damage to a body or space schema that resides in the parietal cortex. However, studies in monkeys have failed to demonstrate any topographic organization of body or space in parietal cortex such as exists in primitive form in primary sensory and visual cortex. Others note that perceptions of external spatial relationships remain constant even as we move our eyes, head, or body, suggesting that continuous computations and transformations of space take place in the parietal cortex. Still others propose simply that parietal cortex participates in a distributed process of continuously shifting and focusing attention. PET studies indicate that parietal, cingulate, and prefrontal cortex are primary nodes in this network. Bilateral systems are normally in balance to direct attention from one side to another. When one side is damaged the other remains unopposed so that symptoms of unilateral neglect would reflect a failure to disengage attention directed by the normal side.

Patients with lesions of the right parietal association cortex behave similarly to those with lesions of the left side in being unaware of their deficit. As patients with Wernicke's aphasia continue to speak but are unaware of the lack of meaning of their speech, so do patients with visuospatial neglect continue to ignore the left world after their deficit is demonstrated to them. Literally speaking, in both situations these patients do not know what they have lost. This raises interesting questions regarding the structure of consciousness in the human brain and the neurobiology of awareness and self-awareness. Patients with pure sensory or motor deficits are aware of their loss and can be instructed with physical therapy to overcome some of their problems. Patients with lesions in association cortex have lost not only important higher brain functions but also the awareness that they are gone. Important aspects of human consciousness reside in the association areas.

FRONTAL LOBE FUNCTIONS

Until recently, the role of the frontal lobes in human behavior eluded precise description. Advances in pathway tracing have led to identification of the major connections of the frontal lobe, and unit recordings of neurons within those pathways in monkeys performing different behaviors have revealed the cortical map of different functional areas. Similarly to the parietal association cortex, the frontal association cortex receives and integrates polymodal sensory information. In addition, however, there is a strong association with the autonomic and limbic systems, which provide information relevant to internal homeostasis of the individual and the emotional context of current and intended events. The frontal lobes analyze information relevant to its bringing reward or punishment, or relevant to its use in achieving future goals, and then make a "go versus no-go" decision to act.

Circuit-Specific Behaviors

Damage to the frontal lobe causes contralateral weakness if motor, premotor, or supplementary motor areas are involved. If the lesion lies anterior to these areas in prefrontal cortex, there is no weakness or sensory loss but rather a complex change in behavior depending on the site of the lesion. Cummings has proposed three circuit-specific syndromes. First, damage to the dorsolateral prefrontal cortex or its projections through dorsolateral caudate causes disorder of executive functions. Symptoms include difficulty in shifting from one mental set to another to make a decision, problems with organizing complex tasks, difficulty with thought generation as in category naming (e.g., names of animals or vegetables), and poor skill on alternating or sequential motor tasks.

An example of difficulty in shifting mental sets can be elicited by the Wisconsin Card Sorting Test. The examiner shows cards to patients that display one to four examples of four different symbols in four different colors. As they are shown the cards sequentially patients are required to sort them into a pile by one criterion, such as the number of symbols shown on each card. While the test is proceeding, the examiner changes the rule for sorting, for example to a particular color, without telling the patient. Patients must discover and obey the new rule by learning whether their new criterion for sorting is right or wrong. Patients with lesions outside the prefrontal cortex learn to shift sorting behavior quickly, but patients with frontal lobe lesions have great difficulty. Some even comment that they knew their response was wrong but made it anyway. Perseveration is a characteristic feature of frontal lobe damage.

PET studies in humans indicate that dorsolateral prefrontal cortex is involved in working memory, becoming activated when subjects are required to shift between two different mental tasks. "Executive functions" are said to reside in this area, since it receives complex information, coordinates it according to a plan, allocates attention to a particular outcome, and initiates action. These functions are disrupted by strokes, tumors, and degenerative processes in this area.

Lesions of the orbitofrontal cortex cause changes in personality, revealing aspects of a second-circuit behavior. A pure syndrome common to all patients is difficult to describe. Most exhibit a disinhibition of behavior compared with their premorbid personality. There is more outspokenness, fewer worries, and less social consciousness regarding the impact of their behavior. Tactlessness and facetiousness may become manifest. Changes in mood occur with more irritability, or there may be an elevation of mood with a fatuous euphoria. Patients lack insight into these shifts in mood. Meningiomas arising from the base of the brain can lead to these changes in personality as they grow and compress orbital frontal cortex.

Medial prefrontal cortex and its connections provide the substrate for a third circuit-specific behavior related primarily to motivation. Bilateral lesions of medial frontal cortex cause apathy as a primary symptom. A meningioma arising from the falx lying between the frontal lobes compresses both medial areas as it grows and causes symptoms of apathy. Apathy reflects damage to the anterior cingulate, a structure that becomes activated in PET studies whenever focused attention is required or novel tasks are performed. Patients retain normal cognitive and motor skills but show a lack of motivation to initiate any particular plan. In contrast to patients with dorsolateral lesions, patients with either orbital frontal or medial frontal lesions perform normally on card sorting tests.

LEARNING AND MEMORY

Learning and memory are terms used in everyday language to mean the acquisition and retention of new information. Neuroscientists use these terms operationally in different experimental paradigms. They are used to describe animal behavior, such as how a rat becomes more efficient over sequential trials in running a maze. They are also employed in studies at the synaptic level, such as how a train of stimuli can permanently facilitate synaptic transmission (Box 6–3). Advances

BOX 6-3   Synaptic Learning and Memory

In 1949, the psychologist Donald Hebb proposed that learning and memory in animals could be the result of an increase in synaptic efficacy. Studies of synaptic events in simple invertebrates like *Aplysia* (sea slug) and *Hermissendra* (snail) as well as in the rodent hippocampus have revealed details of the synaptic events that may underlie memory formation. The basic concept underlying synaptic learning and memory is that afferent stimulation induces changes in synaptic elements that in turn change the response to subsequent stimulation. There can either be facilitation (long-term potentiation [LTP]) or depression (long-term depression [LTD]) of the second response, which can either be short lived (minutes to hours) or permanent. Changes in synaptic efficacy involve both pre- and postsynaptic structures, and different mechanisms occur at different synapses for different neurotransmitters and receptors.

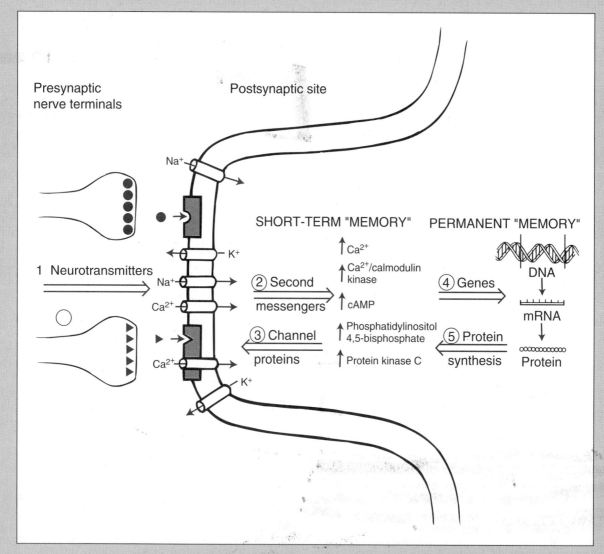

Five events underlie changes in synaptic efficacy. (1) Neurotransmitters bind postsynaptic receptors and induce either an influx in calcium (e.g., NMDA voltage sensitive channels) or an increase in second messengers (e.g., metabotropic receptors and cyclic AMP). (2) Ca^{2+} causes an increase in different secondary messengers in different synapses. (3) Second messengers activate protein kinases, which phosphorylate membrane channels, leading to changes in conductance and membrane potential. These changes alter the efficacy of subsequent synaptic transmission but are short lived. (4) Cyclic AMP (and other second messengers?) activates gene expression. (5) Newly synthesized protein permanently facilitates or dampens receptors, channels, or second messenger enzyme systems. Drugs blocking protein synthesis prevent long-term synaptic memory. Identification of the genes involved in these steps has led to "knockout" experiments in which learning and memory in the whole animal can be explored.

in neuroscience are bringing these two experimental paradigms closer together. For example, there is considerable evidence that specific synaptic activity underlies behavioral learning and memory. Blockade of the glutamate NMDA receptor inhibits maze learning in rats. Drugs that block central muscarinic receptors for acetylcholine (e.g., scopolamine) cause amnesia in humans.

When considering learning and memory systems in humans, it is useful to think of two different types: procedural (implicit) and declarative (explicit). **Procedural learning** is the acquisition of new motor skills, such as hitting a tennis ball, or new cognitive skills, such as learning to read mirror writing. Procedural learning requires learning sessions repeated over time, with each session bringing more speed, accuracy, and efficiency. The processes of procedural learning reside primarily in the motor system, and more specifically in the cerebellum. Studies of simple conditioned responses in animals have found that lesions of the deep nuclei of the cerebellum will block the formation of associations between condition and unconditioned stimuli. Similarly, PET studies in humans learning the classical conditioned eye-blink response show activation of the cerebellum. In everyday life, learning new motor skills is part of the minor adjustments in posture and movement that occur all the time in moving animals. It is innate, unconscious, and largely unavoidable.

Declarative learning is specific to humans, since it involves language and semantic systems. It requires focused attention on auditory and visual stimuli and occurs in seconds, such as learning the name of an object. Information about facts, scenes, and events become stored in the brain and can be recalled and declared upon command. The gathering of new information occurs across cortex, but the hippocampal formation and the dorsal medial nucleus of the thalamus are the two structures necessary for the formation of new declarative memories. These structures seem to act like essential "memory function chips." Damage to these structures causes amnesia in humans and inability to form new declarative memory.

Memory functions in patients can be assessed indirectly or directly. Taking careful mental note of the ease or difficulty with which patients recall details of their illness provides clues about memory functions. Asking patients whether they have noticed any difficulties with memory is useful in the early phase of memory loss, but as the process advances, they will forget that they forget. This situation is typical in the dementias. Direct tests of memory are important when problems are suspected, and screening tests for memory are essential for most elderly patients.

In performing learning and memory tests it is useful to have a model of human memory in mind. Recent memory is defined operationally as the capacity to pay attention to a list of words and to repeat them immediately after hearing them, e.g., "a Mississippi river boat, a hungry dog, and a red balloon." Humans can normally hold seven to nine bits of information on the "scratch pad" of recent memory and retain them there with continuous rehearsal. However, each new word automatically starts the process of encoding within seconds after being heard and continues until it becomes stored in long-term memory. After distracting the patient for 5 or more minutes, the examiner then asks the patient to recall the list of words. The test is performed easily in normal individuals. With aging there is often some difficulty with recall, but it improves with cueing. Normal elderly people will choose the correct response when given a list of alternatives. If there is no recall despite cueing, a disorder in memory registration is likely.

Amnesia Syndromes

Problems with remembering are a characteristic feature of dementing illnesses (Chapter 16). However, a diagnosis of dementia requires finding cognitive deficits in other fields in addition to memory dysfunction, such as difficulty with arithmetic, reading, and visuospatial skills. The Mini-Mental State Examination is a useful tool for surveying deficits across a broad spectrum of higher functions (Box 6-4). Clinicians can easily learn to employ it. Patients with dementia will have deficits in many areas, reflecting a diffuse process of cortical degeneration. The Wechsler Adult Intelligence Scale (WAIS) is a more detailed neuropsychological test for probing abnormalities of cognitive functions.

Amnesia is a severe abnormality in memory function. There are several common etiologies (Table 6-1), but most of them cause damage to one of two neuroanatomical systems. Bilateral damage to the temporal-limbic system due to infection, stroke, or cerebral ischemia following cardiac arrest is common in clinical practice (Box 6-5). Bilateral damage to the dorsomedial nucleus and mamillary bodies is primarily caused by the malnutrition of alcoholism, specifically vitamin B_1 deficiency **(Korsakoff's syndrome)**. In addition to having memory problems, patients with Korsakoff's syndrome typically confabulate, making up answers to questions that they cannot answer.

There are three characteristic features to amnesia. First, there is a global impairment in memory functions. Patients are unable to form new memories based upon either auditory or verbal information, and special tests indicate that the deficit includes the olfactory and somatosensory systems as well. As a result, patients become lost in time, unable to learn the current date or

TABLE 6-1. Neuroanatomy of Amnesia

I. Diencephalon: Medial dorsal nucleus of the thalamus
  A. Trauma: penetrating wound
  B. Tumor: third ventricle cyst; craniopharyngioma
  C. Vascular: anterior communicating artery aneurysm
  D. Metabolic: vitamin B_1 deficiency, Korsakoff's syndrome
II. Temporal lobe: Hippocampus
  A. Vascular: bilateral occlusion of the posterior cerebral arteries
  B. Cardiac arrest: bilateral ischemia of the hippocampus (patient R.B.; Box 6-5)
  C. Infection: herpes simplex encephalitis
  D. Epilepsy: bilateral damage
  E. Surgical removal (patient H.M.; Box 6-5)
III. Unknown, transient
  A. Head trauma: postconcussion
  B. Transient global amnesia

BOX 6-4 The Mini-Mental State Examination*

Each correct answer is given a score of one point for a total possible score of 30 points.

I. **Orientation:** Ask each question without providing clues to the answers: 1. Date. 2. Year. 3. Month. 4. Day. 5. Season. 6. Hospital or clinic name. 7. Floor. 8. City. 9. County. 10. State.

II. **Registration:** Ask the patient to repeat three words. Score the number after the first presentation, but keep saying the words until they are repeated: 11. Rose. 12. Hat. 13. Carrot.

III. **Attention and Calculation:** Ask the patient to subtract 7 from 100 and to keep subtracting 7 from each answer obtained. Do not re-clue with each subtraction. Count each correct subtraction. Alternatively, if patients cannot perform the task, ask them to spell "world" backwards and score the number of letters in correct order: 14. '93.' 5. '86.' 16. '79.' 17. '72.' 18. '65.' Or, alternatively, 14. 'D.' 15. 'L.' 16. 'R.' 17. 'O.' 18. 'W.'

IV. **Recall:** Ask the patient to recall the three words introduced earlier. Do not provide clues: 19. Rose. 20. Hat. 21. Carrot.

V. **Language:**

Naming: Show the patient two items and score one point each: 22. Pencil. 23. Watch.
Repetition: Ask the patient to say "no ifs, ands, or buts." Score one point if the patient repeats correctly after one presentation: 22. Repetition.
Command: Score one point for following each part of a three-step command: 25. Take the paper in your right hand. 26. Fold it in half. 27. Put it in your lap.
Reading: Score one point if the patient reads and follows the written command sentence, "Close your eyes": 28. Closes eyes.
Writing: Patient writes a sentence that contains a subject, a verb, and is sensible. Grammar and spelling are not scored: 29. Writes sentence.

VI. **Visuospatial:** Score one point for copying the intersecting pentangles. Each must contain five sides with an overlapping angle: 30. Draws pentangles.

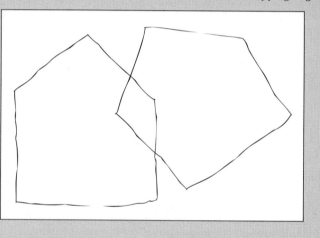

*Modified and reproduced, with permission, from M. F. Folstein, S. E. Folstein, and P. R. McHugh. "Mini-Mental State": A practical method for grading the cognitive state of patients for the clinician. J Psychiatr Res 12:189–198, 1975, Elsevier Science Ltd., Oxford.

note the passing of time. They also become estranged from their circumstances and might continually ask, "what's going on, where am I," only to ask the same question a few minutes later, not having registered the answer.

Second, amnesia affects both the recall of past information, called **retrograde amnesia**, as well as the formation of new memory, called **anterograde amnesia**. Recollection of far distant, long-term memories remains relatively well preserved. Patients can recall distant events and facts learned several months or years prior to their amnesic event (e.g., head trauma, stroke, infection). However, memories formed just prior to the amnesic event are usually affected in varying degrees, consistent with the notion that newly formed memories require a period of processing such as modification of synapses and circuits before they become

permanent. In general, the longer the period of retrograde amnesia is, the worse the prognosis for recovery of memory functions. The greatest deficit in amnesia is in forming new memories. Usually the entire function is lost. No amount of repetition or rehearsal improves performance while amnesia is present. However, the amnesia associated with head trauma or with the syndrome of transient global amnesia (see below) can often end abruptly. When this occurs, patients seem to suddenly wake up to their surroundings, start forming new memories, and are surprised to be told they have literally been awake but unconscious for the period of their anterograde amnesia. The events lost during the period of retrograde amnesia will return just up to shortly before the onset of the amnesic syndrome.

The third feature of amnesia is the preservation of other cognitive functions despite loss of memory. Patients perform normally on tests of other higher functions such as arithmetic, spelling, and visuospatial relationships. Dramatically, within 5 minutes, they will forget having taken the test. Thus, the neocortical systems devoted to these functions are unaffected by pathological processes in the temporal lobe and thalamic systems devoted to memory.

Head trauma is the most common cause of amnesia, but often the injury can seem trivial. It is common, for example, in football and boxing or with a minor blow to the head in an automobile accident. The symptom is manifested following a loss of consciousness of usually less than a few minutes. After recovery from the blow (a "ding"), the patient will be normal upon examination except for memory. The patient will have lost recently formed memories for minutes to hours prior to the blow (retrograde amnesia) and be unable to form new memories. Although full recovery characteristically occurs over hours, the presence of *any* neurological deficit following head trauma requires full evaluation and imaging studies to ensure that there is no intracranial bleeding which could accumulate with time and be fatal.

The exact locus of the lesions that cause transient amnesia from head trauma is unknown. However, the lesions associated with traumatic loss of consciousness have been well studied. Characteristically there are either small hemorrhages deep in the midbrain, diffuse shearing injuries to white matter pathways, or both. If there has been a blow to the front of the head, there is usually bleeding in the tips of the frontal and temporal lobes. This multifocal microscopic injury to the brain is thought to underlie the symptoms of the **posttraumatic syndrome**. In this condition, patients readily regain consciousness but then suffer prolonged headaches, difficulty in focusing and sustaining attention, and problems with diverse cognitive functions that formerly came quite easily, such as reading, doing crossword puzzles, or learning new information. There can be a disruption of normal sleep patterns, nystagmus, and mild ataxia. The postconcussive syndrome can be debilitating and persist for months, but eventual full recovery is the rule. Finally, recurrent head trauma results in cumulative damage to the brain that can cause dementia.

Transient global amnesia is an amnesic syndrome that occurs primarily in people over 60 years of age. Typically there is a rapid onset of memory impairment that persists for several hours and then recedes over 12–24 hours. During the "spell," the patient is confused, repetitively asks what is going on, and is unable to form new memories. A few hours of retrograde amnesia is usually present. Full recovery is the rule, but there will be no memory for the event itself. The syndrome must be distinguished from a stroke or a seizure. The absence of any other neurological abnormality upon examination provides evidence against a stroke, but this must always be suspected in the elderly. The lack of any abnormal movement, posturing, or muscle jerks is evidence against temporal lobe seizures. Patients with recurrent limbic system seizures (partial complex status epilepticus) will manifest major deficits

in all cognitive functions and not just memory. The cause of transient global amnesia is unknown. By inference to other causes of amnesia, it is proposed that there must be a transient disruption of function in the temporal-limbic system or its subcortical projections. A migraine equivalent is one hypothesis. The lack of an increased incidence of stroke following recovery is evidence against a transient ischemic attack as the cause.

MOOD AND EMOTION

Human emotions represent neurophysiological states of activity in cortical, limbic, and subcortical systems that are only now becoming identified and understood. It is useful to analyze human emotional states from two frames of reference. First, it is appropriate to recognize that certain behaviors which humans share with animals have a strong emotional component, such as anger, fear, hunger, and sexual drive. In humans, these emotional states are often associated with internal sensations that arise within the body as well as with changes in heart rate, blood pressure, blood glucose, and secretion of hormones. In the appropriate social and environmental contexts, these states are evoked automatically and unconsciously and result in stereotyped behaviors that have been conserved through evolution, since they are strongly linked to survival. These behaviors are the property of the older parts of the brain—the hypothalamus, basal forebrain, amygdala, and their connections with orbitofrontal, orbitomedial, and anterior temporal cortex.

Humans have brought language to bear upon these states of internal feelings. This provides a second perspective for analysis. Language and culture have allowed dissociation of feelings from both the environmental stimulus and the evoked behavior. Apprehension, anxiety, melancholia, sorrow, euphoria, pleasure, and pain are descriptive terms of emotional states from everyday experience, and they are regularly expressed in music, dance, and art. Furthermore, primitive feelings have become elaborated and refined within cultures into notions of kindness, cruelty, guilt, and altruism. It is commonly said that it is the emotions which add color, flavor, and even meaning to human existence. Analysis of emotions within this cultural domain has spawned many psychological and psychoanalytical schools of thought. Such analysis can be applied descriptively and even therapeutically to individuals experiencing interpersonal conflict and stress. Considered this way, emotions are the property of the neocortex and its influence on the limbic system.

Depression

Depression in humans causes changes in vegetative behaviors as well as internal mental states. **Anhedonia** is the term used to describe the loss of pleasure-seeking behavior. In depression this can encompass loss of interest in eating and in sex as well as in other pleasurable physical activities and social relationships. Patients may lose weight, withdraw from family and friends, and experience changes in sleep-wake patterns.

BOX 6–5 Human Amnesia and the Hippocampus

H.M., a 27-year-old mechanic, had suffered convulsions from childhood that were characterized as temporal lobe seizures with secondary generalization. Since these seizures could not be controlled with medicine, he underwent bilateral temporal lobe surgery on September 1, 1953. The medial aspects of the temporal lobes were removed 8 cm posteriorly from the anterior poles. H.M. awoke from the operation and essentially never formed another new memory. A retrograde amnesia of 2–3 years was also present. In formal neuropsychological testing, he performed well on all tests except those with a memory component. A few years following the operation, his full-scale IQ was 112, slightly improved from 104 preoperatively. There were no deficits in perception, mathematics, abstract thinking, or reasoning. Immediate recall of stories and drawings was below average and his score for learning word associations was zero. Moreover, shortly after completing a portion of the test he could neither recall it nor recognize it if given again.

Follow-up of H.M. over subsequent years revealed a stable deficit. Efforts to improve declarative learning and memory failed. By contrast, procedural learning and memory remained intact. H.M. was shown how to read mirror writing and performed well, but on each encounter he professed he had never seen such writing before. He remained lost in time, usually giving the date as 1953. He did not know where he lived, who took care of him, or what he had eaten for his last meal.

Temporal lobe surgery for epilepsy is an effective therapy. Today MRI and PET scanning along with depth electrode recordings are used to identify the abnormal side. In addition, patients are tested for the lateralization of language and memory functions. Sodium amobarbital is injected into the carotid artery, and its neuropsychological effects are tested as it transiently anesthetizes one hemisphere. This approach assures that only the epileptic temporal lobe is removed and that memory is preserved.

The story of H.M. became widely known in neuroscience for its illustration of the temporal lobe substrate of learning and memory, although there was much debate about whether the hippocampus, amygdala, white matter pathways, or all three were the key mnemonic structures. In 1986 a second seminal case was reported.

R.B., a 52-year-old retired postal worker, underwent his second coronary bypass surgery in September 1978. The postoperative course was extremely complicated with episodes of cardiorespiratory arrest, prolonged hypotension, reoperation, and periods of intubation. Nevertheless he regained health, was discharged from the hospital after 2 months, and lived 5 years longer before dying of cardiac arrest. When R.B. left the hospital, his memory was severely impaired. He repeatedly asked his wife what had just happened, and he could not recall telephone conversations from his children. Like H.M., he tested normally for IQ at 111 (verbal, 108; performance, 114), but memory was severely impaired for learning paired associations, story recall, and diagram recall. Performance of subtests of specific cognitive functions were otherwise normal. There was only a partial loss of memory for the years immediately preceding hospitalization. Afer R.B. died in 1983, his brain was studied in detail. The only abnormalities in the temporal lobes were bilateral lesions restricted to the CA1 subfields of the hippocampus (see figure). This report signified the essential role played by the hippocampus within the temporal lobe for human memory functions.

Continued on next page

In addition, patients have difficulty in thinking, and they verbalize feelings of "mental pain," worthlessness, and guilt. These feelings can come to occupy most of their waking hours. In severe and persistent cases, feelings of hopelessness can lead to suicide.

The neurobiology of human depression is becoming better understood. The catecholamine hypothesis proposes that a deficiency in the synaptic level of catecholamine neurotransmitters underlies the syndrome. Reserpine, a drug that depletes synaptic vesicles of catecholamines, causes a syndrome of behavioral retardation in animals that mimics aspects of human depression. Drugs that block the reuptake of catecholamines generally (e.g., nortriptyline) or specifically block serotonin reuptake (e.g., fluoxetine) are effective antidepressants. These agents increase synaptic levels of biogenic amines. Electroconvulsive therapy is effective in treating severe depression. Experiments in animals show that this treatment increases the synaptic turnover of catecholamines.

Lesions in the prefrontal-limbic system can cause depression. Patients suffering strokes in the prefrontal cortex or the head of the caudate nucleus develop symptoms of depression far more commonly than from strokes elsewhere. The depression is not related to the severity of the stroke. In addition, depression is much more common with left-sided lesions than right-sided ones. Damage to biogenic amine pathways or to critical frontostriatal systems is thought to underlie the mood change. PET studies in patients suffering unipolar depression consistently show a decrease in metabolism in the prefrontal cortex and caudate. Manic-depressive behavior has been reported with lesions of the orbitofrontal cortex and occurs with diseases of the caudate nuclei as well, such as Huntington's disease (Chapter 12).

Obsessive-Compulsive Disorder

The obsessive-compulsive disorder is defined clinically as the presence of recurring, often repugnant thoughts that continuously invade conscious awareness and cannot be willfully stopped. Recurrent ritualistic behaviors, or compulsions, accompany these behaviors. When the compulsions are not performed, patients report intolerable levels of anxiety. An obsession with dirt coupled with compulsive bathing is a common example. In idiopathic cases, the onset usually occurs in childhood or by early adult life. Imaging studies have shown abnormalities in the orbitofrontal and medio-

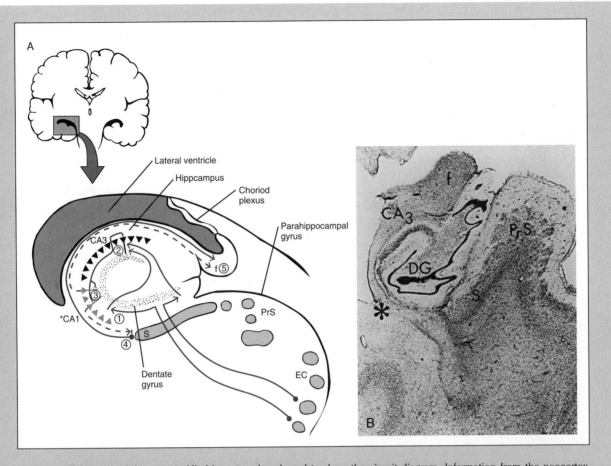

A, The medial aspect of the temporal-limbic system is enlarged to show the circuit diagram. Information from the neocortex comes into the system in the entorhinal cortex (EC), which lies within the parahippocampal gyrus. Neurons in the entorhinal cortex project through five synaptic steps in the hippocampus that result in the formation of new declarative memories in humans: (1) Dentate gyrus (DG) granule cells. (2) CA3 pyramidal neurons. (3) CA1 pyramidal neurons. (4) Subiculum (S). (5) The subiculum neurons and hippocampal pyramidal neurons project down through the fornix (f) to the septum and hypothalamus. *B*, The pathological analysis of the brain from patient R.B. indicated bilateral destruction of the CA1 hippocampal zone (*). Loss of pyramidal neurons and the presence of gliosis can be appreciated. This small lesion effectively interrupted the hippocampal pathways for sequential information processing and caused the amnesic syndrome. PrS, prosubiculum. (Reproduced, with permission, from S. Zola-Morgan, L. R. Squire, and D. G. Amaral. Human amnesia and the medial temporal region: Enduring memory impairment following a bilateral lesion limited to the field CA1 of the hippocampus. J Neurosci 6:2950–2967, 1986.)

frontal cortex and caudate. Since serotonin reuptake inhibitors are effective in treating most patients, it is proposed that an abnormality in serotonin metabolism in prefrontal limbic systems may underlie this disorder. Rarely, strokes or other lesions in these areas can cause these symptoms.

Schizophrenia

Schizophrenia is characterized by abnormalities in thinking, emotion, and movement. Misperceptions, hallucinations, and delusions are characteristic positive symptoms of the schizophrenic psychosis. Changes in mood include apathy and withdrawal from interpersonal relations. Disorders of movement are abnormal posturing and catatonic rigidity. The etiology of the illness is unknown.

Many clinicians have suggested that these abnormalities of behavior reflect dysfunction of prefrontal limbic circuits. At present, two pieces of evidence indirectly support this notion. The mesolimbic dopamine system arising in the ventral midbrain tegmentum projects heavily upon the prefrontal cortex and limbic striatum. Drugs that block the D2 dopamine receptor are potent in relieving psychotic symptoms. Second, some studies using PET scans have found that the prefrontal cortex in schizophrenics does not become activated normally in response to the Wisconsin Card Sorting Test. Neuropharmacological probes and functional imaging studies are expected to provide additional insight into this disorder of higher brain function.

SUMMARY

Damage to the cerebral cortex or limbic system causes loss of the most characteristic of human functions: perception, speech, self-awareness, memory, mood, and future planning. Recognition of specific symptoms and behavioral syndromes leads to identification of the site of the lesion, which can be confirmed by CT or MRI scan. Common disease processes such as stroke, trauma, tumors, and infections disrupt higher functions when they damage specific functional modules. Early detection and prompt treatment are the best hope for restoring function. Localizing the site of such lesions has provided a map of the functional anatomy of the cerebral cortex. This map has been refined and extended by PET and functional MRI imaging in normal people. Use of these imaging studies in patients is providing insight into complex disorders of mood.

Selected Readings

Baxter, L. R. Jr., M. E. Phelps, J. C. Mazziotta, et al. Local cerebral glucose metabolic rates in obsessive-compulsive disorder. Arch Gen Psychiatry 44:211–218, 1987.

Bechera, A., D. Tranel, H. Damasio, et al. Double dissociation of conditioning and declarative knowledge relative to the amygdala and hippocampus in humans. Science 269:1115–1118, 1995.

Corkin, S. Lasting consequences of bilateral medial temporal lobectomy: Clinical course and experimental findings in H.M. Semin Neurol 4:249–259, 1098.

Cummings, J. L. Frontal-subcortical circuits and human behavior. Arch Neurol 50:873–880, 1993.

D'Esposito, M., J. A. Detre, D. C. Alsop, et al. The neural basis of the central executive system of working memory. Nature 378:279–281, 1995.

Folstein, M. F., S. E. Folstein, and P. R. McHugh. "Mini-Mental State": A practical method for grading the cognitive state of patients for the clinician. J Psychiatr Res 12:189–198, 1975.

Mountcastle, V. B. The parietal system and some higher brain functions. Cereb Cortex 5:377–390, 1995.

Raichle, M. E. Visualizing the mind. Sci Am 58–64, (April) 1994.

Tramo, M. J., W. C. Loftus, C. E. Thomas, et al. Surface area of human cerebral cortex and its gross morphological subdivisions: *In vivo* measurements in monozygotic twins suggest different hemisphere effects of genetic factors. J Cognitive Neurosci 7:292–301, 1995.

Zola-Morgan, S., and L. R. Squire. Neuroanatomy of memory. Annu Rev Neurosci 16:547–563, 1993.

Zola-Morgan, S., L. R. Squire, and D. G. Amaral. Human amnesia and the medial temporal region: Enduring memory impairment following a bilateral lesion limited to the field CA1 of the hippocampus. J Neurosci 6:2950–2967, 1986.

COMMON

NEUROLOGICAL

DISEASES

A diagnosis gives a patient a story—a narrative of explanations for symptoms and signs, for why and why now. It also forecasts possible scenarios for the future. Physicians build these stories for and with their patients, enter into them, and help shape them. A knowledge of specific disease processes provides the resource for this exercise. These ten chapters cover the major diseases of the nervous system. Physicians in training come to recognize how their patients exhibit one of the disease processes. They learn to use this knowledge to institute appropriate therapy, to predict and anticipate future events, and to provide education and counseling to their patients and the family. With growing experience, however, physicians also come to recognize that their patients' conditions never *quite* fit textbook descriptions of diseases. Ultimately each patient's narrative proves unique, challenging the physician to blend specific, forever-changing information on diseases with the knowledge and practice of general principles.

CHAPTER SEVEN

MYOPATHY

INTRODUCTION 86

CLINICAL PRESENTATION 86

EVALUATION AND DIFFERENTIAL DIAGNOSIS 86

MUSCULAR DYSTROPHIES 87

    Duchenne-Becker Types 87

    Facioscapulohumeral Dystrophy 89

    Myotonic Dystrophy 89

FAMILIAL PERIODIC PARALYSIS 91

METABOLIC MYOPATHIES 91

MITOCHONDRIAL ENCEPHALOMYOPATHIES 91

    Kearns-Sayre Syndrome 92

    MELAS 92

    MERRF 94

INFLAMMATORY MYOPATHIES 94

    Polymyositis 94

    Dermatomyositis 94

    Inclusion Body Myositis 94

    Retroviral Infection 94

CORTICOSTEROID MYOPATHY 94

SUMMARY 95

INTRODUCTION

Skeletal muscle comprises the greatest bulk of body mass but is little affected by the most prevalent disease processes. Cancer of muscle is exceedingly rare, as are metastases from other malignancies. Atherosclerotic vascular disease does not lead to muscle damage, nor does diabetes mellitus. The diverse diseases that do affect skeletal muscle are primarily inherited defects in muscle membranes or are acquired inflammatory or toxic processes (Table 7–1). A clinician's capacity to diagnose a particular entity is greatly facilitated by experience with a few such cases. The reason lies in the characteristic and memorable pattern of muscle weakness associated with each condition, its effect on particular postures and movements, changes in facial expression, and the patient's response to exercise.

Duchenne-Becker dystrophy and myotonic dystrophy are the most common examples of the muscular dystrophies, and most clinicians in training or general practice will have had experience with these diseases. The inflammatory myopathies are common in adults, and rheumatologists, neurologists, and generalists provide care for these patients. Corticosteroid myopathy is one of the most common causes of weakness in hospitalized patients. Other conditions discussed in this chapter are uncommon but not rare. New findings in several conditions are shedding light on general principles of pathophysiology for systemic diseases as well as muscle disease.

CLINICAL PRESENTATION

Weakness of proximal muscles is the cardinal manifestation of diseases affecting muscle. In adults, this is usually first noted as difficulty in exercising, getting out of a chair, or climbing stairs. Young children have difficulty in standing up from the floor. Weakness of the upper extremities is noted as difficulty in abducting and elevating the arms to comb the hair, shave, or lift an object onto a shelf. Progressive weakness of the pelvic muscles (e.g., gluteus medius, iliopsoas) causes a waddling gait. Weakness of paraspinal muscles can cause difficulty in sitting or holding up the head and can even lead to scoliosis in children. The predilection of genetic and acquired diseases for proximal muscles is not understood. The weakness is usually symmetric in these diseases. There is no pain unless there is direct infiltration of muscle by infection or involvement of adjacent connective tissue or joints. Sensory functions are preserved in pure muscle disease. Reflexes are diminished only in proportion to the degree of weakness.

Several conditions have distinguishing clinical features such as pseudohypertrophy of the calf muscles (Duchenne's dystrophy, Box 7–1) or delayed relaxation of muscle, called myotonia (myotonic dystrophies). Others are notable for effects on other systems such as skin (dermatomyositis), hearing, retina, and heart (Kearns-Sayre syndrome).

EVALUATION AND DIFFERENTIAL DIAGNOSIS

The patient's history provides the first clues toward a diagnosis of muscle disease as the cause of weakness. In children, a developmental delay in reaching motor but not mental milestones suggests muscle disease although the exact moment of onset is difficult to determine. Similarly, in adults the first symptoms of weakness may be overlooked or explained away by the patient or family as fatigue or tiredness. Bilateral weakness does not alert patients to a disease process as readily as focal or unilateral weakness, since comparison of a normal side versus a weak side is not possible. However, the insidious progression of muscle disease eventually interrupts normal postures and movements. During this time, the absence of sensory complaints should direct thinking away from the possibility of a sensorimotor neuropathy (Chapter 9). The absence of weakness that worsens with exercise but improves with rest is evidence against myasthenia gravis as the cause of weakness (Chapter 8).

The distribution of weak muscles provides additional diagnostic clues, and care should be taken to evaluate facial, axial, and girdle muscle strength as well as limb strength. Observation of facial expression, posture, and movement yields important information. Inspection and palpation of weak muscles usually fail to give evidence of the atrophy that is prominent in motor neuropathy. Similarly, fasciculations, fine spontaneous contractions of muscle fibers that would indicate disease of the anterior horn cell (e.g., amyotrophic lateral sclerosis, Chapter 10), will not be found. Finally, stretch reflexes are usually preserved in muscle disease unless the illness is far advanced and the severity of weakness does not allow a tendon jerk response.

The patient's family history is important for identifying other affected and at-risk members who should

TABLE 7–1. Disorders of Skeletal Muscle

Muscular dystrophies
  X-linked recessive
    Duchenne-Becker
    Emery-Dreifuss
  Autosomal dominant
    Myotonic dystrophy
    Facioscapulohumeral
    Scapuloperoneal
    Oculopharyngeal
  Autosomal recessive
    Scapulohumeral
    Limb-girdle
Familial periodic paralysis
  Hypokalemic
  Hyperkalemic
  Hyperthyroid
Metabolic myopathies
Mitochondrial myopathies
  Kearns-Sayre
  MELAS
  MERRF
Inflammatory myopathies
  Infections
  Polymyositis
  Dermatomyositis
  Inclusion body myositis
Toxic myopathies, e.g., due to use of
  Corticosteroids
  Zidovudine (AZT)
  Alcohol
  Many other agents

BOX 7-1 Duchenne Type Muscular Dystrophy (1868)*

Joseph S, residing in Paris, was born well built, of a good constitution, and without any apparent difficulty in the mobility of his limbs. The lower limbs were a bit more developed than the upper. His mother said he was a beautiful baby. No one in the family had been affected with a disease similar to that which he developed. His brother and sister, today aged 14 and 21, are in good health. It was only when attempts were made to teach him to stand and walk at the age of 8 to 10 months that weakness in his lower extremities was noted. If one tried to stand him up, he collapsed. He could not sit a little while in a chair without fatigue, and he cried until he was taken up in someone's arms. He commenced to walk much later than his brother and sister, at the age of 2½ years, and still always needed support. He could not walk except for legs spread apart for lateral balance (swinging gait) and somewhat arched. Toward the age of three years his mother noted that his lower extremities grew in volume. Her attention was first drawn to this by the difficulty in placing his calves in his stockings, which were large enough a short time before. This excessive development of the lower extremities had progressed during 2 years. Since then, the condition of the boy remained stationary until he was presented to me for the first time in 1858 at the age of 7 years.

Here is then what I first observed. The muscles of the lower extremities and the lower spine were so developed and made such a contrast with those of the upper extremities, which were slender, that I immediately made a photograph.... They were firm and even hard, like hypertrophies, and the gastrocnemius and the lumbar spinal (muscles) seemed to bulge through the thinned and distended skin. Therefore I was not a little surprised to learn that these athletic appearing muscles had been lacking such power since birth and had hardly been exercised. All the movements of the lower extremities could be performed, but the strength of each measured individually was very feeble except for extension of the foot on the leg, which had retained great power. If he bent forward when seated he could not straighten up even though the lumbar muscles were greatly distended. On standing, he had to hold to a support to prevent falling. Supported, he could walk, but laboriously, spreading his legs and inclining his trunk with each step to the side of the lower extremity that rested on the ground.... Toward the end of 1862 [age 11] the weakness increased rapidly to the point that the child was obliged to remain constantly in bed or chair. In the first months of 1864 [age 13], the paralysis progressed to involve the upper extremities, where the muscles had not yet increased in volume. Six months later the paralysis was generalized, and movements were almost completely abolished....

*G.B.A. Duchenne. Recherches sur la paralysie musculaire pseudo-hypertrophique, ou paralysie myosclerosique. Archives Generales de Médecine 11:5–25, 179–209, 305–321, 421–443, 552–588, 1868. Translation from R. H. Wilkins and I. A. Brody. *Neurological Classics.* New York, Johnson Reprint Co., 1973, pp. 60–61.

be examined to assure complete case ascertainment. Determining the pattern of genetic transmission often suggests a diagnosis that can be confirmed by molecular genetic tests on blood lymphocytes. Results provide critical information for family counseling. Electromyographic and nerve conduction studies are important for localizing the site of weakness and determining its characteristics. Blood tests for muscle enzymes (e.g., creatine phosphokinase [CPK]), the erythrocyte sedimentation rate (ESR), and specific tests for antibodies

associated with connective tissue diseases can be helpful in particular cases. Muscle biopsy using special histochemical stains can provide diagnostic information. An ECG is an important first step for assessing cardiac muscle.

MUSCULAR DYSTROPHIES
Duchenne-Becker Types

Duchenne-Becker type muscular dystrophy is the most common cause of inherited weakness in children. There are two distinct molecular pathophysiologies and phenotypes for this X-linked form of muscular dystrophy. Both Duchenne's and Becker's dystrophy are allelic variants of abnormalities in the gene for dystrophin located on the short arm of the X chromosome (Xp21). **Dystrophin** is a large, 427-kDa cytoskeletal protein that lies beneath and supports the muscle plasma membrane. Its structure is a hexagonal lattice which is thought to provide stability to the muscle membrane particularly during muscle contraction and relaxation. Dystrophin is absent or markedly reduced (<5%) in Duchenne's dystrophy, whereas it is variably reduced in Becker's dystrophy (commonly 10–30%). Female carriers of Duchenne's dystrophy show a mosaic pattern for the localization of dystrophin on muscle biopsy (Figure 7–1). Patients with Duchenne's suffer a progressive course, usually dying before the third decade. In Becker's, the course is more benign, with half the patients retaining the ability to walk into the late 20's and living much longer.

Duchenne's dystrophy affects 1 in 3300 male births. At least 30% of the cases lack a family history of affected males and are considered new genetic mutations. The high frequency of mutation is due to the mammoth size of the gene—2.3 megabases with 65 exons, more than 10 times larger than most other genes. It thus represents a large target for new mutational events. In Duchenne's it is hypothesized that the deletions cause a shift in the reading frame such that a nonsense codon is created that is read as a "stop" codon for messenger RNA (mRNA). The subsequent transcribed protein is thus greatly truncated and most of it is rapidly removed from the muscle cell.

Males born with Duchenne's have little or no muscle dystrophin and have leaky muscle membranes. The serum level of muscle CPK is elevated at birth and can be used to detect disease. Curiously, many patients do not become weak until 3–5 years of age. The paraspinal, iliopsoas, quadriceps, and gluteal muscles are the first to become affected, and this weakness results in lumbar lordosis, difficulty in standing up, and a waddling gait (Box 7–1). On standing up from a sitting position, the child will flex the trunk, put the hands on the knees, and then push itself up by working the hands up the thighs. This characteristic maneuver is called Gower's sign. The ability to walk is lost between 9 and 12 years of age, and respiratory difficulty and cardiomyopathy develop by the end of the second decade. Death usually occurs by age 20. Dystrophin is also expressed in the brain, but its exact function is unknown. A third of

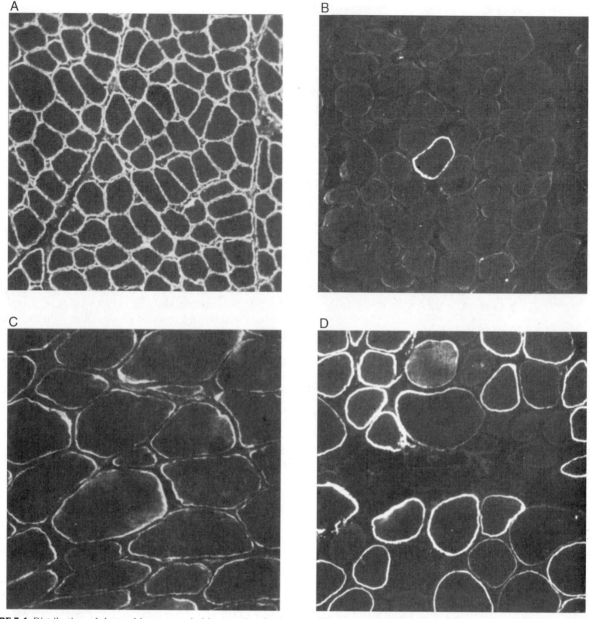

FIGURE 7–1. Distribution of dystrophin on muscle biopsy using the immunofluorescence antibody technique. *A,* Normal distribution under the sarcoplasmic membrane. *B,* Absence of staining in Duchenne's dystrophy except for one fiber. *C,* Patchy distribution of abnormal dystrophin in Becker's dystrophy. *D,* Mosaic pattern in a symptomatic carrier. (Reproduced, with permission from V. Dubowitz. *Muscle Disorders in Childhood.* London, W.B. Saunders Co., 1995, p. 54.)

patients with Duchenne's exhibit mild mental retardation.

The diagnosis of Duchenne's can be made from the typical clinical picture, a myopathic electromyogram, markedly elevated serum CPK level (often greater than 2000 U/L), and muscle biopsy. Biopsies characteristically show variation in fiber size, necrotic and regenerating fibers, and an increase in connective tissue and fat (Figure 7–2). Fat causes pseudohypertrophy of muscles, often most prominent in the calf muscles. Molecular biological techniques are now used for the diagnosis. Immunoblot analysis of muscle allows identification of the size and relative abundance of dystrophin, thus identifying cases and allowing separation

into Duchenne and Becker types. Blood lymphocyte DNA is used for genetic screening by RFLP analysis with intragenic and flanking markers. Prenatal diagnosis analyzes fetal DNA form chorionic villi or cultured cells from amniotic fluid. Southern analysis, polymerase chain reaction or pulse field gel electrophoresis are used.

Therapy is directed at anticipating and treating increasing disability. Contractures develop as the legs weaken and should be counteracted with passive stretching exercises that parents can learn to perform. Splints and braces are important to maintain walking as long as possible. If scoliosis develops, surgery is sometimes recommended to maintain optimum ventila-

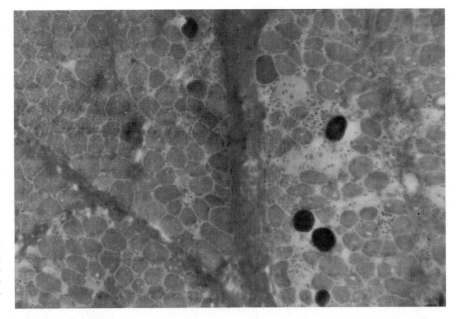

FIGURE 7–2. Muscle biopsy. Duchenne type muscular dystrophy (Gomori's trichrome stain). There are hypercontracted, dark-staining fibers, variation in fiber size, infiltration with histiocytes, and mild endomysial fibrosis. (Courtesy of A. Verity, M.D.)

tion. Corticosteroids have some temporary benefit, but their use is controversial because of their side effects.

Several types of genetic therapy are being tried in Duchenne's dystrophy. In one, myoblasts with a normal dystrophin gene are transplanted into muscles of patients. This strategy has been found to be successful in the *mdx* mouse, which is a model of Duchenne's dystrophy. The myoblasts fuse with the abnormal muscle cells and produce dystrophin. However, problems are associated with delivering myoblasts to all muscle groups, including cardiac muscle, and with achieving sufficient fusion and dystrophin production. A second approach uses a cloned dystrophin gene or gene fragment ("minigene") to achieve the same end. Similar problems of delivery and efficiency remain to be solved. Adenoviruses are being tested as potential vectors for gene delivery.

Patients with Becker's dystrophy illustrate the fact that even a little bit of dystrophin can go a long way. It is hypothesized that the Becker gene deletions do not cause a shift in the reading frame and no premature "stop" codon is formed. The mRNA faithfully transcribes all normal remaining exons. The dystrophin is smaller, and the total amount is reduced, but it apparently can play some role in maintaining a normal sarcoplasma membrane, perhaps by preventing contraction-induced tears. The severity of the clinical disease is probably related both to the total amount of dystrophin present and to the particular segment that is abnormal or missing. Recently, one deletion was found to cause only muscle pain and cramps. Careful genetic study of additional phenotypes may yield important information for potential genetic therapies. Since the gene is so large and the mutation rate is so high, genetic counseling alone has only limited impact on reducing the disease incidence.

Facioscapulohumeral Dystrophy

Facioscapulohumeral dystrophy (FSHD) is an autosomal dominant disorder due to an abnormal gene in the subtelomeric region on the long arm of chromosome 4. The prevalence is approximately 5/100,000 population. The exact molecular genetic defect is the focus of intense research. The disease commonly begins in childhood with perioral or periorbital facial weakness noticed as difficulty whistling or closing the eyes tightly. A horizontal flat smile is typical. There is considerable variability among and within families, but 90% of cases will present before age 20. Weakness of the shoulder girdle and proximal arm muscles causes difficulty in lifting objects early in the course. Forearm and hand muscles are usually spared. Extraocular muscles are not involved. In severe cases, there can be weakness of distal and proximal leg muscles requiring braces or even a wheelchair. More than half the patients have mild sensorineural hearing loss, and a retinal vascular abnormality occurs, rarely with exudative retinal detachment.

Diagnosis of FSHD can be difficult when the family history is uncertain. In completely normal families, nonpaternity and new mutation are considerations. Spinal muscular atrophy, inflammatory myopathies, and metabolic myopathies must be considered in the differential diagnosis. EMG, nerve conduction studies, serum enzyme levels, and muscle biopsies can be used to differentiate these other conditions. A genetic test is anticipated.

Myotonic Dystrophy

Myotonic dystrophy (DM) is the most common type of muscular dystrophy in adults with an incidence of approximately 1/8000 population. It is the result of an autosomal dominant inheritance of a genetic abnormality at 19q13.3. The onset of symptoms usually occurs between ages 20 and 25, but in successive generations of families the disease can present earlier and become more severe, a phenomenon called **anticipation**. In addition, offspring of female patients may have a particularly severe form of congenital myotonic dystrophy with weakness and retardation. This is called **genetic imprinting**, where the sex of the transmitting parent determines a feature of the disease.

The most affected muscles are those of the face with wasting of the frontalis, temporalis, and masseter muscles resulting in the appearance of a long, narrow "hatchet face." Ptosis is commonly present. If severe, patients characteristically tilt their heads backward to see from under their eyelids. The sternocleidomastoids are also weak, adding to this posture. Distal weakness of the hands and feet also occurs. The rate of progression for an individual can only be discovered by examination over time. It is highly variable even among affected members of the same family. Some patients may eventually need help with swallowing and ventilation, whereas others show only mild signs throughout life. The illness also affects other tissues with variable expression of cataracts, heart block, mental retardation, hypersomnolence, gonadal dysfunction, and frontal balding in males.

Myotonia is a characteristic feature, but one that rarely causes complaint or requires treatment. Indeed, many clinicians have noted that patients with myotonic dystrophy rarely seek medical attention. The myotonic phenomenon can be elicited during examination by asking the patient to squeeze his or her hand tightly closed and then to open it rapidly. There is a 3- to 5-second delay and a slower straightening of the fingers. Striking a muscle belly with a reflex hammer also induces a prolonged contraction, called percussion myotonia. During daily activities, patients note that their "stiffness" usually improves after a warm-up period. Cold weather worsens myotonia.

The myotonic disorders are rare in clinical medicine but well studied (Table 7–2). Diverse syndromes have in common abnormalities of muscle membrane channels or their biochemical control. In myotonic dystrophy, there is an abnormality in a protein kinase on chromosome 19, now called myotonin–protein kinase (MT-PK), that is thought to be important in phosphorylating ion channels. The kinase is present in many tissues but is particularly high in skeletal and cardiac muscle. Abnormal phosphorylation of red blood cell membranes was discovered in this disorder long before isolation of the gene. This biochemical defect probably underlies the abnormalities in other tissues as well. A lack of phosphorylation of proteins in the sodium channel may lead to perpetuation of muscle action

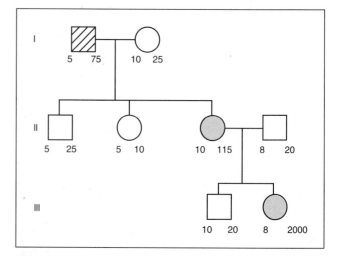

FIGURE 7–3. This stylized pedigree illustrates a family affected with myotonic dystrophy. The numbers underneath each member indicate the number of CTG repeats within the gene for MT-PK on each copy of chromosome 19. Open symbols indicate normals, solid symbols individuals with the disease. Hatched symbols indicate a member that is only mildly affected. The pedigree illustrates the instability of the length of the repeats, which change from one generation to the next. The affected member in the third generation was born with severe weakness.

potentials and contraction. This situation is readily identified by EMG where repetitive decrementing discharges can be induced simply by moving the recording needle and irritating muscle membrane.

The exact cause of the abnormality in myotonin protein kinase is likely related to an unstable trinucleotide (cytosine, thymidine, and guanosine [CTG]) that is located in the 3' untranslated region of the gene. In normal people there are between 5 and 35 repeats of CTG. In mildly affected patients there are more than 50, and in severe cases there may be thousands. A genetic probe for the sequence of DNA containing the trinucleotide repeat can be used for diagnosis. Of note, as in other "trinucleotide diseases" (Box 12–2), the length of the repeats expands in families over successive generations, accounting for anticipation. Rarely, there may be a reduction in the length of the repeats with amelioration of the disease in the next generation. Marked amplification of repeats during meiosis in women may underlie the phenomenon of imprinting, in which the offspring of a female patient is born with particularly severe disease (Figure 7–3). Amplification can also occur during spermatogenesis in myotonic dystrophy. The mechanism of these changes is under investigation. Presumably the length of the repeats influences the translation of adjacent sequences coding for myotonin–protein kinase. With longer repeats there would be lower kinase levels in tissues.

Treatment of patients with myotonic dystrophy is usually directed first at distal weakness of hands and feet. Lightweight splints and braces can be helpful. Difficulties with swallowing or ventilation can occur late in the illness in severe cases and require attention. Myotonia rarely needs treatment, but in selected cases

TABLE 7–2. Genetic Classification of the Myotonias

Type of Disease	Locus
Sodium channel diseases	17q
Hyperkalemic periodic paralysis	
Paramyotonia congenita	
Myotonia fluctuans	
Protein kinase–related diseases	19q
Myotonic dystrophy	
Chloride channel diseases	7q
Thomsen's myotonia congenita	
Becker's myotonia congenita	

phenytoin is the drug of choice, since quinine and procainamide can aggravate heart block. A cardiac pacemaker should be considered if there is prolongation of the PR interval over time, or if syncope occurs. Cataract surgery is needed when posterior lens opacities develop.

FAMILIAL PERIODIC PARALYSIS

Acute weakness of muscle can be caused by inherited disorders of the muscle membrane. These have been described clinically in relationship to changes in serum potassium, i.e., *hypo-* and *hyper*kalemic periodic paralysis. These rare disorders are quite dramatic. A typical case would be that of a young man who develops focal or asymmetric muscle weakness when resting after a period of activity. Occasionally generalized weakness can develop. In the hypokalemic variety, the episode usually occurs at night, often after a carbohydrate meal. Potassium moves into muscle cells in response to the action of insulin, and serum potassium falls below 3.0 meq/L. Paralysis can last from a few hours to a few days. Cranial nerve muscle, ventilation, and cardiac and smooth muscle are rarely affected. During weakness the muscle membrane is hypopolarized, and nerve stimulation fails to elicit a muscle action potential. The potential recovers with potassium treatment. Once recognized, the episodes can be prevented by supplemental oral potassium.

Hyperkalemic periodic paralysis is due to point mutations in the gene for the voltage-dependent sodium channel located on chromosome 17q. The point mutations cause amino acid substitutions in the membrane spanning domain near the cytoplasmic surface. It is hypothesized that under high potassium conditions a change in tertiary structure of the channel occurs that results in delayed inactivation of the sodium current. There is persistent channel opening during prolonged depolarization. Muscle weakness comes on during periods of rest after exercise and is associated with serum potassium levels above 5.0 meq/L. Episodes usually last less than an hour. Myotonia is rarely associated with this condition. However, amino acid substitutions at other sites of the channel cause paramyotonia congenita. In this condition, hyperkalemia or cold can induce focal myotonia and weakness. These two disorders can be diagnosed by means of a potassium load and can be prevented by an acidifying diuretic such as acetazolamide.

METABOLIC MYOPATHIES

This class of disorders is caused by genetic defects in enzymes associated with energy metabolism, particularly the metabolism of carbohydrates and lipids. Abnormalities in enzymes involved in glycogenolysis (e.g., myophosphorylase), glycolysis (e.g., phosphofructokinase, phosphoglycerate kinase), and lipid transport (carnitine palmitoyltransferase [CPT]) are examples. These disorders are inherited as autosomal recessive, typically begin in childhood or adolescence, and show a preponderance of males. The most characteristic presentation is exercise intolerance, with the appearance of fatigue and cramps and, rarely, dark-colored urine due to muscle breakdown and myoglobinuria. Serum glucose and muscle glycogen are particularly important fuels during the early phase of exercise. Disorders of carbohydrate metabolism prevent the metabolism of glucose as an energy source in muscle. By contrast, exercise intolerance in patients with CPT deficiency does not occur until after 45 minutes. During prolonged exercise, the muscle switches toward metabolism of serum fatty acids for fuel, but this is prevented when there is a deficiency of fatty acid transport in CPT deficiency. Special biochemical tests and histochemical tests in muscle are required for diagnosis.

MITOCHONDRIAL ENCEPHALOMYOPATHIES

The mitochondrial encephalomyopathies are a group of heterogeneous illnesses caused by, or partially related to, defects in mitochondrial genes. Although the clinical diseases have been described for some time, their basic biochemical pathophysiology has come under study only in the last decade. These studies are revealing new insights into disease mechanisms as well as new information about normal aging.

Compared with nuclear DNA (3 million kb), mitochondrial DNA (mtDNA) is small with 16.5 kb in a circular, double-stranded molecule (Figure 7–4). This molecule encodes 2 ribosomal RNAs, 22 transfer RNAs and 13 of the 67 protein subunits of the respiratory chain complexes. There is very little noncoding sequence. There are several molecules per mitochondrion, and as there are thousands of mitochondria in muscle cells and neurons, there are many thousands of copies of mtDNA per cell. When a pathological mutation occurs in mtDNA, it will affect only a small amount of the total. The cell would thus contain both normal (wild type) and mutated mtDNA, a condition called heteroplasmy. The pathological consequences of the mutated mtDNA thus depend on its relative abundance. A threshold effect exists for pathological changes, and a dose effect for the onset and severity of symptoms. Mutations in mtDNA accumulate in nondividing cells and may play a role in aging. Mutations that occur in a female's eggs would have a serious consequence on the offspring, since all mitochondria come from the mother. Mutated maternal mtDNA is differentially distributed throughout the developing embryo into somatic tissues. Differences in this distribution, in the local rate of mitochondrial replication, and in the rate of oxidative phosphorylation could all play a role in the diversity of the clinical phenotypes.

The three disorders discussed below have abnormalities of skeletal muscle in common, but there is considerable variation and even overlap among them. The use of special stains on muscle biopsy (Mallory's trichrome stain or succinic dehydrogenase histochemistry) usually, but not always, reveals accumulations of abnormal mitochondria, giving a characteristic appearance called "ragged red fibers" (Figure 7–5*A*). To ob-

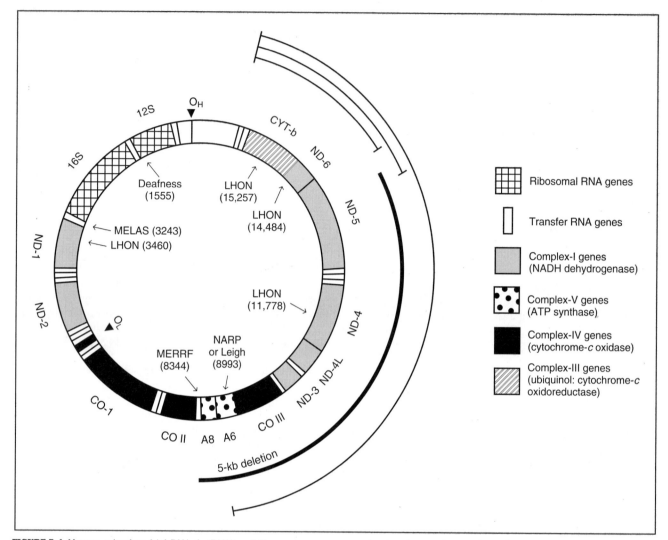

FIGURE 7–4. Human mitochondrial DNA (mtDNA) and the most common associated pathogenetic mutations. Point mutations in structural and protein-coding genes are shown inside the circle, with the clinical phenotype indicated and the nucleotide position of the mutation shown in parentheses. The position of the most common single deletion, which is 5 kb long, and the multiple deletions are indicated by the arcs outside the circle. MERRF, myoclonic epilepsy with ragged red fibers; NARP, neuropathy, ataxia, and retinitis pigmentosa; Leigh, maternally inherited Leigh disease; LHON, Leber's hereditary optic neuropathy; MELAS, the syndrome of mitochondrial encephalomyopathy, lactic acidosis, and stroke-like episodes. O_H denotes the origin of heavy-stranded and O_L the origin of light-stranded DNA replication. CYT-*b*, apocytochrome-*b* subunit; ND-1, -2, -3, -4, -5, and -6, NADH dehydrogenase subunits; CO I, II, and III, cytochrome-*c* oxidase subunits; 12S and 16S, ribosomal RNA subunits; A6 and A8, ATPase subunits. The large open space at the top (which includes O_H) is the noncoding D (displacement) loop. (Reproduced, with permission, from D. R. Johns. Mitochondrial DNA and disease. [Seminars in Medicine of the Beth Israel Hospital, Boston.] N Engl J Med 333:638–644, 1995.)

tain a secure diagnosis in atypical cases, it is necessary to analyze lymphocyte or muscle mtDNA.

Kearns-Sayre Syndrome

The Kearns-Sayre syndrome (KSS) is characterized by progressive external ophthalmoplegia, pigmentary degeneration of the retina, heart block, ataxia, and elevated CSF protein; onset occurs before the age of 20 years. In some cases there can be sensorineural hearing loss, diabetes mellitus, and hyperparathyroidism. The prognosis is poor, and most untreated patients die of cardiac arrest before age 40. The basic defect lies in deletions in mitochondrial DNA. Mutations are sporadic and are thought to occur in the zygote and do not

become part of a viable germ cell line. There is no established pattern of inheritance for most cases. To explain the different clinical features, it is hypothesized that different tissues either have different proportions of abnormal mitochondria or accumulate them at different rates.

MELAS

MELAS (mitochondrial encephalopathy, lactic acidosis, and stroke-like episodes) is a disorder that presents in childhood and can be devastating in its full form. There is often a history of migraine-like headaches. Lactic acidosis occurs at rest. Strokes usually occur in the parietal or occipital cortex, without identi-

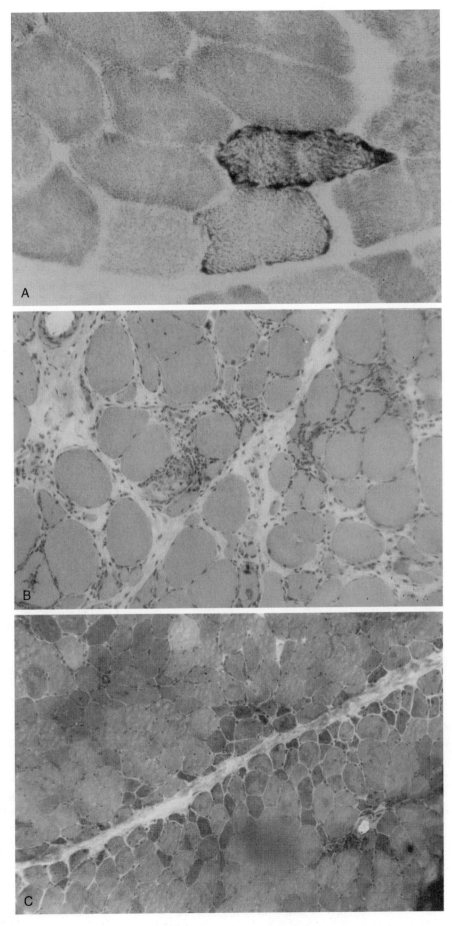

FIGURE 7-5. Muscle biopsies. *A*, Mitochondrial myopathy—ragged red fiber. The special stain for succinic dehydrogenase shows an increased number of mitochondria and displacement of them to the periphery of the muscle cell below the plasma membrane. *B*, Polymyositis (hematoxylin-eosin stain). There is prominent infiltration of lymphocytes and histiocytes with fiber necrosis. *C*, Dermatomyositis (Gomori's trichrome stain). Degeneration of fibers is most prominent at the edge of the muscle fascicle (perifascicular atrophy) as seen by the variability in staining. (Courtesy of A. Verity, M.D.)

fiable provocative factors. In a majority of patients, a point mutation has been found at base pair 3243 in the mitochondrial leucine tRNA gene. However, there are other patients with this defect who do not have strokes but rather variable combinations of myopathy, ataxia, deafness, progressive external ophthalmoplegia, and diabetes, with different ages of onset. Not all have ragged red fibers on muscle biopsy. The presence of other factors interacting with this genetic defect is likely but unknown.

MERRF

MERRF (myoclonic epilepsy with ragged red fibers) is also a relatively nonspecific syndrome with combinations of myoclonus, myopathy, cerebellar ataxia and dysmetria, optic atrophy, hearing loss, and dementia. In these cases, an A to G transition is present at position 8344 in the mitochondrial lysine tRNA gene. There is some correlation of symptoms with the proportion of abnormal mitochondria.

INFLAMMATORY MYOPATHIES
Polymyositis

Polymyositis is an immune-mediated inflammatory disease of muscle fibers. In adults, the illness presents subacutely or insidiously after the age of 50 years. In children, it occurs between 5 and 15 years and is usually more acute. The hallmark is proximal muscle weakness: neck (head droop), shoulders, upper arms, trunk, and thighs. Extraocular muscles are always spared. Distal musculature of the extremities is involved in less than 25% of cases. Dysphagia and dysarthria may occur from involvement of pharyngeal and laryngeal muscles. In adults there is past or present evidence of other connective tissue disease (e.g., rheumatoid arthritis, lupus erythematosus, progressive systemic sclerosis) in 15–20% of cases. Elevated serum CPK and a myopathic electromyogram are characteristic but nonspecific. The diagnosis rests upon muscle biopsy showing direct infiltration of muscle fibers with lymphocytes (CD8+ cytotoxic T cells) and macrophages, and the development of fiber necrosis (Figure 7–5B). The considerable diversity among the T cell populations invading muscle of patients suggests that there is likely more than one antigenic cause for polymyositis.

Dermatomyositis

Dermatomyositis causes a similar clinical picture to polymyositis with regard to muscle weakness but is distinguished by a rash. A purplish-blue discoloration occurs in a butterfly distribution over the cheeks, nose, and eyelids. An erythematous or maculopapular rash can also appear over the elbows, knees, or shins and precede, follow, or be concomitant with the muscle weakness. The muscle biopsy in dermatomyositis shows a perivascular inflammatory response with B cells and macrophages. Electron microscopic studies suggest that immune–mediated injury to the endothelium is a primary event. IgG, IgM, and complement can be found

in the walls of arterioles and venules. These findings indicate a major role for humoral immunity in the pathophysiology, whereas cellular immunity plays the dominant role in polymyositis. The muscle shows atrophy of fibers at the periphery of the fascicle (perifascicular atrophy) consistent with an ischemic process secondary to vascular occlusions within muscle (Figure 7–5C).

Patients with either polymyositis or dermatomyositis can have systemic manifestations including fever, fatigue, weight loss, and cardiac, pulmonary, or gastrointestinal abnormalities. Intestinal necrosis with ulceration and perforation has occurred in acute, severe cases. Of special note is the high incidence of cancer found in patients with dermatomyositis, particularly in the older age groups. Tumors of lung, breast, and ovary are the most common and should be tested for in these patients. Corticosteroids with or without azathioprine is the treatment for these immune-mediated diseases and is continued for years.

Inclusion Body Myositis

Inclusion body myositis causes insidiously progressive proximal muscle weakness in adults over age 50. Serum CPK can be normal or only slightly elevated, suggesting a clinical picture similar to amyotrophic lateral sclerosis (ALS) rather than myopathy. EMG and muscle biopsy reveal distinguishing features. On light microscopy, vacuoles containing membranous material, groups of atrophic fibers, and endomysial inflammation secure the diagnosis. Treatment with doses of the corticosteroids that are useful in polymyositis do not prevent progression of this disease.

Retroviral Infection

Retroviral infection can also cause myositis. Both HIV and HTLV-1 infection can be associated with a polymyositis syndrome. In AIDS, muscle weakness can be an early or late manifestation of HIV infection. In addition, the simultaneous occurrence of myelopathy or neuropathy can cause weakness and confuse the picture. Finally, zidovudine (AZT) treatment in AIDS has been found to cause mitochondrial damage in muscle in some patients after prolonged therapy. EMG, serum enzyme measurements, and muscle biopsies may be helpful in sorting out the cause of weakness in these patients. Some patients respond to cessation of AZT and others to nonsteroidal antiinflammatory agents or corticosteroids.

CORTICOSTEROID MYOPATHY

Long-term treatment of patients with high-dose corticosteroids (particularly dexamethasone) is known to cause proximal weakness, principally of quadriceps muscles. There is type II fiber atrophy on biopsy, and clinical wasting can be prominent. Serum CPK is usually normal. Occasionally it can be difficult to determine whether corticosteroids or the primary disease process for which steroids are being used (e.g., inflammatory myopathy or connective tissue disease) is responsible. Elevated muscle enzymes favor a primary disease process, but a repeat biopsy may be necessary in some cases. Recovery from steroid myopathy can take several months.

SUMMARY

Inherited disorders of muscle membranes and metabolic processes present as characteristic patterns of weakness in children and young adults. Specific genetic tests are becoming available for many of these. The Duchenne-Becker type dystrophy is the most common and is due to mutations in the large dystrophin gene on the X chromosome. Dystrophin and related glycoproteins stabilize the sarcoplasmic membrane and its relationship to the extracellular matrix. Defects in genes for muscle membrane ion channels have been found to cause myotonic dystrophy and periodic paralysis. Inherited disorders of mitochondrial DNA cause weakness and a great variety of other organ symptoms. The pathophysiology of these disorders is only now being understood. Inflammatory and toxic myopathies commonly present in adult years as causes of weakness. Specific treatment for these conditions can stabilize and occasionally improve a patient's condition.

Selected Readings

Brooke, M. H. *A Clinician's View of Neuromuscular Diseases.* Baltimore, Williams & Wilkins, 1986.
Brouwer, O. F., C. Wijmenga, R. R. Frants, and G.W. Padberg. Facioscapulohumeral muscular dystrophy: The impact of genetic research. Clin Neurol Neurosurg 95:9–21, 1993.
Caskey, C. T., A. Pizzuti, Y.-H. Fu, et al. Triplet repeat mutations in human disease. Science 256:784–789, 1992.
DiMauro, S., and C. T. Moraes. Mitochondrial encephalomyopathies. Arch Neurol 50:1197–1208, 1993.
Engel, A. G., and K. Arahata. Mononuclear cells in myopathies. Hum Pathol 17:704–721, 1986.
Hoffman, E. P., and L. M. Kunkel. Dystrophin abnormalities in Duchenne/Becker muscular dystrophy. Neuron 2:1019–1029, 1989.
Lotz, B. P., A. G. Engel, H. Nishino, et al. Inclusion body myositis. Brain 112:727–747, 1989.
Ptacek, L. J., K. J. Johnson, and R. C. Griggs. Genetics and physiology of the myotonic muscle disorders. N Engl J Med 328:482–489, 1993.

CHAPTER EIGHT

MYASTHENIA

GRAVIS

INTRODUCTION 97

CLINICAL PRESENTATION 97

PATHOPHYSIOLOGY 97

IMMUNOPATHOLOGY 100

EVALUATION AND DIFFERENTIAL DIAGNOSIS 102

TREATMENT 104

SUMMARY 105

INTRODUCTION

Myasthenia gravis (MG) is an autoimmune disease of the neuromuscular junction in which antibodies bind the acetylcholine receptor and disrupt neuromuscular transmission. It characteristically causes fatigue and weakness of cranial nerve and proximal muscles. It was first described clinically by the physiologist and clinician Thomas Willis in 1672:

At this time I have under my charge a prudent and honest Woman, who for many years hath been obnoxious to this form of spurious *Palsie*, not only in her Members, but also in her tongue; she for some time can speak freely and readily enough, but after she has spoke long, or hastily, or eagerly, she is not able to speak a word, but becomes as mute as a Fish, nor can she recover the use of her voice under an hour or two.

—Thomas Willis. *De Anima Brutorum.* Oxford, Theatro Sheldoniano, 1672. Reproduced, with permission, from H. R. Viets. A historical review of myasthenia gravis from 1672 to 1900. JAMA 153:1274, 1953. Copyright 1953 American Medical Association.

CLINICAL PRESENTATION

Myasthenia affects women more than men between the ages of 20 and 40 years and men more than women between 50 and 70 years. It commonly starts with intermittent periods of double vision and ptosis, reflecting weakness of extraocular and eyelid muscles. These muscles eventually become involved in almost all cases. In about 15% of cases, the illness remains restricted clinically to these muscles alone (Table 8–1). During examination, the diplopia can be localized to defects at the neuromuscular junction, since the abnormal pattern of eye movements does not fit clinical characteristics of either a simple central lesion in oculomotor pathways or a peripheral lesion of cranial nerves III, IV, or VI. In particular, the eye movements are disconjugate and the weakness of individual eye excursions will often fluctuate during an examination. The presence of fatigability can usually be appreciated when the patient is unable to sustain an upward gaze and one or both eyelids droop. The pupils are not affected.

With involvement of other cranial nerve muscles, there may be difficulty in smiling and flattening of the face (the myasthenic sneer) or problems with closing

TABLE 8–1. Clinical Stages in Myasthenia Gravis*

I	Ocular myasthenia
IIA	Mild generalized myasthenia with slow progression; no crisis; drug-responsive
IIB	Moderate generalized myasthenia; severe skeletal and bulbar involvement, but no crisis; drug response less than satisfactory
III	Acute fulminating myasthenia; rapid progression or severe symptoms with respiratory crisis and poor drug response; high incidence of thymoma; high mortality
IV	Late severe myasthenia, same as III but progression over 2 years from class I to II

*Data from K. E. Osserman. *Myasthenia Gravis.* New York, Grune & Stratton, 1958, p. 80.

the eyes, pursing the lips, sticking out the tongue, whistling, speaking, chewing, or swallowing. The presence of diplopia, dysarthria, and dysphagia is characteristic. However, these clinical features are usually subtle, intermittent, and asymmetric at onset. One patient may have difficulty closing the jaw, using the hand to prop it up, while another may become fatigued during conversation and have slurred or nasal speech. In elderly men, problems with swallowing are a characteristic presentation that may be overlooked until tests for an esophageal tumor or stricture prove negative.

Weakness of the limbs is more marked proximally than distally, with patients having difficulty combing their hair, shaving, arising from a chair, or climbing stairs. Fatigability can be demonstrated by progressive weakness during repetitive forward arm abductions. Neck extensors can be involved and cause difficulty in holding up the head. Breathing problems can develop from involvement of intercostal muscles and the diaphragm, necessitating intubation to support ventilation (the "myasthenic crisis"). Usually there is no muscle atrophy until late in the disease in severe cases when there has been chronic weakness and disuse. Reflexes are preserved. Coordination and sensation are normal. Spontaneous remissions lasting up to a year have been reported in up to 20% of untreated cases, but relapses are common and the course in any one case is difficult to predict at onset (Box 8–1).

PATHOPHYSIOLOGY

At the normal neuromuscular junction at rest, there is continuous release of acetylcholine from the synaptic terminal as individual vesicles randomly bind to the presynaptic membrane and release their contents. Acetylcholine diffuses across the synaptic cleft and binds to the receptor, causing an allosteric conformational change in its structure and opening up a central cationic channel (Figure 8–1). External sodium diffuses down its concentration gradient through this channel, causing a transient change in the postsynaptic potential. This potential remains localized to the junctional endplate and is called the miniature end-plate potential (MEPP). Measurement of the amplitude of the MEPP is an estimate of the number of activated receptors by a quantum of acetylcholine. Acetylcholine diffuses off the receptor and is subsequently inactivated by the enzyme acetylcholinesterase in the postsynaptic folds.

When an action potential comes down the motor axon and invades the synaptic terminal, it causes an increased influx in calcium resulting in enhanced binding of vesicles and the release of approximately 100 quanta of acetylcholine. The amount released binds with approximately 100,000 acetylcholine receptors. This number is more than enough to cause the endplate potential to exceed the threshold of activation and trigger an action potential. The excess activation of receptors is a "safety factor," guaranteeing muscle contraction with each nerve impulse. The muscle action potential spreads out across the muscle membrane, invades the transverse tubular system, and initiates calcium influx and muscle contraction.

BOX 8-1   A Clinical History of Myasthenia Gravis

Clear case descriptions of myasthenia began to be collected and published with increasing frequency around the turn of the century. The following is an abstracted and abridged version of case 4 from E. F. Buzzard's 1905 publication (The clinical history and *post-mortem* examination of five cases of myasthenia gravis. Brain 28:438–483. By permission of Oxford University Press). In this article, he drew attention to abnormalities of the thymus and to lymphorrhages (infiltrates of lymphocytes) in muscles and suggested that there may be "some toxic, possibly auto-toxic, agent which has a special influence on the proto-plasmic constituent of voluntary muscle..."

H.B., a 40 year old schoolmaster, sought medical atten-tion for recurring weakness in October 1899. He had enjoyed good health until age 32 when he noticed weak-ness of his little and ring finger after sawing wood, but this speedily recovered. The weakness recurred after playing the organ, and his right index finger would occasionally drop. In 1893 he occasionally saw double, and this trouble recurred in 1894. About this time his voice, after speaking a few minutes, would acquire a nasal character. His right eyelid, too, tended to droop. In the summer of 1897 he felt weakness in his lips and tongue, and spoke through his nose. After speaking some time the voice would become feeble. He again saw double. In the vacation he walked eight or ten miles a day without fatigue for several days. After this his right leg became weak. He found that he frequently had to stop and rest it for a few minutes, after which he could go on walking. In October 1898, whilst suffering from catarrh, he had difficulty in coughing and clearing his throat, and also in swallowing. In January 1899, his right arm was so weak that he could not brush his hair or write upon the blackboard, but after two days' rest he was able to move the arm quite well. At Easter 1899, he again had ptosis of the right lid, which persisted in varying degree since. In June he gave up work. Diplopia and masticatory difficulty were then his chief troubles, but from time to time he also suffered from dyspnoea, especially after exertion or emotion. After a considerable rest his symptoms almost entirely disappeared.

Upon examination in October 1899 his face was some-what expressionless and there was right sided ptosis. Intelli-gence was not impaired. After speaking a little his speech became slower, laboured, and indistinct. It was noticeable that the chest expanded less and less with each succeeding breath. Diplopia was present only on extreme lateral devia-tion to the right, and then only if the eyes were maintained for some considerable time in this position. The optic discs, hearing, smell and taste were normal. He was unable to open his eyes widely, and if he looked steadily upwards at an object held above his line of vision, his upper lids would gradually droop lower and lower until the eyes were almost closed. The pupils reacted perfectly to light and on convergence. Upon first inspection the palate symmetri-cally rose on phonating the letter A: gradually as he re-peated the phonation, the movements became less and less marked, and finally hardly raising the palate was ob-served. He was quite unable to raise the eyebrows and wrinkle the forehead, and could only frown slightly. He could whistle and show his teeth but movement of the upper lip was feeble. The tongue was protruded straight, promptly, and to its full extent. It was symmetrical, and the movements were good, but easily exhausted.

The movements of the upper extremities were feeble, the right more so than the left. The ready way in which the muscles of the hand became fatigued was demonstrated by asking him to button and unbutton his waistcoat repeat-edly. He could raise his arms above his head, but could not maintain them in this position for more than half a minute. If requested to lift his arms quickly above his head several times in succession he did this, but at each effort the arms were lifted less high, and after doing this seven or eight times they could not be lifted at all, but hung at his sides. After a rest of from thirty to sixty seconds they could be lifted nearly as high as they were at first. All movements of the lower extremities were well and power-fully performed, but the right leg especially was easily fatigued. There was no muscle atrophy or fibrillary twitchings.

No disturbances of cutaneous sensibility could be ascer-tained. The arm-jerks were present, feeble. The knee-jerks were present and equal and not depressed. No ankle clonus was present. The plantar reflex was a sluggish flexor response.

The patient left the hospital in the early part of 1900, but remained more or less in the same condition for the next years. Every few weeks he would suffer from severe paroxysms of dyspnoea, and he ultimately died of respira-tory failure on January 24, 1904, at 45 years of age.

In myasthenia, the *pre*synaptic structures and events of neuromuscular transmission are normal (Figure 8–2). On the *post*synaptic side, the number of recep-tors is often reduced to less than a third of normal by the autoimmune process (see below). This was discov-ered by using radiolabeled α-bungarotoxin (a snake venom that irreversibly binds to the receptor) *in vitro* and counting the radioactivity bound to neuromuscular junctions of patients compared with controls. With a reduction in receptor number there is a proportional reduction in the size of the MEPPs at rest and a de-crease in the safety factor during neuromuscular trans-mission.

Weakness in myasthenia correlates with the reduc-tion in the number of receptors; during a volitional effort insufficient receptors are available to activate the required number of muscle fibers to sustain a full mus-cle contraction. Normally with repeated muscle con-tractions, there is a natural "rundown" in the amount of released acetylcholine, but because of the safety factor, sufficient receptors still become activated to sus-tain maximum contraction. In patients, any fall in re-leased acetylcholine can result in a further loss of acti-vated fibers, since the number of receptors is marginal. In addition, repetitive contraction can lead to receptor desensitization. These two processes underlie the phe-nomenon of fatigability of individual muscles in myas-thenia. With repeated movement or sustained effort, there is increasing weakness. With rest, there is resensiti-zation of the receptors as well as reestablishment of acetylcholine balance on the presynaptic side. Muscle strength gradually recovers.

Approximately 75% of patients have abnormalities of the thymus gland. Of these, 15% have a thymoma, while most of the others have hyperplasia. The thymus is implicated in the cause of myasthenia because lym-phocytes extracted from the thymus have a higher reac-tivity to the acetylcholine receptor than do peripheral

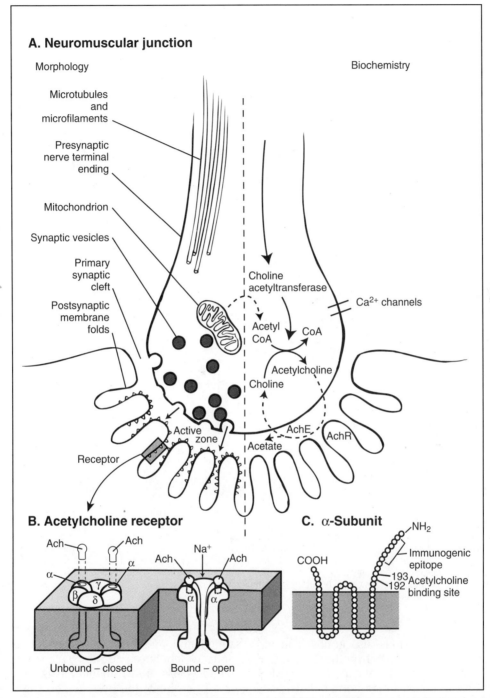

A. Neuromuscular junction

Morphology

Biochemistry

Microtubules and microfilaments

Presynaptic nerve terminal ending

Mitochondrion

Synaptic vesicles

Primary synaptic cleft

Postsynaptic membrane folds

Choline acetyltransferase

Ca²⁺ channels

Acetyl CoA

CoA

Acetylcholine

Choline

Active zone

AchE

AchR

Acetate

Receptor

B. Acetylcholine receptor

Ach

Ach

Na⁺

Ach

Ach

α

α

β

γ

δ

α

α

Unbound – closed

Bound – open

C. α-Subunit

NH₂

COOH

Immunogenic epitope

193 192 Acetylcholine binding site

FIGURE 8–1. Diagram of the neuromuscular junction, acetylcholine receptor (AchR), and its α-subunit. *A,* At the neuromuscular junction, acetylcholine is synthesized and packaged into quanta in synaptic vesicles. These are released spontaneously at low rates, causing postsynaptic miniature end-plate potentials (1 mV amplitude) after binding with the acetylcholine receptor. During stimulation of the motor nerve, there is an increased influx of calcium, which facilitates the release of as much as 100 quanta. Acetylcholine binds with more than enough receptors (the safety factor) to initiate a muscle action potential (10 mV amplitude, surface electrode). AchE, acetylcholinesterase. (Adapted from J. C. Keesey. Electrodiagnostic approach to defects in neuromuscular transmission. AAEE minimonograph No. 33. Muscle Nerve 12:613–626, 1989. Copyright 1989 by John Wiley & Sons, Inc. Reprinted by permission of John Wiley & Sons, Inc.) *B,* The acetylcholine receptor is situated on the apex of postsynaptic folds at the extremely high density of 10,000/μm². There are five subunits per receptor in the stoichiometry of α2, β, δ, μ. The peptide units have considerable homology and are thought to come from one ancestral gene that has evolved into four. The molecular masses of the peptides range from 40,000 to 60,000, and each has four α-helix transmembrane spanning domains. *C,* Each α-subunit binds a molecule of acetylcholine at residues 192–193. The main immunogenic region is adjacent to the binding site. When two molecules of acetylcholine bind with the receptor, the central cationic channel opens and Na⁺ moves intracellularly, creating the end-plate potential.

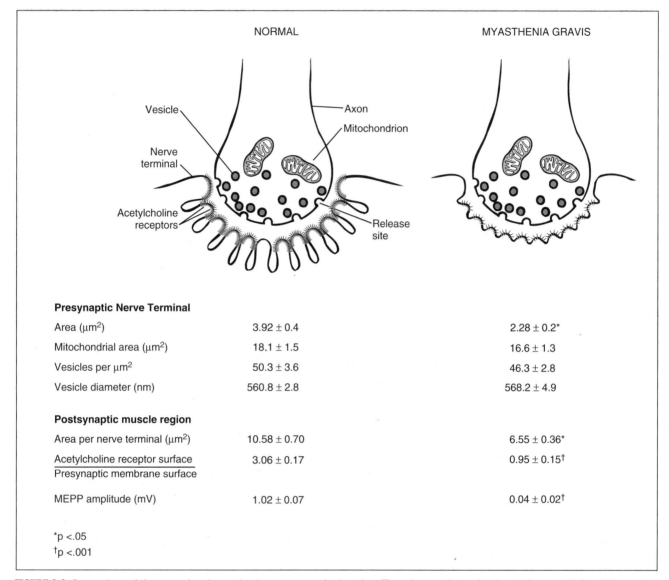

	NORMAL	MYASTHENIA GRAVIS
Presynaptic Nerve Terminal		
Area (μm^2)	3.92 ± 0.4	2.28 ± 0.2*
Mitochondrial area (μm^2)	18.1 ± 1.5	16.6 ± 1.3
Vesicles per μm^2	50.3 ± 3.6	46.3 ± 2.8
Vesicle diameter (nm)	560.8 ± 2.8	568.2 ± 4.9
Postsynaptic muscle region		
Area per nerve terminal (μm^2)	10.58 ± 0.70	6.55 ± 0.36*
Acetylcholine receptor surface / Presynaptic membrane surface	3.06 ± 0.17	0.95 ± 0.15†
MEPP amplitude (mV)	1.02 ± 0.07	0.04 ± 0.02†

*$p < .05$
†$p < .001$

FIGURE 8–2. Comparison of the normal and myasthenic neuromuscular junction. There is a modest reduction in the overall size of the motor terminal but no change in vesicle size or density. There is a simplification of the postsynaptic membrane with loss of folds, reduction in the area of the receptor membrane, and consequently reduction in MEPP amplitude (see also Fig. 8–4). (Data from T. Santa, A. G. Engel, and E. H. Lambert. Histochemical study of neuromuscular junction ultrastructure. Neurology 22:71–82, 1972, and from A. E. Engel, J. M. Lindstrom, E. H. Lambert, and V. A. Lennon. Ultrastructural localization of the acetylcholine receptor in myasthenia gravis and in its experimental autoimmune model. Neurology 27:307–315, 1977.)

blood lymphocytes. The thymus also contains myoid cells, which, according to one hypothesis, are the source of the antigenic stimulus that causes the disease. A larger percentage of patients than normal individuals has evidence of other autoimmune disease, including thyroiditis, lupus erythematosus, and rheumatoid arthritis.

IMMUNOPATHOLOGY

In 1973, Patrick and Lindstrom fortuitously discovered that injection of acetylcholine receptor molecules from the electric eel into rabbits caused weakness with characteristics identical to myasthenia gravis (Box 8–2). There was a decremental response to repetitive nerve

stimulation, and the weakness could be overcome with antiacetylcholinesterase drugs. Since then the immune pathogenesis of myasthenia has been well established, and it is one of the best studied examples of autoimmune disease in humans.

Almost all patients have circulating IgG antibodies to human limb acetylcholine receptor subunits. Patients with focal ocular myasthenia probably have antibodies to unique epitopes on extraocular muscle receptors. It is known that patients have their own characteristic antibody response, which can be quite heterogeneous. There are many antibodies—B cell clones—directed against many epitopes. Antibodies to the α-subunit are most common, perhaps because there are two subunits in each receptor. The acetylcholine binding site is just

BOX 8-2   Experimental Autoimmune Myasthenia Gravis

Up until 1973 there was debate as to whether myasthenia gravis was a disease of the presynaptic or the postsynaptic side of the neuromuscular junction. In that year, J. Patrick and J. Lindstrom published their results of injecting rabbits with acetylcholine receptor purified from the electric organ of *Electrophorus electricus* (Autoimmune response to acetylcholine receptor. Science 180:871–872, 1973). After two or more injections of 0.3–0.4 mg of receptor in complete Freund's adjuvant over 3–4 weeks, the rabbits developed flaccid paralysis. The weakness could be temporarily reversed by anticholinesterase medicines such as edrophonium (Tensilon) or neostigmine, and electrophysiological studies revealed characteristics similar to the human disease. These findings were readily reproducible in mice, rats, and other animals, and it became possible to explore and compare clinical and pathological features of MG with EAMG (experimental allergic myasthenia gravis). The autoimmune hypothesis of myasthenia as a disease of the postsynaptic acetylcholine receptor was soon accepted.

In contrast to experimental allergic encephalomyelitis (EAE; Box 14–2) as a disease model for multiple sclerosis, EAMG became recognized as reproducing nearly all the features of the human disease once acetylcholine receptor antibodies became established as the main pathogenetic mechanism in experimental animals and humans. Yet it must be emphasized that the exact cause, or causes, for initiating the abnormal cellular immunity in multiple sclerosis (MS) and the abnormal humoral immunity in MG remain unknown.

EAMG is a biphasic illness. An acute phase occurs between 7 and 11 days following injection and is characterized by mononuclear infiltration of neuromuscular junctions with splitting away of postsynaptic junctional folds and phagocytosis of membrane and receptors. Acetylcholine receptor antibodies are just beginning to rise at this time. Cellular inflammation in human myasthenia has only recently drawn attention. A mild mononuclear cell infiltration into junctions can be found on biopsy in up to a third of specimens, but this requires special searching and electron microscopy (Figure 8–3C). The cells have not been well characterized in EAMG or MG.

The chronic phase of the experimental illness begins 2 weeks later when the neuromuscular junctions show an absence of inflammatory cells but a simplification of the postsynaptic membrane and a severe reduction of receptors. There is a reduction of MEPP amplitude and the muscle compound action potential—features typical of MG. The animals are weak and can develop a relapsing course or progress to death.

EAMG provides a system for testing potential new therapies. Many of these are directed at developing specific approaches to selectively blocking the immune response against the acetylcholine receptor without causing a more widespread immune suppression. Two approaches have been developed against T cells. In the first, a fusion protein was genetically engineered that combined interleukin 2 (IL-2) with the toxic portion of diphtheria toxin. T lymphocytes express IL-2 receptors when activated and would take up the fusion protein and be destroyed. When the fusion protein was given at the time of immunization, the primary acetylcholine receptor antibody response was blocked by 50%, but the treatment had no effect once the disease became established.

The second approach targets T lymphocytes that recognize acetylcholine receptor antigens on the surface of antigen-presenting cells. This strategy uses B lymphocytes as "guided missiles" to present digested peptides of the acetylcholine receptor within their MHC II domain, but the B cells are treated first with a fixative. As a result, the T cells recognize the antigen but do not become activated. A state of anergy is induced in the acetylcholine receptor–specific T cells, but all other aspects of cellular immunity remain normal. This strategy is being tested in animals.

Oral tolerization is another therapeutic strategy under investigation. Antigens given orally to animals can have a suppressive effect on the later induction of autoimmunity from antigen injections. This has been found in collagen-induced arthritis, autoimmune uveoretinitis, insulin-dependent diabetes, and experimental allergic encephalomyelitis (Box 14–2). If Lewis rats are fed *Torpedo* acetylcholine receptor, their subsequent immune response to injected receptor is blunted. They develop lower levels of antibody and do not become weak. The mechanism of oral tolerization is unknown, but scientists have suggested it may involve clonal deletion or specific activation of CD8+ suppressor T cells.

---

proximal to the major immunogenic region on the α-subunit, which suggests how antibody binding can block receptor activation during neuromuscular transmission (Figure 8–1). Some patients also have antibodies to the ε-subunit. This is expressed only during development, prior to nerve innervation. The presence of such antibodies suggests that there may be antigenic sites for the disease other than adult skeletal muscle, perhaps in the thymus.

Whereas some antibodies block the active acetylcholine site, others form cross linkages and clustering of receptors that lead to an increase endocytosis and receptor degradation. Studies *in vitro* indicate a two- to three-fold increase in receptor degradation in myasthenia. Antibody binding can also invoke the complement cascade as another mechanism of receptor damage. Myasthenia can be passively transferred to mice with these serum antibodies.

Biopsies of patients with myasthenia typically show simplification of the postsynaptic receptor with loss of folds and a reduction in the area of the end-plate receptor membrane (Figure 8–3). Immunohistochemical stains have been used to identify IgG and complement on the receptors. Only rarely have biopsies demonstrated inflammatory cells. Some scientists suggest that appreciation of cellular infiltrates may be a sampling error and that an inflammatory response may be an early but brief component of the pathological proc-

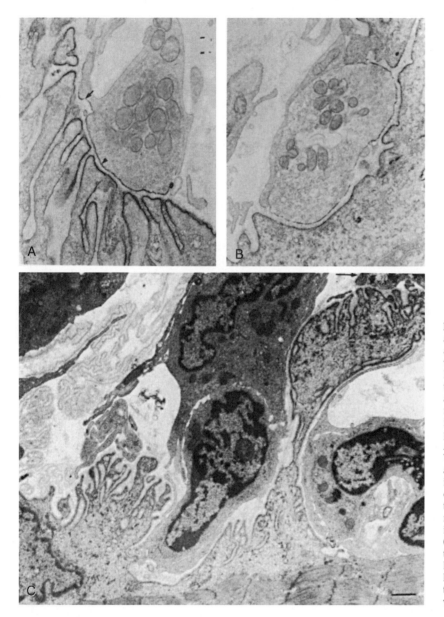

FIGURE 8–3. The neuromuscular junction in myasthenia. Electron micrographs ($\times$22,300) in *A* and *B* are stained with peroxidase conjugated with α-bungarotoxin to localize the acetylcholine receptors. *A*, There is extensive staining of the apex and adjacent membrane of the postsynaptic folds. *B*, The postsynaptic membrane in myasthenia is greatly simplified with sparse staining of receptors. (*A* and *B* are reproduced, with permission of Little, Brown and Company, from A. E. Engel, J. M. Lindstrom, E. H. Lambert, and V. A. Lennon. Ultrastructural localization of the acetylcholine receptor in myasthenia gravis and in its experimental autoimmune model. Neurology 27:307–315, 1977.) *C*, A macrophage appears to be pinching off a segment of the postsynaptic membrane. Mononuclear cell infiltrates are mild in myasthenia and are usually found in only 6–33% of junctions even with careful examination. (Reproduced, with permission of Little, Brown and Company, from R. A. Maselli, D. P. Richman, and R. L. Wollman. Inflammation at the neuromuscular junction in myasthenia gravis. Neurology 41:1497–1504, 1991.)

ess as occurs in experimental autoimmune myasthenia gravis in animals. The role of monocytes and macrophages found in muscle biopsies in acute cases remains to be determined (Figure 8–3*C*).

T helper (CD4+) lymphocytes play an important role in myasthenia. It is thought that they are responsible for processing receptor antigens presented to them by macrophages or dendritic cells in the thymus. These T cells subsequently stimulate B cells to produce antibodies. T cells and their cytokines are probably not directly involved at the neuromuscular junction. Both patients and controls have T cells that respond to acetylcholine receptor stimulation, but the response in patients is more robust and individual cell lines can be propagated for experimental investigation. It has been found that these patients' cells can respond to more than 30 antigenic sites on the receptor. In addition, there does not appear to be a restricted expression of the T cell receptor. These and other findings indicate that myasthenia is a T cell–dependent antibody-mediated autoimmune process. Antibodies to CD4+ T cells have been used therapeutically to block myasthenia in experimental animals, and treatments in patients have begun.

EVALUATION AND DIFFERENTIAL DIAGNOSIS

Acetylcholine receptor antibodies are found in the serum of 85% of patients with MG, and a positive test is specific for diagnosis. Solubilized human limb muscle acetylcholine receptor labeled with ^{125}I–α-bungarotoxin is the antigen used in the test. A small number of patients without antibodies probably reflect an insensitivity of the test. Some of these antibody-negative patients have ocular myasthenia, and the epitopes that are attacked on the receptors on these muscles may not be present in the receptor assay. Serum from other so-called antibody-negative patients has been found to bind acetylcholine receptors of cultured muscle cells and accelerate their degradation. For these reasons, it is likely that all myasthenic patients produce antibodies, some of which are not measured by present assays. The absolute level of antibody does not correlate with severity of the disease. Some patients may have a large concentration of antibodies against epitopes on the receptor that do not interfere with acetylcholine binding, whereas others may have a low concentration of potent blocking antibodies.

Pharmacological testing with anticholinesterase medicine can often assure a diagnosis. Drugs that inhibit acetylcholinesterase at the neuromuscular junction cause a build-up of acetylcholine, resulting in the activation of more receptors for a longer period of time, which causes stronger muscle contractions. Edrophonium (Tensilon) has a rapid onset, has a 5-minute duration of action, and can be given intravenously. A 2-mg test dose is given to gauge potential effects, followed after 5 minutes by 4–8 mg. If there is definite improvement in a weak muscle, the test is considered positive.

Clinical neurophysiological testing is important in helping to localize the cause of a patient's weakness to the nerve, neuromuscular junction, or muscle (Chapter 2). In myasthenia, tests of motor nerve conduction velocity and the electromyogram are normal. Two special tests may be abnormal in MG and are useful if antibody titers are normal—the repetitive nerve stimulation test and single-fiber electromyography (EMG).

Supramaximal repetitive stimulation of a motor nerve at low frequencies of 2–4 Hz results in repetitive compound muscle action potentials measured on skin of the same size and configuration in normal people. In myasthenic patients, the first action potential is normal or near normal, but the subsequent three to five potentials fall off (Figure 8–4A). A greater than 10% decrement is accepted as abnormal. The explanation for the fall-off is related to the reduction of the safety factor in myasthenia. With a reduced number of receptors, the normal reduction in released acetylcholine with repetitive stimulation successively activates fewer receptors so that end-plate potentials do not attain threshold and fewer muscle fibers fire. The test is abnormal in 65% of patients with myasthenia if both distal and proximal muscles are tested.

Single-fiber EMG is a more sensitive test than repetitive nerve stimulation when performed by an experienced electromyographer. Abnormalities in myasthenia are seen in Figure 8–4B. This test also probes the reduction in receptors by recording the variable speed and success of a motor neuron to fire two of its muscle fibers near the recording electrode. Normally both muscle fibers fire in a relatively fixed time relationship with repetitive stimulation. In myasthenia there is delay between the firing of the fibers, causing an increase in variability in the timing of the response between the two fibers, a phenomenon called jitter. If jitter is severe, the second fiber may not fire at all, a phenomenon called blocking. Single-fiber EMG is abnormal in all

patients with definite myasthenia and in up to 90% of patients with mild disease.

Given the availability of sensitive and specific tests, the diagnosis of myasthenia gravis can usually be made with assurance in typical cases. Nevertheless, certain other conditions should be considered at the time of first evaluation. When there is weakness of cranial nerves, an MRI scan of the head should be obtained to rule out compressive lesions. **Graves' disease** should be considered when there are abnormalities of eye movements even in the absence of exophthalmos. Hyperthyroidism alone can also cause weakness, and patients should be evaluated for thyroid function. A search for other conditions associated with myasthenia would include a chest CT scan for thymoma and tests for autoimmune disorders such as rheumatoid arthritis and lupus erythematosus.

Botulism is a rare condition of neuromuscular poisoning caused by the toxin of *Clostridium botulinum* bacteria. Clusters of cases have occurred from eating improperly sterilized canned foods. Typically there is onset of ophthalmoplegia with dilated pupils within 12–24 hours after ingestion. Cranial nerve and somatic muscle weakness follow, occasionally with difficulty breathing leading to respiratory paralysis. The toxin is extremely potent, and as little as 0.05 mg can be fatal in 24 hours. The toxin binds to the presynaptic membrane and inhibits acetylcholine release. In this case repetitive nerve stimulation causes an increase in release of acetylcholine and an improvement in muscle contraction, just the opposite of myasthenia. Recovery from botulinum poisoning is very slow because it requires synthesis of new membrane and sprouting.

The **Lambert-Eaton myasthenic syndrome** resembles myasthenia gravis in that weakness can become worse after prolonged exercise. Proximal muscles are most often involved, and eye muscles and cranial nerves are affected in a minority of cases. Cholinergic synapses in the autonomic nervous system are also affected, so patients may experience dry mouth, blurred vision, impotence, and decreased sweating. In addition, tendon reflexes are often diminished or absent. The cause of the syndrome is an autoantibody to a voltage-sensitive calcium channel protein on the presynaptic nerve terminal membrane that is associated with acetylcholine release. When an action potential invades the terminal, there is a reduced amount of calcium influx and thus a reduction of the amount of acetylcholine released. Of note, in contrast to myasthenia, maximal muscle contraction or tetanic nerve stimulation will greatly improve neuromuscular transmission for a short period of time. The block of the calcium channel can be overcome by these techniques, briefly restoring synaptic levels of calcium available to facilitate transmitter release.

The majority of patients with the Lambert-Eaton myasthenic syndrome are men who have an oat cell carcinoma of the lung. It is thought that the oat cell is derived from a neuroectodermal line, since it carries many neuronal markers including calcium channels. Apparently antibodies directed against the tumor's calcium channel cross-react with sites at peripheral cholin-

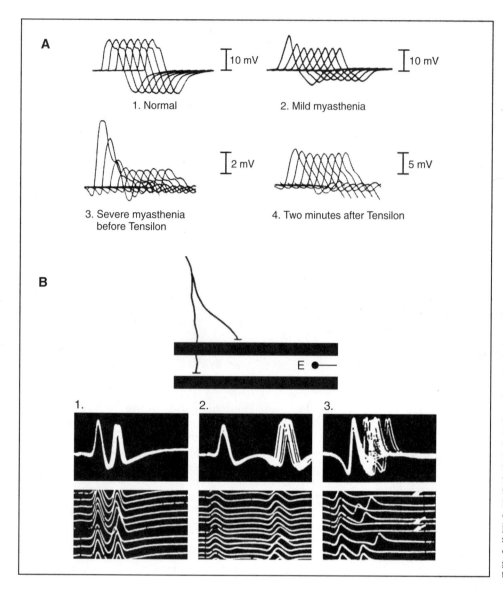

FIGURE 8–4. Electrophysiological tests for myasthenia. *A,* The repetitive nerve stimulation test in a normal person (1) shows no decrement in the compound muscle action potential when the nerve is stimulated at 3/s. The myasthenic patient may show a mild (2) or marked (3) decremental response that is largely corrected by anticholinesterase medication (4). (Reproduced, with permission, from R. P. Lisak and R. L. Barchi. *Myasthenia Gravis.* Vol II of Major Problems in Neurology. Philadelphia, W.B. Saunders Co., 1982.) *B,* The single-fiber EMG records the timing of the response of two muscle fibers in the same motor unit (lower tracings). In the normal condition (1), the fibers fire in almost the same time interval with each nerve stimulus. In myasthenia (2 and 3), there may be a delay or even failure of response (arrows in 3) in one of the fibers. When the tracings are superimposed with the time locked to the action potential of the first fiber, the variability of the second fiber becomes obvious. This variability is called jitter. (Reproduced, with permission, from E. Stalberg. Clinical electrophysiology in myasthenia gravis. J Neurol Neurosurg Psychiatry 43:627, 1980.)

ergic synapses. Patients require surgery of the tumor and immunosuppression. Other patients without oat cell tumors often have autoimmune disorders.

A variety of **drugs** can interfere with neuromuscular transmission and cause weakness in normal people and aggravate myasthenic weakness in patients. These include the curare-like neuromuscular blocking agents used in surgery and intensive care units. Aminoglycoside antibiotics are also known to aggravate weakness in myasthenia and should be avoided.

TREATMENT

In general, patients with myasthenia do better when they pace their daily activities, rest frequently, and eat well-balanced meals high in potassium. They should take care to avoid infections, heat, and undue stress. They should be provided with the list of drugs that can make their weakness worse and that should be avoided, including anesthetics, muscle relaxants, antiarrhythmics, and aminoglycoside antibiotics. Con-

tinuous therapy with good functional outcome is the standard practice today.

Anticholinesterase medication is helpful in nearly all myasthenic patients. Pyridostigmine is the most commonly used preparation and is usually started in doses of 30 mg every 4 hours with food (Table 8–2). Patients should be told that not all muscles will respond in the same way, with some improving while others remain seemingly resistant or even weaker. The medicine has a peak effect 1–2 hours after administration and wears off 2–3 hours later. Patients should be encouraged to keep a log of their response to the medicine during the day, noting improvement as well as side effects. Individual doses can be used for particular situations, such as extra medication before meals for patients with weakness chewing or swallowing.

Thymectomy is recommended for patients between puberty and age 60. Although a prospective randomized study has not been done on this procedure, a retrospective computer-matched analysis of 80 operated patients and unoperated controls indicated a significant

TABLE 8-2. Treatment of Myasthenia Gravis

Drug	Dose (mg/d)	Onset	Side Effects
Anticholinesterase			
Pyridostigmine	90–480 (in four divided doses)	30 minutes	Twitching, salivation, abdominal cramps, diarrhea
Immunosuppressive			
Prednisone	20–60 (switching to every other day after 1 month)	2–3 weeks	Hypertension, obesity, osteoporosis, diabetes, cataract
Azathioprine	100–250	3–12 months	Leukopenia, thrombocytopenia, neoplasia

benefit. Remissions occurred in 35% of the surgical group compared with 8% of controls. Long-term survival was also better in the surgical group with 85% versus 58% survival at 20 years. The benefit of the operation often is not evident for several years. Pathological analysis of the thymus reveals a tumor in up to 15% of patients. In the majority of the others, there is hyperplasia of reactive germinal lymphoid centers, indicating ongoing antibody production. The mechanism of the benefit of thymectomy may relate to removal of the myoid cells as the source of antigen, removal of thymic B cells as the source of antibody, or removal of some thymic abnormality in immune tolerance.

Immunosuppression is required for most patients at some time during their illness. Many patients do best on long-term or permanent immunosuppression. Prednisone and azathioprine are the drugs most commonly used (Table 8–2).

At times of acute worsening, such as during infections, during pregnancy, or in association with surgery, it may be useful to perform plasmapheresis. This process removes serum antibodies to the acetylcholine receptor, and some patients report improved strength with the first treatment. Two to four liters of plasma can be exchanged during a treatment. During the next 48 hours there is equilibration with antibodies from extracellular fluid throughout the body, so it is useful to repeat the treatment every 2 days for four or five exchanges. The benefit is temporary because antibodies return to their pretreatment level within a month, and on occasion there is a rebound overshoot. Intravenous immunoglobulin (IVIG) can also be given as a temporary treatment to avoid myasthenic crisis. The effect of this treatment may be to bind and inactivate circulating pathogenetic antibodies. A 5-day course of 0.4–1.0 g/kg/d has been reported to induce improvement starting in 10 days and lasting several months.

Specific immunotherapies are now in experimental trials. Most of these were designed and tested in experimental animals (Box 8–2). Anti-CD4+ antibodies have been found effective in one trial, but this treatment broadly depresses immune function. Oral tolerization with the acetylcholine receptor has proved effective in experimental animals if it is given before

immunization. A strategy to induce *in vivo* T lymphocyte tolerance to the receptor is under evaluation. These types of therapies are promising, since so much is known about the antigen and the cellular and antibody response.

SUMMARY

Myasthenia gravis is a T cell–dependent antibody-mediated autoimmune disease of the neuromuscular acetylcholine receptor. Weakness and muscle fatigability occur generally in young women and older men, and abnormalities of the thymus are characteristic. Thymectomy, anticholinesterase medication, and immunosuppression are effective therapies and promise patients good functional activity and a normal life span. Further research promises specific immune therapy that will block individual steps in the pathogenesis of the disease.

Selected Readings

Buckingham, J. M., F. M. Howard, Jr., P. E. Bernatz, et al. The value of thymectomy in myasthenia gravis: A computer-assisted matched study. Ann Surg 184:453–458, 1976.

Buzzard, E. F. The clinical history and *post-mortem* examination of five cases of myasthenia gravis. Brain 28:438–483, 1905.

Drachman, D. B. Myasthenia gravis. (Medical Progress.) N Engl J Med 330:1797–1810, 1994.

Engel, A. E., M. Mitsuhiro, E. H. Lambert, et al. Experimental autoimmune myasthenia gravis: A sequential and quantitative study of the neuromuscular junction ultrastructure and electrophysiologic correlations. J Neuropathol Exp Neurol 35:569–587, 1976.

Engel, A. E., J. M. Lindstrom, E. H. Lambert, and V. A. Lennon. Ultrastructural localization of the acetylcholine receptor in myasthenia gravis and its experimental autoimmune model. Neurology 27:307–315, 1977.

Keesey, J. C. Electrodiagnostic approach to defects in neuromuscular transmission. AAEE minimonograph No. 33. Muscle Nerve 12:613–626, 1989.

Maselli, R. A., D. P. Richman, and R. L. Wollman. Inflammation at the neuromuscular junction in myasthenia gravis. Neurology 41:1497–1504, 1991.

Patrick, J., and J. Lindstrom. Autoimmune response to acetylcholine receptor. Science 180:871–872, 1973.

Penn, A. S., D. P. Richman, L. Ruff, and V. A. Lennon (eds.). Myasthenia gravis and related disorders: Experimental and clinical aspects. Ann N Y Acad Sci 681:1–125, 1993.

Viets, H. R. A historical review of myasthenia gravis from 1672 to 1900. JAMA 153:1273–1280, 1953.

CHAPTER NINE

PERIPHERAL

NEUROPATHY

INTRODUCTION 107

CLINICAL PRESENTATION 107

EVALUATION AND DIFFERENTIAL DIAGNOSIS 109

NERVE INJURY 110

ENTRAPMENT NEUROPATHIES 111

    Carpal Tunnel Syndrome 111

    Ulnar Nerve Entrapment 111

    Meralgia Paraesthetica 111

    Peroneal Palsy 112

DIABETES MELLITUS 112

IMMUNE SYSTEM–MEDIATED NEUROPATHIES 112

    Guillain-Barré Syndrome 112

    Chronic Inflammatory Demyelinative Polyneuropathy 114

    Multifocal Motor Neuropathy 114

    Paraproteinemias 114

HEREDITARY NEUROPATHIES 114

    Charcot-Marie-Tooth Disease 114

    Familial Amyloid Polyneuropathy 115

INFECTIOUS NEUROPATHIES 115

    Human Immunodeficiency Virus (HIV) 115

IDIOPATHIC POLYNEUROPATHY 116

TREATMENT 116

SUMMARY 116

INTRODUCTION

Peripheral neuropathy is commonly encountered in clinical medicine. A large number of inherited and immune system–mediated diseases affect the peripheral nerves specifically, and many systemic, metabolic, and toxic conditions can involve the peripheral nerves as part of their protean manifestations. Although the peripheral sensory, motor, and autonomic nerves are relatively simple histologically, they nevertheless are some of the largest cells in the body (Figure 9–1). For example, the sensory nerve to the foot sends its central axon to the nucleus gracilis in the upper cervical spinal cord, thus spanning a distance of more than 80% of the body's length. The cell body of this nerve located in the dorsal root ganglion must support the structure and metabolism of the nerves' projections in their furthest extent. This involves synthesizing and transporting macromolecules and organelles to the cells' central and peripheral terminal fields. The size and length of peripheral nerve cells make them vulnerable to metabolic, toxic, and traumatic injuries.

CLINICAL PRESENTATION

Patients with peripheral neuropathy commonly seek medical attention for changes in sensation or strength. The diagnostic exercise for the physician is the same as for diseases of the central nervous system (Chapter 2). The most important steps are a careful history followed by examination. Localization of the abnormalities and consideration of mechanisms of pathophysiology reduce the numerous etiological possibilities to a few hypotheses that can be pursued by laboratory testing. A step-by-step approach to the diagnosis is the most secure method (Box 9–1).

Patients with disorders of sensation often complain of numbness, tingling, and pain. The latter may be described as "deep," "aching," "burning," or "sharp." These symptoms can indicate involvement of different classes of fibers and different pathophysiological processes (Chapter 4). It is important to record the patient's own words rather than to use terms such as "paresthesia" or "dysesthesia." This approach allows an easier and more direct vocabulary for following disease progression or response to therapy over time.

The clinical history and examination can help determine whether "numbness" is due to a disorder of large myelinated fibers or of small, thinly myelinated and unmyelinated fibers. Disorders of large fibers (e.g., immune-mediated demyelinative neuropathies) often cause a painless numbness and diminished sensation to light touch and vibration in addition to weakness. Disorders affecting small fibers (e.g., diabetes and amyloidosis) can cause diminished sensation to touch, pinprick, and temperature. Small-fiber neuropathies are frequently painful owing to spontaneous or irritative discharges in damaged or regenerating fibers. The pain is usually "burning" (C fibers) or "prickling" (Aδ fibers) and localized to the area of sensory loss. By contrast, injury to roots or large nerve trunks causes deep aching pain that is relatively poorly localized (e.g., plexus neuropathies, sciatica).

BOX 9-1 Clinical Approach to Peripheral Neuropathy

Goals
(1) Determine the syndromic classification (Table 9–1).
(2) Establish the pattern (Figure 9–1) and/or the anatomic localization (Table 9–2).
(3) Evaluate the pathophysiological process (Table 9–3).
(4) Determine the etiology (Table 9–4)

Clinical History
(1) Define and explore the symptoms.

   Numbness: touch/proprioception versus pain-temperature
   Pain: burning versus prickling versus aching versus lightning
   Weakness: proximal versus distal; flaccid versus stiff or spastic
   Autonomic features: faintness, sweating, impotence, bowel and bladder incontinence

(2) Determine the time versus intensity of the symptoms: acute, subacute, relapsing, chronic.
(3) Explore the family history for weakness, difficulty in walking, and sensory loss.
(4) Review the medical history for symptoms of systemic diseases, diabetes mellitus, hypothyroidism, arthritis, rash, fever, etc.
(5) Evaluate each drug being used, including vitamins and food supplements.
(6) Review the history for exposure to toxins, especially organic solvents.

Physical Examination
(1) Determine the type, pattern, and localization of sensory loss: touch threshold, pin prick, temperature, vibration, and position sense.
(2) Determine the presence, location, and pattern of muscle weakness.
(3) Determine if autonomic functions are involved: skin moisture, color, turgor, orthostatic changes in blood pressure.
(4) Test all reflexes.

Spontaneous discharges in large fibers cause tingling sensations in the dermatomal distribution of the nerve. A common example of this principle occurs when trauma to the ulnar nerve behind the elbow causes brief tingling in the fourth and fifth fingers. High-frequency discharges in large fibers can also cause brief, intense "sharp" or "electrical" pain that is highly localized. This occurs characteristically above the upper lip in trigeminal neuralgia (tic douloureux) and in the extremities following nerve injury. In addition, abnormalities of large fibers can cause loss of position sense at the joints. This leads to difficulties with balance and a wide-based ataxic gait when it affects the legs, or tremor when it affects the upper extremities (e.g., syphilitic tabes dorsalis and chronic inflammatory demyelinating polyneuropathy [CIDP]). Occasionally there is spontaneous movement of the fingers when the arms are outstretched with the eyes closed—a sign of

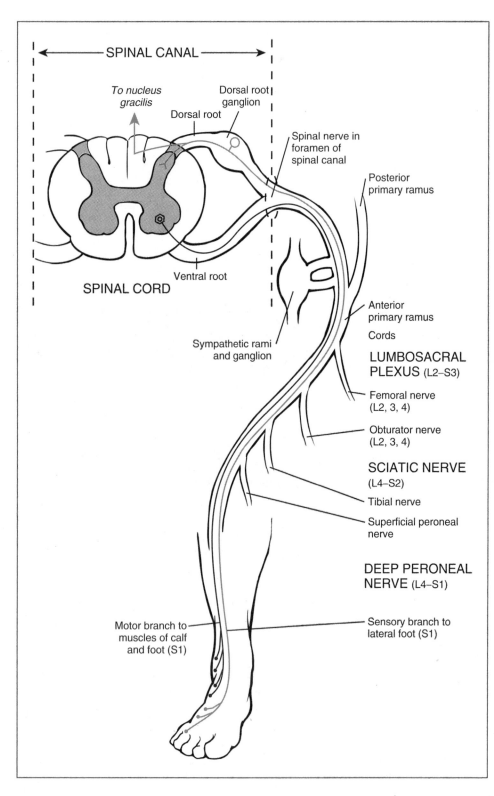

FIGURE 9-1. Anatomy of a peripheral nerve (S1 fibers to the foot). The components of a peripheral nerve include the sensory fibers whose cell bodies lie in the dorsal root ganglia, the motor fibers from the motor neurons in the anterior horn of the spinal cord, and autonomic fibers. Ten to fifteen dorsal and ventral root pairs from adjacent spinal cord segments come together to form the numbered cervical (C1–8), thoracic (T1–12), lumbar (L1–5), and sacral (S1–5) nerves that innervate dermatome and myotome body segments, traveling to these destinations through cords, plexuses, and peripheral nerves. Disease processes can affect nerve cell bodies and roots within the spinal canal (e.g., toxic, infectious, and metabolic diseases), peripheral nerve (e.g., entrapment and trauma), or myelin sheath (i.e., immune-mediated disease) distally. The longest nerve cells are the most vulnerable such that symptoms of damage often begin with sensory loss and weakness in the feet.

sensory ataxia called pseudoathetosis. Pure examples of large and small fiber sensory loss are not as common as metabolic and toxic conditions that cause variable loss of all somatic sensations: light touch and pressure, vibration, position sense, and pain-temperature.

Distal weakness is common in peripheral neuropathy. As discussed below, some disorders can cause pure motor neuropathy (e.g., multifocal motor neuropathy)

or a clinical picture in which rapidly ascending weakness dominates (e.g., Guillain-Barré syndrome). Weakness almost always begins in the feet, reflecting the vulnerability of the longest nerves. A patient may complain of stumbling, discovered on examination to be due to weakness in ankle flexion. There will also be difficulty in spreading the toes, indicating weakness of intrinsic muscles of the feet, muscles innervated by the body's longest motor nerves. As the illness progresses and shorter nerves become involved, the proximal leg muscles will weaken at about the same time as the hands become affected. Difficulty in spreading the fingers is an early sign of peripheral nerve weakness in the upper extremities.

When denervation of muscle occurs, characteristic electrical changes begin after approximately 2 weeks. Positive sharp waves and fibrillations are found with needle electromyography (EMG; Chapter 3), but these changes are not appreciated on clinical examination. Muscle atrophy occurs with chronic denervation owing to loss of trophic factors when the nerve's axon is damaged. This can be appreciated by inspection and palpation of muscles after chronic denervation of 4–6 months.

In weakness due to peripheral neuropathy, muscle tone is decreased and reflexes are diminished or totally abolished. The loss of the ankle jerk, or Achilles reflex, is an early sign of peripheral neuropathy. Reflexes rarely return with recovery from neuropathy. This is probably due in part to the alteration in conduction velocity that occurs with remyelination of large, fast conducting fibers subserving the stretch reflex. The synchrony of the volley becomes dispersed, preventing a uniform contraction of a sufficient number of muscle fibers to create a jerk response.

Dysfunction of the autonomic nervous system occurs when small unmyelinated fibers are affected (e.g., in amyloidosis and diabetes). Orthostatic hypotension is the most common manifestation, but patients can also experience impotence (men), dry skin, abnormal pupillary reactions, changes in bowel motility (e.g., nocturnal diarrhea), and bladder atony with incontinence. Abnormalities of autonomic and small sensory fibers can lead to trophic changes of the skin with discoloration, loss of hair and skin turgor, nail changes, skin ulcers, and deformities of joints.

EVALUATION AND DIFFERENTIAL DIAGNOSIS

Physicians are aided in their diagnosis of peripheral neuropathies by consideration of the classification

TABLE 9-1. Classification of Peripheral Neuropathy by Clinical Syndrome

Clinical Syndrome	Common Example
Acute ascending paralysis	Guillain-Barré syndrome
Subacute/chronic sensorimotor polyneuropathy	Metabolic and toxic disorders (Table 9–4)
Familial chronic sensorimotor polyneuropathy	Charcot-Marie-Tooth disease (Table 9–6)
Relapsing polyneuropathy	Chronic inflammatory demyelinating polyneuropathy (CIDP), porphyria, HNPP
Predominately motor neuropathy	Guillain-Barré syndrome, CIDP, multifocal motor neuropathy
Predominately sensory neuropathy	Sjögren's syndrome, cancer, vitamin B_{12} deficiency, leprosy
Autonomic neuropathy	Amyloidosis, diabetes, alcoholism, acute pandysautonomia

TABLE 9-2. Classification of Peripheral Neuropathy by Anatomical Site

Anatomical Site	Common Example
Cranial nerve	III, IV, or VI: Diabetes V: Tic douloureux VII: Bell's palsy
Multiple cranial nerves	Meningeal spread of cancer, sarcoidosis
Mononeuropathy	Entrapment neuropathy (Figure 9–2)
Mononeuropathy multiplex	Diabetes, polyarteritis nodosa
Nerve root	Cervical and lumbar disk herniation, neurofibroma
Plexus	Idiopathic brachial plexus neuropathy, diabetes, cancer
Symmetric distal polyneuropathy	Metabolic and toxic etiologies (Table 9–4)

of these disorders by clinical syndrome (Table 9–1), anatomical site (Table 9–2), topography (Figure 9–2), and pathophysiological mechanism (Table 9–3). There are more than 50 different causes of peripheral neuropathy when all the genetic disorders and numerous toxins and drugs that have been reported to cause neuropathy are included. Common causes are listed in Table 9–4. Occasionally it is necessary to consult comprehensive lists found in reference texts before an individual diagnosis can be assured.

Laboratory tests are an essential part of patient evaluation in most cases. Nerve conduction studies are used to localize the site of a conduction block (e.g., entrapments), describe the distribution and severity of a polyneuropathic process, and determine the presence and severity of demyelination or axonal destruction. EMG helps localize the site of weakness to a nerve root, peripheral nerve, neuromuscular junction, or muscle either locally or extensively. Blood tests are important in searching for metabolic, inflammatory, endocrinological, and immune causes (Table 9–5). Lumbar punctures are occasionally helpful in confirming infectious (e.g., syphilis, Lyme disease, cytomegalovirus [CMV]) or neoplastic etiologies or when an elevated protein is found (e.g., Guillain-Barré syndrome, CIDP, diabetes). Nerve biopsies are indicated for those cases in which vasculitis, amyloidosis, or carcinomatous infiltration are suspected but cannot otherwise be determined. At pres-

TABLE 9-3. Classification of Peripheral Neuropathy by Pathophysiological Mechanism

Pathology	Common Example
Demyelination	Guillain-Barré syndrome, CIDP
Axonal "dying back"	Metabolic etiologies, toxins (e.g., arsenic), and drugs (e.g., vincristine)
Segmental demyelination and axonal loss	Diabetes
Wallerian degeneration	Nerve transection
Compression	Entrapment (e.g., carpal tunnel syndrome)
Ischemia and infarction	Polyarteritis nodosa
Inflammation or infiltration	Leprosy, CMV, lymphoma

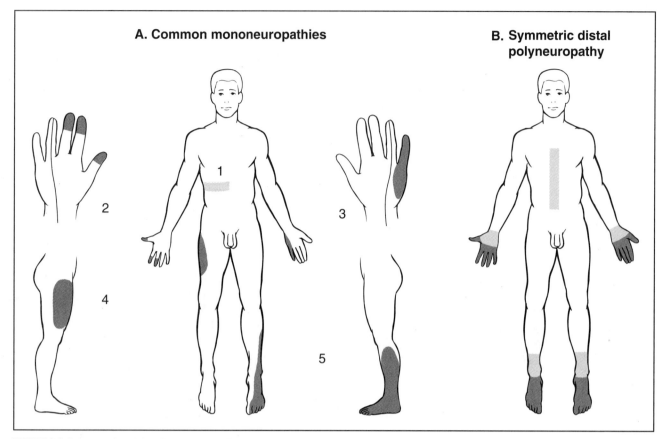

A. Common mononeuropathies

B. Symmetric distal polyneuropathy

FIGURE 9–2. Patterns of peripheral neuropathy. The dark shading indicates loss of pinprick sensation. The light shading indicates a decrease in appreciation of light touch. *A,* Common mononeuropathies include (1) the dermatomal rash and pain of herpes zoster, (2) the carpal tunnel syndrome due to entrapment of the median nerve, (3) ulnar neuropathy, (4) meralgia paresthetica due to entrapment of the lateral cutaneous nerve of the thigh, and (5) peroneal palsy due to compression of the common peroneal nerve at the neck of the fibula. *B,* Symmetric distal polyneuropathies cause loss of sensation in a stocking-glove distribution on the feet and hands. Loss of sensation in a shield pattern on the chest reflects dysfunction of the ends of the longest thoracic nerves.

ent, approximately 10–20% of cases cannot be precisely diagnosed. The more common causes of neuropathy are considered below.

NERVE INJURY

Trauma that results in a severed nerve causes instant anesthesia and flaccid weakness. If the distal portion of the nerve is stimulated electrically immediately after the accident, the conduction velocity will be normal and muscle will be activated. However, as axoplasmic transport from the cell body is interrupted, the distal portion begins to undergo dissolution of both the axon and myelin sheath in a process called wallerian degeneration. In addition, muscle fibers deprived of trophic input will begin to degenerate. Schwann cells proliferate upon injury, and there is an increase in factors in the extracellular matrix that promote and guide neurite growth cones: laminin, tenascin, and the neuronal cell adhesion molecule. It is thus important to surgically reconnect or bridge together the proximal and distal ends of a nerve to provide a distal albeit damaged and cluttered pathway for axonal growth. If reanastomosis is successful, axons growing at rates between 0.1 and 1.0 mm/d will eventually reinnervate terminal fields. However, with reanastomosed severed

nerves and even crushed or compressed nerves, the degree of reinnervation is usually incomplete, especially at distant sites. In addition, the pattern of reinnervation can be abnormal. For example, following compression of cranial nerve VII (Bell's palsy), regenerating fibers headed toward the mouth (orbicularis oris) can become abnormally directed to the eye (orbicularis oculi). As a result, when the patient smiles the eye will wink. Anomalous reinnervation in an extremity is not as critical functionally where large groups of muscles act in synergy.

When a nerve is crushed or compressed acutely, there will likely be a local block of action potentials with resultant distal sensory loss and weakness. Large myelinated fibers are the most vulnerable to compression injury, since myelin is often stripped from its axon. Preservation of small fibers usually leaves some cutaneous sensation intact, although patients will describe it as abnormal. Surgery is not indicated when the nerve retains its continuity. Over a few hours to a few days, the local contusion and edema associated with the injury resolve and conduction through the area is restored for those nerves that were not directly damaged. Two to six weeks are required for remyelination and restoration of conduction block. If weakness persists beyond several months, damage to axons can be as-

TABLE 9-4. Classification of Peripheral Neuropathy by Etiology

Metabolic Causes
Diabetes mellitus
Hypothyroidism
Acromegaly
Uremia
Alcoholism
Vitamin deficiencies: B_1, B_2, B_3, B_6, B_{12}
Malabsorption
Porphyria

Toxic Causes
Drugs, e.g., vincristine, cisplatin, nitrofurantoin
Heavy metals: arsenic, lead, thallium
Organic compounds, e.g., hexane, acrylamide, organophosphates

Infections
Leprosy
HIV, CMV
Herpes zoster
Lyme disease

Immune or Inflammatory Causes
Demyelinative disease: Guillain-Barré syndrome, CIDP
Multifocal motor neuropathy
Paraproteinemias, e.g., myeloma, monoclonal gammopathy
Carcinomatous sensory neuropathy

Ischemia
Vasculitis, e.g., polyarteritis nodosa

Genetic Causes
Charcot-Marie-Tooth syndromes: 17p11.2, 1q22, 1p, Xq13.1
Familial amyloid polyneuropathies

---

sumed and recovery will occur only after the process of axon regrowth reaches its destination. For example, the weakness of the foot that results from injury to the sciatic nerve at its emergence below the gluteal fold at

TABLE 9-5. Laboratory Tests in Peripheral Neuropathy*

Blood tests, commonly helpful
　CBC
　Chemistry panel
　Fasting blood glucose
　Erythrocyte sedimentation rate (ESR)
　Antinuclear antibody (ANA)
　Thyroid function tests
　Serum protein electrophoresis
　Immunoelectrophoresis (IEP)
Blood tests, for specific conditions
　Lyme antibody titer (history of exposure and skin rash)
　Rheumatoid factor (history of joint pain or suspicion of vasculitis)
　Hu antibody (for diagnosis of carcinomatous sensory neuropathy)
Urine tests, for specific conditions
　Heavy metals (history of exposure and clinical profile)
　Immunoelectrophoresis (rarely positive when serum IEP is normal)
Cerebrospinal fluid
　For diagnosis of infections and inflammatory conditions and cancer
　Helpful in Guillain-Barré syndrome, CIDP, and diabetes when protein is elevated
Nerve biopsy
　For diagnosis of vasculitis, tumor infiltration, amyloidosis, dysproteinemia, sarcoidosis, and leprosy when other tests are inconclusive

---

*Laboratory tests are not routinely ordered for every patient but are selected to explore or confirm etiological hypotheses. The clinical profile usually guides the choice of specific tests.

---

the back of the hip will take 1–2 years to resolve. Sprouting from local intact fibers will also help advance recovery.

ENTRAPMENT NEUROPATHIES

When peripheral nerves become compressed in fibro-osseous tunnels or by overlying ligaments or tendons, intermittent and then permanent symptoms will develop. There are numerous sites for possible compression, but four conditions are particularly common (see below and Figure 9–2). In any particular case, clues should be investigated for possible causes. Occasionally there is underlying diabetes, acromegaly, uremia, hypothyroidism, or a paraproteinemia. A recent gain in weight might be implicated, or repeated trauma from a particular posture or activity. A family history would indicate the rare condition of "hereditary neuropathy with liability to pressure palsy" (HNPP, chromosome 17p11.2; see below).

Carpal Tunnel Syndrome

In the carpal tunnel syndrome, the median nerve becomes compressed at the wrist in its osseous tunnel. This condition is more common in women, particularly during late pregnancy. Patients typically feel pain and tingling at night, often extending up into the forearm. Examination in the earliest stages is usually normal, but with advanced compression there is sensory loss at the tips of the first and middle fingers and weakness of the abductor pollicis and opponens pollicis muscles. Percussion over the carpal tunnel may produce tingling in the first two fingers (Tinel's sign). Nerve conduction studies should be done on both hands to localize the conduction block. Since the condition is often self-limiting, simple wrist splints are commonly tried for several months before proceeding to surgery.

Ulnar Nerve Entrapment

Ulnar nerve entrapment at the elbow can occur after a fracture, with repeated trauma, or with arthritis. Numbness and sensory loss occur in the fourth and fifth digits, and weakness develops in the intrinsic and interosseous muscles of the hand manifested as difficulty in spreading the fingers. In advanced cases, the fourth and fifth fingers develop a claw-like deformity with extension at the metacarpal phalangeal joint and flexion at the proximal interphalangeal joint. Muscle wasting can be seen in the hypothenar eminence and first dorsal interosseous muscle. Avoidance of resting on the elbows and other forms of trauma is important. Surgery in mild cases is controversial.

Meralgia Paraesthetica

Meralgia paraesthetica is the common name used for the syndrome caused by entrapment of the lateral cutaneous nerve of the thigh where it passes under the attachment of the inguinal ligament to the iliac crest. An irritative, burning sensation develops over the anterolateral part of the thigh. It is aggravated in different positions, commonly becoming worse upon standing but decreasing with walking. Both decreased sensation and hyperpathia can be appreciated on examination. There is no weakness. Weight loss, avoidance of tight belts, and an occasional injection of a local anesthetic can be helpful. Patients are reassured to learn the condition is benign and self-limited.

Peroneal Palsy

Peroneal palsy is caused by entrapment of the peroneal nerve between the neck of the fibula and the insertion of the peroneus longus muscle. Weakness of the tibialis anterior muscle with a resultant footdrop is the characteristic finding. Weakness of the extensor hallucis longus (extension of the great toe) and the peroneal muscles (eversion of the foot) are also present. Sensory loss over the dorsal part of the foot is usually mild. Trauma to the leg, or the practice of crossing the weakened leg over the opposite knee, is sometimes present in the history. The use of a lightweight footdrop support that fits into the shoe is important to prevent tripping while the nerve recovers. Four to twelve months is the usual course.

DIABETES MELLITUS

Diabetes is the most common cause of neuropathy in the United States and presents in different clinical patterns: distal sensorimotor neuropathy, mononeuropathy, mononeuropathy multiplex, autonomic neuropathy, and lumbosacral plexopathy. Similarly to most metabolic and toxic causes of neuropathy, the most common clinical syndrome is symmetric distal polyneuropathy. Loss of sensation in the feet is the most frequent symptom with a diminution of superficial touch, pinprick, and vibratory sensation in a stocking distribution found on examination. Ankle jerks are depressed or lost. A mild weakness of dorsiflexion of the large toe and ankle may be present. This clinical picture can worsen with poor diabetic control over time. Numbness and weakness can extend up the legs and involve the hands as well. Sensory loss on the anterior midline of the abdomen can occur as a reflection of involvement of the distal parts of the thoracic nerves. Small, thinly myelinated and unmyelinated fibers can become involved, with the development of burning dysesthetic pain, skin and joint changes, and autonomic dysfunction.

Diabetes can also affect large nerves either singly or at multiple sites (mononeuropathy multiplex). The third and the sixth cranial nerves are commonly affected as isolated palsies, and patients present with diplopia. The third nerve palsy begins with pain behind the eye in half of the cases, followed by ptosis and extraocular paralysis in 24 hours. The cause is infarction from an endoneurial vessel. Parasympathetic pupilloconstrictor fibers traveling on the outer side of the nerve are spared. By contrast, compression of the third nerve by an aneurysm of the adjacent posterior communicating artery regularly causes paralysis and dilatation of the pupil (Chapter 5).

Vascular ischemia or infarction of large nerves or cords of the lumbosacral plexus causes pain and focal asymmetric weakness in the legs. The pain is often severe and precedes the weakness by several days. Weakness of the quadriceps, iliopsoas, and hip adductors is common, with atrophy developing later (diabetic amyotrophy). Sensory loss is a minor component. Weakness of the legs is usually unilateral or asymmetric. Bilateral symmetric weakness implies either muscle disease (lower motor neuron syndrome; Chapter 3) or spinal cord disease (upper motor neuron syndrome).

The cause of neuropathy in diabetes is related to protracted hyperglycemia. Excessive glycosylation of proteins in the endothelium of capillaries and larger vessels is thought to underlie the damage. Glycosylated proteins may be resistant to degradation and turn over more slowly, leading to reduplication of the basement membrane, thickening of the vascular wall, and disruption of the blood-nerve barrier with endoneurial edema. Chronic hyperglycemia may also affect the metabolism and function of the neuron, Schwann cell, and axon directly. Pathologically nerves show both segmental demyelination and loss of axons. Controlled clinical studies indicate that intensive insulin treatment to control blood glucose greatly reduces the incidence of neuropathy. Insulin-like growth factors have been found to stimulate peripheral nerve regeneration in animals with experimentally induced diabetic neuropathy.

IMMUNE SYSTEM–MEDIATED NEUROPATHIES

Autoimmunity is thought to play a role in several different kinds of peripheral neuropathies (Table 9–4). Several can be recognized clinically (Guillain-Barré syndrome, CIDP), whereas others require serological testing (paraproteinemias, carcinomatous sensory neuropathy) or special electrophysiological study (multifocal motor neuropathy with conduction block). Convincing proof for autoimmunity requires demonstration of abnormal activated T cells or serum antibodies localized to sites of disease and passive transfer to animal or *in vitro* experimental systems. Passive transfer has been accomplished for the Guillain-Barré syndrome. Other conditions show either specific serum antibodies or immune-mediated inflammation on biopsy. Plasma exchange and intravenous immunoglobulin (IVIG) have proved effective in treating these neuropathies, further substantiating an immune-mediated pathophysiology.

Guillain-Barré Syndrome

The Guillain-Barré syndrome typically presents as an acute ascending motor paralysis. Cases can occur at any age, and an antecedent stimulus for autoimmunity can often be found. Commonly the weakness will begin several weeks after a nonspecific viral syndrome, mumps, measles, Epstein-Barr (EB) virus infection (infectious mononucleosis, hepatitis), *Mycoplasma* pneumonia, or *Campylobacter jejuni* enteritis. HIV, Hodgkin's disease, and surgery have also been identified as precedent conditions. The overall incidence is one to two new cases per 100,000 population per year. Although weakness is the most characteristic abnormality, patients often report back or leg pain and tingling numbness as the first complaints. Most patients reach their nadir by 4 weeks with weakness of all four extremities and the face. Reflexes are absent. Up to a third of patients will require mechanical support for ventilation when vital capacity drops below 15–20 mL/kg. Respiratory failure can progress rapidly, and vital capacity should be followed closely in weak patients to plan for intubation. Autonomic involvement manifested by instability of heart rate and blood pressure occurs in advanced cases.

Laboratory studies become abnormal after a week of illness with elevation of CSF protein without pleocytosis. The presence of inflammatory cells in the spinal fluid suggests another diagnosis such as AIDS, Lyme disease, or carcinomatous meningitis. Slowed nerve conduction studies indicative of demyelination can be found in nerve roots (F wave test; Box 9–2) within a week and in peripheral nerves after that time. Pathological studies have found macrophage and lymphocyte infiltration of nerve roots, cranial nerves, and in peripheral nerves (Figure 9–3). Serological studies have shown elevation of antimyelin antibodies in up to a third of cases, but tests for serum antibodies are neither routinely indicated nor clinically helpful.

Treatment of patients with plasma exchange for 2 weeks or longer ameliorates the disease process and is standard therapy. IVIG may also be beneficial and is in clinical trials. Complete recovery with rehabilitation can be anticipated for the majority of patients in 3–6 months. A poorer outcome is indicated for the elderly, those with rapid progression of the disease, and those requiring prolonged ventilatory support.

There are several variations on this typical presentation. One subgroup will experience weakness of only the pharyngeal, cervical, and brachial muscles. Another subgroup will have only ophthalmoplegia, ataxia, and areflexia—a triad called Miller Fisher syndrome. Interestingly, serum antibodies to a myelin epitope heavily represented on the oculomotor nerve (GQ_{1b}) have been found in this syndrome, but in Guillain-Barré syndrome only when there are extraocular palsies. An axonal variant of Guillain-Barré syndrome is well recognized by characteristic changes on electrophysiological tests: normal nerve conduction studies with a reduction of the compound muscle action potential. In these cases, there is profound weakness with denervation and atrophy of muscles. The course is usually protracted with incomplete recovery of distal muscle strength. Seasonal epidemics of acute motor axonal neuropathy have been identified in children in northern China.

BOX 9-2 Nerve Conduction Studies

Peripheral motor and sensory nerves can be studied electrically to determine properties of nerve roots, axons, and myelin sheaths. Nerve conduction velocities are commonly measured as a test of the integrity of the myelin sheath on the largest axons. Motor conduction velocities are usually measured in the median, ulnar, and lateral popliteal nerves using surface recording electrodes over the abductor pollicis brevis, abductor digiti minimi, and extensor digitorum brevis muscles, respectively. Normal values are available for most nerves relative to age and sex and typically run between 45 and 80 m/s. Adult values are reached by 4 years of age and slow only slightly with advancing age. Sensory action potentials (latency and amplitude) are measured by stimulating the index and little fingers and measuring the median nerve and ulnar nerve responses at the wrist.

As an example, the ulnar nerve can be stimulated at the wrist, forearm, or above the elbow while the compound muscle action potential is recorded over the hypothenar eminence (Figure 3–3). The conduction velocity can then be computed between these points to determine if there is a slowing compared to normal controls matched for age and sex. A delay in the distal latency between the wrist and the muscle indicates abnormalities of the distal axon or its myelin sheath. This abnormality is typically due to a metabolic or toxic etiology. A uniformly slowed nerve conduction velocity suggests an inherited demyelinative process (e.g., Charcot-Marie-Tooth IA), while a slowed conduction velocity with temporal dispersion and focal block (see below) indicates a nonuniform, acquired demyelinative disease process (e.g., Guillain-Barré syndrome, CIDP). Focal slowing across a specific segment indicates local demyelination due to trauma or compression (e.g., ulnar neuropathy from entrapment behind the elbow). Conduction velocities measure the health only of the largest myelinated fibers. Diseases of anterior horn cells or axons cause weakness, but motor nerve conduction studies will be near normal limits since there is no demyelination.

Axonal neuropathies can be identified by a decrease in the magnitude of the nerve action potential which is a sum of all individual fiber action potentials. The compound action potential amplitude drops in proportion to axon loss. This can be measured directly by recording over sensory or motor nerves. In motor neuron disease and axonal neuropathies, there also is a reduction in the compound muscle action potential (CMAP) following stimulation of a motor nerve. Changes in CMAP over time can be used to follow disease progression or response to therapy. Measurement of amplitudes is difficult when demyelination is present because of temporal dispersion of the signal, which flattens out owing to slowing of some of the fibers.

Conduction through the proximal nerve root can be measured by the F wave test. Stimulation of a motor nerve causes retrograde deplorization of a small number of anterior horn cells. Upon discharge, these send a subsequent volley of action potentials back down to muscle. A second muscle potential will be evoked following the muscle potential caused by the original anterograde stimulus. The difference in the timing of the two is a measure of conduction through proximal roots. This test is abnormal in the early phase of Guillain-Barré syndrome and other radiculopathies.

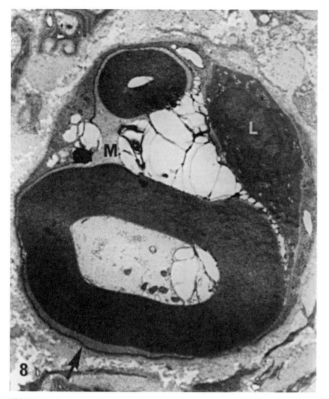

FIGURE 9–3. Acute demyelinating polyneuropathy—Guillain-Barré syndrome. A lymphocyte (L) lies within the basement membrane of a nerve fiber showing early myelin breakdown. Bubbling dissolution of the myelin membrane is seen adjacent to the lymphocyte and a macrophage (M). A tongue of cytoplasm of the macrophage has penetrated and lifted away part of the myelin sheath (arrow). × 8200. (Reproduced, with permission of Williams & Wilkins, from J. W. Prineas. Acute idiopathic polyneuritis. Lab Invest 26:133–147, 1972.)

Chronic Inflammatory Demyelinative Polyneuropathy

Chronic inflammatory demyelinative polyneuropathy (CIDP) typically begins in adults between 40 and 60 years of age with progressive or relapsing weakness. Asymmetric proximal weakness of the legs is common, with depression or absence of all tendon reflexes. Weakness of neck flexors is often present, but the face is generally less involved. The illness is usually painless, with sensory loss of the large fiber type and diminution of vibratory and position sense. Nerve conduction studies showing slowed velocities are required for diagnosis. CSF protein is commonly elevated. The illness can occur in isolated or idiopathic form and also in association with AIDS, monoclonal gammopathies, or rarely CNS demyelinating disease. Immunosuppression with corticosteroids, plasma exchange, or IVIG results in large and unequivocal improvement, but treatment is required for many years.

Multifocal Motor Neuropathy

Multifocal motor neuropathy (MMN) is an uncommon cause of weakness that usually begins in young adults, particularly men. It is important to differentiate this neuropathy from motor neuron disease (e.g., amyo-

trophic lateral sclerosis), since immunosuppressive treatment is effective. Patients typically present with progressive, asymmetric lower motor neuron–type weakness of distal muscles with depressed or absent reflexes. The upper extremities commonly are affected, and cramps and fasciculations can occur. Sensation is normal. The diagnosis rests on electrophysiological evidence of focal areas of slowed nerve conduction and partial block of motor nerves. Patients commonly have elevated levels of antibodies to membrane glycolipids (anti-GM_1 antibodies), but these are nonspecific, being found in the Guillain-Barré syndrome, CIDP, and a small percentage of cases of ALS. Treatment with IVIG is effective in the short term, and immunosuppression with cyclophosphamide can induce sustained improvement.

Paraproteinemias

Paraproteinemias must be searched for in cases of undiagnosed sensorimotor peripheral neuropathy. Finding a monoclonal gammopathy in the serum or immunoglobulin light chains (Bence Jones protein) in the urine would prompt a full hematological evaluation in search of multiple myeloma or other bone marrow dyscrasia (osteosclerotic myeloma, Waldenstrom's macroglobulinemia, amyloidosis). Occasionally a monoclonal gammopathy (IgM > IgG > IgA) is found as the sole abnormality of the immune system. Its significance to the neuropathy is uncertain, prompting the name "monoclonal gammopathy of undetermined significance" (MGUS). However, careful analysis of patients with IgM gammopathy reveals a high proportion with antibodies to myelin-associated glycoprotein (MAG) and nerve biopsies have found IgM deposits within areas of myelin splitting, suggesting a pathophysiological role for this antibody. Plasma exchange is effective in some patients with these forms of neuropathy.

HEREDITARY NEUROPATHIES
Charcot-Marie-Tooth Disease

The Charcot-Marie-Tooth (CMT) neuropathies are the most common forms of hereditary sensorimotor neuropathy. Described clinically in 1886 by Charcot and Marie and separately by Tooth, these neuropathies are now known to be a diverse group of genetic diseases primarily affecting peripheral Schwann cell myelin proteins (Table 9–6). The overall prevalence is 1/2500 population. The common presentation is symmetric weakness and wasting of the foot and calf muscles. The foot typically shows a high arch with hammer toes ("club foot") and is turned in owing to weakness of the peroneal muscles. Patients may complain of difficulty in running or of abnormal appearing feet rather than of weakness. This lack of complaint probably reflects the slow progression of the abnormality and adaptation by the patient. Many do not seek medical attention at all. Similarly, sensory complaints are rare, although objective evidence of deficits can be found on examination. Late in the course, the intrinsic muscles of the hands become weak.

TABLE 9–6. Charcot-Marie-Tooth Neuropathies (Hereditary Motor and Sensory Neuropathies)

Neuropathy	Phenotype	Locus	Gene	Mechanism
CMT type I				
CMT 1A	Demyelinative neuropathy, palpably enlarged nerves	17p11.2–12	PMP22 Compact myelin protein	Duplication or point mutations
CMT 1B	Demyelinative neuropathy	1q22–23	P0 Compact myelin protein	Point mutations
CMT 1C	Demyelinative neuropathy	Undetermined		
CMTX	Demyelinative neuropathy (males)	Xq13.1	CX32 Nodes of Ranvier	Point mutations
CMT type II				
CMT 2A	Neuronal, late onset, mild	1p36	Undetermined	Unknown
CMT III (Dejerine-Sottas)				
CMT 3A	Demyelinative neuropathy, severe, childhood	17p11.2–12	PMP22	Point mutations
CMT 3B	Demyelinative neuropathy, severe, childhood	1q22–23	P0	Point mutations
Hereditary neuropathy with pressure palsies				
HNPP	Demyelinative neuropathy, recurrent entrapment neuropathies	17p11.2–12	PMP22	Deletion—reciprocal of CMT 1A, point mutations

There are many variations in the phenotypic expression of these neuropathies, despite similar genetic abnormalities. For example, different point mutations in the gene for PMP22, a protein involved in the compact structure of peripheral myelin, can cause severe childhood-onset demyelinative neuropathy (CMT 3A, Dejerine-Sottas disease), recurrent entrapment neuropathies, or classical CMT. The biochemical mechanisms underlying these differences remain to be explained. Conversely, different genetic abnormalities can cause the same clinical abnormality, e.g., point mutations in the genes for PMP22 and P0 (another myelin protein). The relationship between CMT 1A and hereditary neuropathy with pressure palsy (HNPP) is particularly informative. A crossover event during meiosis apparently underlies both disorders. In CMT 1A, approximately 70% of cases have a duplication of a 1.5-megabase segment in the PMP22 gene. In HNPP, the same segment is deleted. These two phenotypically different neuropathies are thus reciprocal expressions of a transformation abnormality at the same locus. In CMT 1A, there may be overexpression of the protein or a fragment. The nerves are palpably enlarged and show proliferation of Schwann cells and myelin in an "onion bulb" formation. In HNPP, the nerves are not enlarged but are unusually sensitive to pressure, causing focal demyelination. DNA testing for these neuropathies is becoming available. At present there are no specific therapies.

Familial Amyloid Polyneuropathy

Familial amyloid polyneuropathy (FAP) presents primarily as a peripheral sensory and autonomic neuropathy with loss of pain and temperature sensation in the feet, orthostatic hypotension, problems with bowel motility, and urinary incontinence. Identification of amyloidosis by biopsy in a family pedigree secures the diagnosis. Amyloid is the generic name given to proteins that are birefringent when examined histologically with polarized optics. The proteins assume an insoluble β-pleated sheet configuration owing to changes in their structure. To date, point mutations in the genes for three different proteins have been identified in different families: transthyretin, apolipoprotein A1, and gelsolin. Defects in transthyretin, the thyroxine transport protein (formerly called prealbumin), are the most common. Transthyretin amyloid can deposit in the heart (cardiomyopathy) and gastrointestinal tract as well as in peripheral nerves. The protein is synthesized in the liver, and several patients with severe neuropathy have been successfully treated by liver transplantation.

INFECTIOUS NEUROPATHIES

Infections of peripheral nerves are uncommon in the United States except in patients with AIDS. Worldwide, infections with leprosy or *Trypanosoma cruzi* (Chagas' disease) are the most common infectious causes of peripheral neuropathy.

Human Immunodeficiency Virus (HIV)

Patients infected with HIV commonly develop peripheral neuropathy when CD4 counts fall below 200, the level used to define AIDS. The prevalence of AIDS neuropathy ranges between 30% and 50% depending on whether mild findings are included in surveys. There are several different syndromes. The most common presentation occurs late in AIDS as a distal, symmetric, predominantly sensory neuropathy with pain. Electrophysiological studies indicate axonal degeneration. The cause is unknown, and treatment is symptomatic.

Cytomegalovirus (CMV) commonly causes infections in AIDS patients and can present as a rapidly progressive, painful paraparesis. The virus invades Schwann cells of the lumbosacral plexus and cauda equina, causing aggressive inflammation. Flaccid weakness, loss of sensation below a dermatomal level, and urinary retention can occur. Lumbar puncture reveals pleocytosis, elevated protein, and low glucose. Syphilis and lymphomatous meningitis are less common but can give the same clinical picture. CMV infection is treated with intravenous ganciclovir.

Herpes zoster radiculitis occurs in 10% of AIDS patients and is common in all patients with immunosuppression. In addition, demyelinating neuropathy (Guillain-Barré syndrome) and vasculitis can occur, and if a specific diagnosis can be secured, appropriate treatment should be instituted. Finally, treatment of AIDS patients with the antiviral agent 2',3'-dideoxycytidine (ddC) can cause a toxic, painful, peripheral sensorimotor neuropathy. Development of this neuropathy limits the usefulness of this agent.

IDIOPATHIC POLYNEUROPATHY

Detailed evaluation of patients with neuropathy leads to a definitive diagnosis in 85–90% of cases. After blood work, electrophysiological study, evaluation of latent genetic causes (e.g., CMT 2A), and quantitative evaluation of nerve biopsy, patients remain for whom a diagnosis cannot be made. The typical patient is more than 50 years old and male and has a symmetric, distal sensorimotor neuropathy. In some, the sensory dysfunction predominates, but for a few weakness is more troublesome. Dysesthetic pains are usually mild. Electrophysiological studies and biopsies reveal a chronic axonal-type neuropathy. Follow-up of these patients is important, since a few will be found to have a malignancy or a paraproteinemia, usually within a year. Occult alcoholism may also become evident. For the majority, their course will remain stable or only very slowly progressive, and symptomatic treatment of pain or a footdrop brace will be helpful.

TREATMENT

The first principle of therapy for peripheral neuropathy is to provide primary treatment of the underlying cause (discussed briefly above). Symptomatic treatment is important in all cases. Peripherally acting (e.g., NSAID) and centrally acting (e.g., tricyclic antidepressant) analgesics are helpful for painful neuropathies, and anticonvulsants provide relief when lightning or electrical pains are present in addition (Chapter 4). When weakness is present, physical therapy exercises can provide useful ways to avoid developing contracture by means of passive range-of-motion stretching as well as active exercises. Splints and braces help maintain useful function for patients with wristdrop (radial nerve palsy) or footdrop (peroneal nerve palsy). Nerve growth factors that have proved efficacious in experimental animals for stimulating nerve regeneration are now in clinical trials and promise new approaches for helping patients with peripheral neuropathy due to a wide variety of causes.

SUMMARY

Peripheral neuropathy is a common clinical malady for which there are many causes. The clinical history and examination go a long way in reaching a specific etiological diagnosis. Classifying a particular patient's findings by syndrome and anatomical site aids in selecting appropriate laboratory tests. Once the etiological diagnosis is in hand, effective treatment can be started for nerve entrapments, diabetes mellitus, immune-mediated neuropathies, toxins, infections, and metabolic causes. Symptomatic treatments for pain and weakness will help restore useful function for most patients. Nerve growth factors offer the promise of primary treatments to stimulate nerve regeneration.

Selected Readings

Albers, J. W., and J. J. Kelly. Acquired inflammatory demyelinating polyneuropathies: Clinical and electrodiagnostic features. Muscle Nerve 12:435–451, 1989.

Chaudry, V., A. M. Corse, D. R. Cornblath, et al. Multifocal motor neuropathy: Response to human immune globulin. Ann Neurol 33:237–242, 1993.

Chiba, A., S. Kusunoki, H. Obata, et al. Serum anti-GQ1b IgG antibody is associated with ophthalmoplegia in Miller Fisher syndrome and Guillain-Barré syndrome: Clinical and immunohistochemical studies. Neurology 43:1911–1987, 1993.

The Diabetes Control and Complications Trial Research Group. The effect of intensive treatment of diabetes on the development and progression of long-term complications in insulin-dependent diabetes mellitus. N Engl J Med 320:977–986, 1993.

Dyck, P. J., W. L. Litchy, K. M. Kratz, et al. A plasma exchange versus immune globulin infusion trial in chronic inflammatory demyelinating polyneuropathy. Ann Neurol 36:838–845, 1994.

Dyck, P. J., P. K. Thomas, J. W. Griffin, et al (eds.). *Peripheral Neuropathy*, 3rd ed. Vols. 1 and 2. Philadelphia, W.B. Saunders Co., 1993.

Giannini, C., and P. J. Dyck. Ultrastructural morphometric abnormalities of sural nerve endoneurial microvessels in diabetes mellitus. Ann Neurol 36:408–415, 1994.

Lupski, J. R., P. F. Chance, and C. A. Garcia. Inherited primary peripheral neuropathies: Molecular genetics and clinical implications of CMT1A and HNPP. JAMA 270:2326–2330, 1993.

Mcleod, J. G., R. R. Tuck, J. D. Pollard, et al. Chronic polyneuropathy of undetermined cause. J Neurol Neurosurg Psychiatry 47:530–535, 1984.

Mendell, J. R. Chronic inflammatory demyelinating polyradiculoneuropathy. Annu Rev Med 44:211–219, 1993.

Nobile-Orazio, E., E. Manfredini, M. Carpo, et al. Frequency and clinical correlates of anti-neural IgM antibodies in neuropathy associated with IgM monoclonal gammopathy. Ann Neurol 36:416–424, 1994.

Thomas, P.K. (ed.). Neuromuscular disease: Nerve. Curr Opin Neurol 7:367–415, 1994.

CHAPTER TEN

AMYOTROPHIC LATERAL SCLEROSIS

AND THE MOTOR NEURON DISEASES

INTRODUCTION 118

CLINICAL PRESENTATION 118

PATHOLOGY 120

PATHOPHYSIOLOGY 123

EVALUATION AND DIFFERENTIAL DIAGNOSIS 123

DIAGNOSIS 123

TREATMENT 124

SUMMARY 125

INTRODUCTION

Amyotrophic lateral sclerosis (ALS) is a degenerative disease of motor neurons in the spinal cord, brain stem, and cerebral cortex of adults that causes progressive weakness and wasting, leading inexorably to death in 2–5 years in the majority of cases. The cause is unknown. Credit is given to Charcot (1869) for describing the clinical-pathological correlations of the illness, and in France the disease is known as Charcot's disease (Box 10–1). In England it is known as motor neuron disease, a term that is also used in the plural to indicate the wide variety of illnesses and conditions that can injure motor neurons (Table 10–1).

The criteria for making a diagnosis of ALS include the presence of both lower and upper motor neuron signs and symptoms (Table 10–2). Lower motor neuron signs include weakness, atrophy, fasciculations, and electromyographic evidence of denervation and reinnervation. Upper motor neuron signs include increased tone; hyperactive reflexes; glabellar, snout, or suck reflexes in the face; clonus; Babinski's sign; and Hoffmann's sign. Patients who have only lower motor neuron signs are more accurately classified as having **progressive muscular atrophy**. In this latter condition, when only spinal cord motor neurons are involved, the disease is called **progressive spinal muscular atrophy**. If only cranial nerve muscles are involved, it is known as **progressive bulbar palsy**.

Pure lower motor syndromes are less common than ALS in adults. In addition, many patients who present with pure lower motor findings at the time of their first examination develop upper motor neuron signs with the passage of time. Additionally, when these pure cases have been examined pathologically there is often evidence of more widespread disease in both upper and lower motor neuron systems than was appreciated clinically. Nevertheless, it is important to identify patients with progressive muscular atrophy clinically and follow them closely, since the long-term prognosis can be more favorable than for ALS (Figure 10–1).

CLINICAL PRESENTATION

ALS typically begins between the ages of 50 and 60 years, affecting men more than women in a ratio of

---

BOX 10-1 Lectures on the Diseases of the Nervous System

DELIVERED AT LA SALPETRIERE

J. M. Charcot
1881*

I shall try, gentlemen, to summarize, in a few lines, the symptomatological characters of *amyotrophic lateral sclerosis*, considered in what may be called its normal conditions.

1. Paresis, without anesthesia, of the upper extremities, accompanied by rapid emaciation of the muscular masses and often preceded by numbness and formication. Spasmodic rigidity seizes, at a given period, on the paralyzed and wasted muscles and determines permanent deformations by contracture.
2. The lower extremities are invaded in their turn. In the first instance, appears a paresis, without anesthesia which, promptly advancing, causes standing and walking to be, in a short time, impossible. To these symptoms is added a spasmodic rigidity which, at first intermittent, next becomes permanent and sometimes complicated with *tonic spinal epilepsy*. The muscles of the paralyzed limbs only become atrophied in the course of time, and never to the same extent as those of the upper extremities.

    The bladder and rectum are not affected; there is no tendency to the formation of bedsores.
3. A third period is constituted by the aggravation of the preceding symptoms and by the appearance of bulbar symptoms.

    These three phases follow each other, in a short space of time. Six months or a year after the invasion all the symptoms have accumulated, and become more or less strongly marked. Death supervenes at the end of two or three years, on an average, owing to the bulbar symptoms.

    Such is the rule; but the chapter of anomalies, it is well understood, is also in existence. These latter, however, are few in number and change nothing essential in the picture which I have just traced. Thus, the disease, in certain cases, begins by the lower extremities; again, it may be confined, at the beginning, either to one upper, or to one lower extremity; occasionally, it remains limited, for some time, to one side of the body, under a hemiplegic form. Finally, in two cases, it began by bulbar symptoms.

    The *prognosis*, up to the present, is of the gloomiest. There does not exist, so far as I am aware, a single example of a case where, the group of symptoms just described having existed, recovery followed. Is this doom final? The future alone shall decide.

    It remains for me now, gentlemen, to collate the lesions with the symptoms, and to seek, in a short essay of *pathological physiology*, the bond which unites them together.

1. The paresis which appears, at the beginning, and the permanent contractures which after a brief delay succeed it are, unquestionably, dependent on the symmetrical and lateral sclerosis.
2. The paresis and contracture precede the atrophy; that is clinically established. Hence, there is reason to admit that the lateral sclerosis, to which they are due, is produced before the lesion of the anterior grey substance with which the amyotrophy is unquestionably connected.

---

*J. M. Charcot. Lectures on the diseases of the nervous system. Lecture XIII, On amyotrophic lateral sclerosis. Symptomatology. Published under the auspices of the library of the New York Academy of Medicine by Hafner Publishing Co., New York, 1962, pp. 202–203.

TABLE 10-1. The Motor Neuron Diseases*

Genetic

Infantile spinal muscular atrophy, e.g., Werdnig-Hoffmann disease: autosomal recessive, 1 in 25,000 births, fatal in 2 years

Juvenile or chronic childhood spinal muscular atrophy, e.g., Kugelberg-Welander syndrome: autosomal recessive, chromosome 5, onset before 3 years of age, variable progression

X-linked spinal-bulbar muscular atrophy, Kennedy's syndrome: excess triplet repeats in the androgen receptor gene, adult onset, gynecomastia, testicular atrophy

Distal spinal muscular atrophy: dominant or recessive, predominately feet or hands, in different families, localized

Hereditary spastic paraplegia: dominant or recessive, early or late adult onset, progressive lower extremity spasticity with or without other signs

Familial ALS: 10% of all cases, 20% of which have defect in SOD gene on chromosome 21, indistinguishable from sporadic ALS (see text)

Acquired

Amyotrophic lateral sclerosis
Progressive spinal muscular atrophy
Progressive bulbar muscular atrophy
Monomelic or segmental amyotrophy
Poliomyelitis
Toxins (?): lead, mercury, aluminum
Paraneoplastic or immunologic (?): plasma cell dyscrasia, lymphomas

*There are more than 80 different descriptions of genetic forms of motor neuron disease. Molecular genetic studies in the future will help redefine many of these. This abbreviated list identifies the more comon conditions seen clinically.

approximately 2 to 1. Ten percent of cases begin before age 40 and another 10% after age 70. The disease is progressive from onset with approximately 50% survival at 3.5 years, 25% at 5 years, and <10% at 10 years. The pace of the illness must be determined in each case. It cannot be predicted at onset but usually is evident by 1–2 years. Considering the implications of a diagnosis of rapidly progressive degenerative disease without primary treatment, it is important to note the existence of even a few long-term survivors (Box 10–2).

Weakness commonly begins asymmetrically in an extremity. For example, a patient may note difficulty with small movements of the hand as in turning a key, or clumsiness of a leg while jogging. Muscle cramps in the leg are not uncommon. Occasionally a patient will report a feeling of numbness in the limb, but direct

TABLE 10-2. Diagnostic Criteria for ALS (World Congress of Neurology, 1990)

Definite ALS

Upper and lower motor neuron signs in bulbar and two spinal regions, or upper and lower motor signs in three spinal regions (classic/Charcot)

Probable ALS

Upper and lower motor neuron signs in two regions with upper motor neuron signs in a region rostral to lower motor neuron signs

Possible ALS

Upper and lower motor neuron signs in one region, or upper motor neuron signs in two regions

Suspected ALS

Lower motor neuron signs in two regions (progressive muscular atrophy)

sensory examination remains normal. Patients come to recognize the numbness as a sensation of weakness or heaviness rather than of insensitivity to touch. Some patients will also note muscle wasting, and others will remark upon muscle "twitchings," which are discovered clinically to be fasciculations—the spontaneous discharges of injured motor units. Inspection and testing the limb in the early stages will often reveal a normal muscle adjacent to a weak one, especially in an affected hand. Patients may comment that the weakness remains confined to one extremity, progressively involving adjacent muscles. Clinical testing and EMG will likely reveal more widespread evidence of disease, and in typical cases the illness will become symmetric over time.

ALS can begin with involvement of bulbar muscles with weakness, atrophy and fasciculations of the tongue, and difficulty in speaking or swallowing. The face can become flat. These findings can give the appearance of pure lower motor neuron involvement unless there are increased reflexes at the same site, such as a hyperactive jaw jerk, an increased gag reflex, or the presence of a suck or snout reflex. Some patients will have an increased tendency to laugh or to cry seemingly without provocation. This symptom is called "pseudobulbar palsy" to indicate upper motor neuron dysfunction. Extraocular movements are spared in almost all patients.

As described by Charcot (Box 10–1), ALS can remain in one limb or on one side of the body for a period of time as a hemiparesis. Additionally, it can cause lower motor neuron weakness in the hands and upper motor neuron weakness in the legs—a particular clinical picture that suggests local cervical cord compression. Rarely, the diaphragm and muscles of ventilation can be affected disproportionately near the onset, portending a grave prognosis. In all cases, there is preservation of sensation and autonomic nervous system function, factors that probably account for the relative lack of bedsores in these patients. Bladder and bowel sphincter function also remains normal.

The majority of patients maintain normal mental function to the end. However, detailed neuropsychological testing reveals evidence of impairment in immediate visuospatial memory, visual attention, and verbal fluency in some patients. These deficits may reflect abnormal frontal lobe function and correlate with a decrease in cerebral blood flow in the medial prefrontal cortex. PET studies show depressed functional activity in most frontal cortical areas which project into the corticospinal tract or which are connected to primary motor cortex (Figure 10–2). Pathological studies have found degenerating fiber pathways from motor cortex into these areas. These studies emphasize several points. First, it is often necessary to perform functional tests of a system—either motor or cognitive—in order to appreciate dysfunction. Second, functional deficits are manifestations not only of the local area of primary pathology but of the disruption of activity this causes through its extended circuits.

Anterior horn cells of the spinal cord also degenerate in a variety of other diseases, including parkinson-

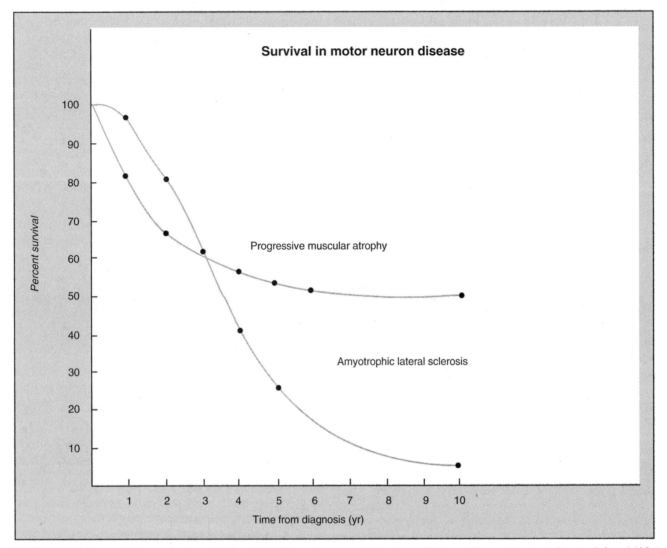

FIGURE 10-1. Patient survival from the time of diagnosis is different for pure anterior horn cell disease (progressive muscular atrophy) and ALS. This finding probably represents intrinsic differences in the pace of the two disease processes rather than a special lethal effect of the upper motor neuron lesion in ALS. (Data from D. W. Mulder and F. H. Howard, Jr. Patient resistance and prognosis in amyotrophic lateral sclerosis. Mayo Clin Proc 51:537–541, 1976, and from A. Chio, F. Brignolio, M. Leone, et al. A survival analysis of 155 cases of progressive muscular atrophy. Acta Neurol Scand 72:407–413, 1985.)

ism, Alzheimer's disease, Creutzfeldt-Jakob disease, Lewy body disease, and pure frontal lobe dementia. How to interpret these dementing illnesses with "amyotrophy" is unclear. They may represent an aggressive manifestation of a degenerative process that more commonly remains confined to one area or system or be a manifestation of a particular host mechanism, or even be an entirely separate disease. At present these cases are noted by specialists but are not well understood.

Familial ALS accounts for approximately 10% of the cases where autosomal dominant inheritance is evident. Molecular genetic studies have found that in 20% of these families there is an abnormality on chromosome 21 in the gene for the enzyme Cu,Zn superoxide dismutase (SOD1). This enzyme catalyzes the dismutation of the toxic superoxide anion $O_2^{\cdot}$ to O_2 and H_2O_2. To date, 11 missense mutations have been found in 13 different families with ALS. Studies of mutant enzymes indicate that they produce *more* H_2O_2 than

normal—a gain of function. It is believed that an increase in H_2O_2 could lead to cumulative cytotoxicity of cells over time and neural degeneration. Excess oxidative stress might underlie sporadic (90%) ALS cases as well. In familial ALS, the onset of the disease occurs 2–3 years earlier than in sporadic ALS and the sex ratio is equal between men and women.

PATHOLOGY

The principal pathological findings in ALS are degeneration and loss of motor neurons in the cortex, brain stem, and spinal cord. There is massive loss of large pyramidal Betz's cells in layer V of the precentral gyrus of the motor cortex with mild reactive gliosis. Marchi's stains of secondarily degenerating axons show involvement of corticocortical and transcallosal pathways from the motor cortex, as well as corticospinal projections through the internal capsule, pons, medulla,

BOX 10-2   Clinical Variability in Motor Neuron Disease: Lou Gehrig* and Stephen Hawking†

On June 1, 1925, 21-year-old Lou Gehrig started at first base for the New York Yankees. For the next 14 years he never missed a game—2130, a record for the most consecutive games played that was not broken until 1995. He was known as the "iron horse of baseball." He had a lifetime batting average of .340, hit 493 home runs, and won the most valuable player award for the American league four times. In 1938, his last complete season, he had an "off" year, hitting "only" 29 home runs and had "only" 107 runs batted in. In spring training of 1939, he did not exhibit much power at the plate, and his movements at first base lacked their usual smoothness. After eight games of the 1939 season, he asked his manager to be benched. He never played baseball again. Six weeks later he visited the Mayo Clinic where the diagnosis of ALS was obvious. The public was told that he had a chronic form of poliomyelitis and would not be able to play baseball. He was a shy and introverted man and never discussed his diagnosis. Over the next 2 years, there was progressive weakness of the limbs with eventual difficulty in swallowing and ventilation. He died on June 2, 1941, at age 38. When the nature of his illness became known, the lay public adopted the name "Lou Gehrig disease" for ALS.

Stephen Hawking developed weakness and clumsiness in 1962, in his third year at Oxford, and underwent diagnostic testing one year later while at Cambridge at age 21. He was told he had an incurable disease that could be fatal in a few years.

My dreams at that time were rather disturbed. Before my condition was diagnosed, I had been very bored with life. There had not seemed to be anything worth doing. But shortly after coming out of hospital, I dreamt that I was going to be executed. I suddenly realized that there were a lot of worthwhile things I could do if I were reprieved. Another dream that I had several times was that I would sacrifice my life to save others. After all, if I was going to die anyway it might as well do some good.

But I didn't die. In fact, although there was a cloud hanging over my future, I found to my surprise I was enjoying life in the present more than I had before. I began to make progress with my research, I got engaged and married, and I got a research fellowship at Caius College, Cambridge.

Stephen Hawking's motor neuron disease progressed more slowly than typical of ALS, probably indicating progressive muscular atrophy, or pure lower motor neuron disease. In writing of his illness, he chronicles the progressive steps that occurred over many years' time, including moving into an electric wheelchair, having a tracheostomy, requiring full-time nurses, and adapting to a speech synthesizer for communication. He and his wife had three children and his professional career in theoretical physics expanded successfully despite progressive weakness. Today he holds Isaac Newton's chair as the Lucasian Professor of Mathematics at Cambridge University. He is renowned for his work on the quantum mechanics of black holes and theories on the origin and fate of the universe. His popular book, *A Brief History of Time*, has sold more than 5.5 million copies.

*Morton Nathanson. *Classics in Neurology*. Lou Gehrig: A brief commentary. Neurology 36:1349, 1986.
†Stephen Hawking. My Experience with ALS. In *Black Holes and Baby Universes, and Other Essays*. New York, Bantam Books, 1993.

and spinal cord. Degenerating corticifugal fibers can also be traced into terminal fields in the basal ganglia, thalamus, midbrain, and pons where mild gliosis can be recognized. In the medulla, neuronal loss is most readily demonstrated in the hypoglossal nuclei, dorsal

motor nucleus of the vagus, and nucleus ambiguus. Lesser degrees of degeneration can also be found in cranial nerve nuclei of V, VII, and rarely III.

In typical cases, the spinal cord shows severe degeneration and loss of anterior horn cells at all levels

FIGURE 10-2. A decrease in regional functional activity in the cortex of patients with ALS has been found by studying blood flow changes with positron emission tomography (PET). The highlighted areas were significantly ($p < 0.05$) depressed compared with controls. These areas receive projections from primary motor cortex where there is loss of pyramidal neurons, and they also send projections into the corticospinal tract. Abnormal activity here may correlate with abnormal upper motor neuron function and subtle abnormalities of cognitive function as well. The areas include lateral premotor cortex (LP), the sensorimotor cortex (SMC), the superior parietal lobule (SPL), the inferior parietal lobule (IPL), the medial parietal cortex and paracentral lobule (MP), the supplemental motor area (SMA), and the anterior insula (INS). (Reproduced, with permission of Oxford University Press, from J. J. M. Kew, P. N. Leigh, E. D. Playford, et al. Cortical function in amyotrophic lateral sclerosis: A positron emission tomography study. Brain 116:655–680, 1993.)

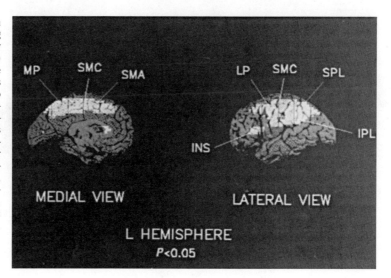

(Figure 10–3C). There is degeneration of the corticospinal tract, both the lateral and anterior segments, seen as pallor with a myelin stain (Weigert's) or as a positive reaction with a stain for myelin breakdown products (Marchi's; Figures 10–3A and B). The myelin breakdown is secondary to the death of the parent neurons and axonal degeneration. Degeneration is found in the dorsal columns in 10% of sporadic cases of ALS but in up to 80% of familial cases. The ventral roots exiting the cord show severe loss of large myelinated fibers but relative sparing of smaller myelinated and thinly myelinated fibers, indicating the selective destruction of alpha motor neurons and preservation of gamma motor neurons and sympathetic fibers. Neuromuscular junctions are abnormal. Many show a decrease in or absence of nerve terminals thought to reflect degeneration of one motor neuron with sprouting and reinnervation from another. Electrophysiological analysis of neuromuscular transmission reveals a decrease in quantal release from these nerve terminals. Muscle biopsies typically reveal neurogenic group fiber atrophy, with abnormal muscle fibers surrounded by healthy ones (Figure 10–3D).

Studies of anterior horn cells have been hampered owing to the advanced stage of patients coming to autopsy. Often there are too few neurons left to study. In short, rapid cases, it has been possible to conclude that the degenerative process is not accompanied by retrograde chromatolysis, inflammation, or neuronophagia. Neurons become pale, atrophic, and shrunken and disappear. Many show a small cytoplasmic eosinophilic body called a Bunina body whose chemistry is unknown. Viral particles have not been identified. Some neurons show accumulations of neurofilaments—structures called spheroids—in the proximal portion of axons. Interestingly, these are a prominent part of the neuropathology of hereditary canine spinal muscular atrophy of Brittany spaniels. Spheroids are not unique to motor neuron disease pathology, however. Immunohistochemical studies in ALS have found an increase in ubiquitin immunoreactivity in anterior horn

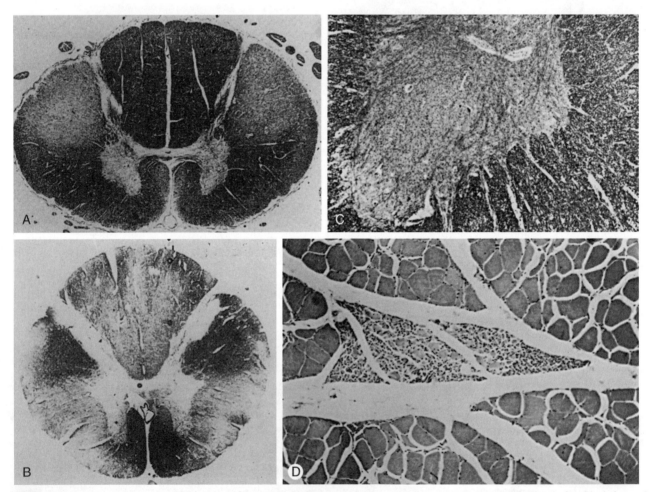

FIGURE 10–3. The neuropathology of ALS is characterized by loss of motor neurons in the cortex, brain stem, and spinal cord. A, Loss of corticospinal neurons in the cortex results in degeneration of the crossed lateral corticospinal tract and the uncrossed ipsilateral ventral spinal tract seen here as pallor with a Weigert myelin stain, or (B) as a positive reaction product using the Marchi preparation for myelin debris. C, This ventral horn of the lumbar spinal cord is almost totally devoid of motor neurons (Luxol fast blue/cresyl violet, ×40). (A, B, and C are reproduced, with permission, from B. Brownell, D. R. Oppenheimer, and J. Trevor Hughes. The central nervous system in motor neuron disease. J Neurol Neurosurg Psychiatry 33:338–357, 1970.) D, Muscle biopsies can reveal muscle fibers of a motor unit undergoing atrophy while neighboring units remain healthy. (Reproduced, with permission, from J. T. Hughes. Pathology of amyotrophic lateral sclerosis. In L. P. Rowland [ed.]. Human motor neuron diseases. Adv Neurol 36:72, 1982.)

cells and some cortical cells. Ubiquitin is a protein that participates in ATP-dependent, lysosome-independent proteolysis of cellular proteins. An increase in ubiquitin-labeled proteins also occurs in other degenerative disease such as the Lewy bodies of Parkinson's disease. The chemical nature of the ubiquinated protein in ALS cells is unknown.

PATHOPHYSIOLOGY

Intense investigation has focused on neurotropic viruses as a possible cause of ALS, especially because of the affinity of the poliovirus for anterior horn cells. Nevertheless, epidemiological data, serological analysis, and the direct study of pathological tissue with electron microscopy and molecular biological techniques have failed to provide convincing evidence of a viral etiology. Toxins remain of interest as an explanation for clusters of the disease in the Mariana islands (Guam), the Kii peninsula of Japan, and southwest New Guinea. Unproved hypotheses have focused on heavy metals (lead, mercury, aluminum), nutritional deficiencies (calcium and magnesium deficiency coupled with excess aluminum), and potential excitotoxins found in sources of food, e.g., β-N-methylamino-L-alanine (BMAA) in the cycad plant eaten by the Chamorro Indians in Guam. Interestingly, as these areas become more developed, the incidence of cases in younger people has decreased. Finally, some investigators propose an immunological hypothesis, pointing to a high prevalence of paraproteins, antibodies to membrane gangliosides, and antibodies to L-type calcium channels in patients. However, no benefit has been derived from immunosuppressive therapy.

Considerable attention is now focused on the biochemical pathophysiology of neuronal death. One study has reported an abnormally low level of glutamate transport in the spinal cord and motor cortex of patients with ALS. It is proposed that accumulation of extracellular glutamate could lead to excitotoxicity of motor neurons. Studies of familial ALS have drawn attention to biochemical pathways important in detoxifying internally generated oxygen radicals. At present it is unclear why motor neurons alone are so susceptible to this type of damage, although the Betz cells of the cortex and the anterior horn cells of the spinal cord are some of the longest cells in the body. Of note, an inherited deficiency in hexosaminidase A can cause damage to anterior horn cells. Hexosaminidase A is a housekeeping enzyme similar to Cu,Zn superoxide dismutase (see above). Spinal muscular atrophy is one of the phenotypic expressions of hexosaminidase A deficiency. In this rare autosomal recessive disease, there is a deficiency in the metabolism of GM_2 gangliosides, which accumulate in alpha motor neurons and other cells.

EVALUATION AND DIFFERENTIAL DIAGNOSIS

There are no specific tests for ALS. Muscle enzymes (e.g., creatine phosphokinase [CPK]) can be modestly elevated in serum as a nonspecific reflection of muscle breakdown. CSF is normal. It is important to perform MRI of the brain to rule out cranial nerve lesions in cases of isolated bulbar palsy, and MRI of the cervical spine to rule out spondylosis, syrinx, or tumor when the findings could be explained by disease localized to the cervical cord. Spastic paraplegia beginning insidiously in the mid-30's should prompt a careful family history for evidence of familial spastic paraplegia for which there is evidence for linkage on chromosomes 2 and 14. In pure cases of lower motor neuron syndrome, testing for antiganglioside antibody in the serum is important to rule out immune-mediated motor neuropathy (Chapter 9).

Clinical neurophysiological testing is important to characterize the nature of weakness; localize it to the anterior horn cell, nerve, neuromuscular junction, or muscle; and determine the pattern of distribution in the rest of the body. In ALS there are fibrillations and fasciculations on electromyographic testing of muscles, indicating neuronal degeneration and irritability of the anterior horn cells. There is a decrease in the interference pattern—the number of muscle action potentials activated during maximal voluntary effort. However, individual muscle action potentials become larger, longer, and more complex in configuration as a sign of reinnervation (Figure 10–4). Single-fiber EMG will reveal an increase in fiber density as a reflection of an increase in the number of individual single fibers innervated by the same motor neuron recorded within the radius of the microelectrode. This is a characteristic finding in ALS. Nerve conduction studies remain normal in ALS.

DIAGNOSIS

Diagnosis must be approached with great care, since there is no curative treatment for ALS and the prognosis includes increasing disability and death within a few years in the majority of cases. MRI and electrophysiological testing supplement clinical skills in defining both upper and lower motor neuron disease. When these are present and no other process is evident, the diagnosis is secure.

In dealing with individual patients, it is best to delay a final diagnosis until all tests have been completed and other possibilities excluded. The area of greatest clinical difficulty arises in cases in which lower motor neuron signs and symptoms dominate the picture and the evidence for upper motor neuron dysfunction is less obvious. Since a pure lower motor neuron disease will diminish reflexes, some clinicians feel that the presence of strong or increased reflexes in a limb where there is weakness and atrophy is sufficient evidence for both upper and lower motor neuron dysfunction. If there is absence of sensory loss and there are motor signs in other limbs or the bulbar muscles, the diagnosis would be secure for most clinicians. The presence of increased muscle tone, especially in the lower extremities, can also be an important finding. This is a matter of clinical judgment rather than of absolute certainty. Other clinicians require the presence of abnormal upper motor neuron signs such as clonus, Babinski's or

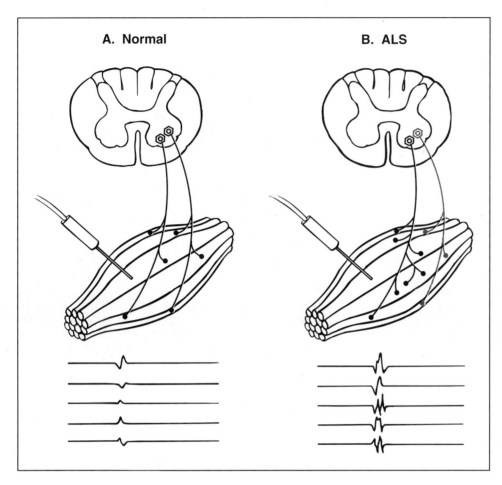

A. Normal

B. ALS

FIGURE 10–4. Electromyographic signs of reinnervation in ALS. Degeneration of one nerve and reinnervation of neuromuscular junctions by an adjacent nerve are characteristic in ALS. The degenerative process eventually overcomes any effect of reinnervation, and weakness develops. When reinnervation occurs, a nerve will excite more muscle fibers than normal over a greater distance, causing the muscle action potential to be larger, longer, and more complex than normal, as illustrated by the stylized single-fiber EMG recordings.

Hoffmann's sign, snout or suck reflexes, or loss of superficial abdominal reflexes to conclude that there is upper motor neuron dysfunction. Strict diagnostic criteria are used when patients are entered into clinical trials (Table 10–2).

For most patients, neuroimaging of the brain and spinal cord is required to rule out compressive or intrinsic lesions. Nerve conduction studies of motor nerves are important for excluding immune-mediated demyelinating motor neuropathies (Chapter 9). Tests for thyroid function should be performed, since hyperthyroidism can cause weakness and fasciculations. A condition called "benign fasciculations" can cause alarm because of the similarity of the muscle twitching to ALS. In this condition, there is no atrophy or weakness.

TREATMENT

Although ALS is incurable, an effective treatment plan will maximize the quality of the remainder of life. Management involves physical, occupational, nutritional, speech, and respiratory therapy. A frank but sensitive discussion of morbidity and mortality with the patient and appropriate family members is an important first step when the diagnosis is secure. On the one hand, it is important to analyze individual disease progression and its implications. On the other hand, it is important not to remove all possible hope. Because time is short, patients should be encouraged not to postpone activities that would bring pleasure while they can enjoy them, such as exercise, travel, and vacations. Physical and occupational therapy are important from the start to maximize mobility and strength, identify treatable disabilities, provide orthotic devices (e.g., footdrop braces, wrist splints), and develop a plan to respond to changing needs (e.g., cane, walker, wheelchair). Attention to nutrition is important for all patients, aiming at 1500–2000 calories per day. When bulbar symptoms impair swallowing, nasogastric feeding or a percutaneous feeding gastrostomy should be considered. Most patients prefer the latter, since it avoids irritation of the nose and pharynx and is more acceptable cosmetically. Some relief is available for respiratory fatigue. Providing intermittent positive pressure ventilatory assistance at night for patients with bulbar or respiratory weakness can bring great comfort and is easy to manage. When patients eventually develop increasing respiratory failure, the physician should discuss the possible use of permanent home ventilation, its benefits, efficacy, costs, and burdens to the family.

Several medications are helpful in the treatment of common symptoms. Baclofen or diazepam is useful for severe spasticity. Quinine is helpful for treating muscle cramps. Pain related to immobility is best treated with passive movement exercises. Narcotic analgesics are helpful with advancing paralysis. Patients who have difficulty swallowing will often derive benefit from medicines that dry secretions. Amitriptyline, propantheline, or transdermal scopolamine can be helpful in this regard.

Treatment with growth factors is in clinical trials (Box 10–3). Both ciliary neurotrophic factor (CNTF) and brain-derived growth factor (BDNF) have been found to prevent the death of anterior horn cells in experimental animals. Insulin-like growth factor (IGF-1) is under consideration for trial. Riluzole, an agent that blocks glutamate neurotransmission, modestly prolongs survival in patients. Determination of the best factor or combination of factors represents an important new line of therapeutic investigation. As further basic research reveals fundamental mechanisms of neuronal death, possible new strategies for intervention may be revealed.

SUMMARY

Amyotrophic lateral sclerosis is the most common form of motor neuron disease in adults causing both

---

BOX 10-3 Experimental Models of Motor Neuron Disease

Animal models of neurological disease are important tools for developing and testing new therapies. In the last 10 years, animal models and potential new therapies for motor neuron disease have developed side by side. The history of this field dates to the discovery and purification of nerve growth factor (NGF) by Victor Hamburger, Rita Levi-Montalcini, and Stanley Cohen at Washington University, for which the latter two won the Nobel prize in 1986. NGF is a peptide made in the skin, blood vessels, and sympathetically innervated glands. During development, it is retrogradely transported to cell bodies upon innervation where it is responsible for keeping sympathetic neurons alive. The sympathetic nervous system does not develop in an embryo given antibodies to NGF. A family of growth factor peptides and their receptors have been identified and cloned; there is both specificity and some overlap in their functions.

Factor	kd	Tissue Source	Receptor	Tissue Target
NGF	13	Skin, vessels, glands, hippocampus, cortex	trkA	Sympathetic and sensory (pain) cells, cholinergic basal forebrain cells
BDNF	13.5	Hippocampus, cerebellum, muscle, skin, other	trkB	Motor neurons, cholinergic basal forebrain cells
NT-3	13.6	Hippocampus, cerebellum, muscle, periphery	trkC	Nodose and sympathetic ganglia, proprioceptive neurons
NT-4/5	14	CNS and periphery	trkA/trkB	Motor neurons, ganglia
CNTF	22	Schwann cells, astrocytes	CNTF Receptor a	Diffuse: motor, sensory, sympathetic, and central neurons
GDNF	40	Glia	?	Dopaminergic cells, motor neurons

In testing these peptides for biological activity, it was soon discovered that ciliary neurotrophic factor (CNTF) and brain-derived growth factor (BDNF) were potent in protecting motor neurons from programmed cell death as well as from injury. Both sustain motor neurons grown in culture, and both prevent retrograde degeneration of axotomized motor neurons in the facial nucleus of the neonatal rat. CNTF promotes nerve terminal sprouting in adult mice and prevents degeneration of motor neurons in the pmn/pmn mouse model of progressive motor neuronopathy. Disruption of the CNTF gene causes progressive motor neuron degeneration. BDNF is retrogradely transported from muscle to motor neurons, whereas CNTF is not. Applied to the cut end of the sciatic nerve, BDNF prevents retrograde death of motor neurons. In contrast to CNTF experiments, however, knockout experiments of either the BDNF gene or the trkB receptor gene in mice failed to cause any abnormality of motor neurons. Used together, CNTF and BDNF have a synergistic effect on neurons in culture and an enhanced protective effect on the survival of motor neurons in the *wobbler* mouse—a genetic model of spinal muscular atrophy.

Despite these optimistic experiments in animals, the use of these agents to treat human ALS faces several obstacles. First, there is no evidence that ALS is a disease of neurotrophic factor deficiency. Thus, any benefit will likely be symptomatic rather than to reduce the primary disease process. Second, the success in animal studies occurred largely during developmental periods of growth, less so in adults. Third, the half-life of systemically administered peptides is often only a few minutes, and although they will have access to the lower motor neurons, they will not likely reach upper motor neurons. Finally, preliminary results from clinical trials with CNTF have revealed side effects of a flu-like syndrome impairing functional performance of patients. Despite these obstacles, the neurotrophins are potent compounds and further tests searching for clinical efficacy are proceeding.

The identification of the gene responsible for one form of familial ALS has allowed development of additional animal models. To date, 11 unique mutations in the gene for Cu,Zn superoxide dismutase have been found in patients with inherited ALS (see text). Transgenic mice have been prepared using clones of some of these abnormal genes. One of these with a glycine-to-alanine substitution at position 93 was found to overproduce the abnormal enzyme in brain and cause degeneration of anterior horn cells. This remarkable experiment reveals the potency of molecular techniques. Within 3 years of localization, the abnormal gene has been characterized and introduced into animals for the exploration of new therapies.

upper and lower motor neuron degeneration. Patients characteristically develop fatigue, weakness, wasting, fasciculations, and cramps, without sensory loss or major changes in cognition. Combined clinical and laboratory tests are available to make the diagnosis over a short period of time. A small number of patients have pure progressive muscular atrophy as a manifestation of motor neuron disease. Although the cause of sporadic ALS is unknown, new information from genetic cases has revealed abnormalities in the metabolism of oxygen radicals. This finding is providing new directions in research and potential therapies. The study of experimental animals with motor neuron degeneration has revealed the potency of growth factor therapy, and clinical trials in humans are in progress. Continuous care of a patient and support of the family are important to maximize quality of life.

Selected Readings

Barinaga, M. Neurotrophic factors enter the clinic. Science 264:772–774, 1994.

Bensimon, G., L. Lacomblez, and V. Meininger. A controlled trial of riluzole in amyotrophic lateral sclerosis. N Engl J Med 330: 585–591, 1994.

Brownell, B., D. R. Oppenheimer, and J. Trevor Hughes. The central nervous system in motor neuron disease. J Neurol Neurosurg Psychiatry 33:338–357, 1970.

Clatterbuck, R. E., D. L. Price, and V. E. Koliatsos. Ciliary neurotrophic factor prevents retrograde neuronal death in the adult central nervous system. Proc Natl Acad Sci USA 90:2222–2226, 1993.

Gurney, M. E., H. Pu, A. Y. Chiu, et al. Motor neuron degeneration in mice that express a human Cu,Zn superoxide dismutase mutation. Science 264:1772–1775, 1994.

Kew, J. J. M., P. N. Leigh, E. D. Playford, et al. Cortical function in amyotrophic lateral sclerosis: A positron emission tomography study. Brain 116:655–680, 1993.

Koliatsos, V. E., R. E. Clatterbuck, J. W. Winslow, et al. Evidence that brain-derived neurotrophic factor is a trophic factor for motor neurons in vivo. Neuron 10:359–367, 1993.

Leigh, P. N., H. Whitwell, O. Garofalo, et al. Ubiquitin-immunoreactivity in intraneuronal inclusions in amyotrophic lateral sclerosis. Brain 114:775–788, 1991.

Rosen, D. R., T. Siddique, D. Patterson, et al. Mutations in Cu/Zn superoxide dismutase gene are associated with familial amyotrophic lateral sclerosis. Nature 362:59–62, 1993.

Rothstein, J. D., L. J. Martin, and R. W. Kuncl. Decreased glutamate transport by the brain and spinal cord in amyotrophic lateral sclerosis. N Engl J Med 326:1464–1468, 1992.

Smith, M. C. Nerve fiber degeneration in the brain in amyotrophic lateral sclerosis. J Neurol Neurosurg Psychiatry 23:269–282, 1960.

Stalberg, E. Electrophysiological studies of reinnervation in ALS. In L. P. Rowland (ed.). Human motor neuron diseases. Adv Neurol 36:47–59, 1982.

CHAPTER ELEVEN

PARKINSON'S DISEASE

AND THE

MULTIPLE SYSTEM ATROPHIES

PARKINSON'S DISEASE 128

   Introduction 128

   Clinical Presentation 128

   Pathology 130

   Pathophysiology 131

   Evaluation and Differential Diagnosis 131

MULTIPLE SYSTEM ATROPHIES 134

PROGRESSIVE SUPRANUCLEAR PALSY 135

   Treatment 135

SUMMARY 137

PARKINSON'S DISEASE
Introduction

Parkinson's disease is characterized by symptoms of bradykinesia, rigidity, and resting tremor that begin between ages 40 and 70 years and progress over a 10- to 20-year time course. Men and women are affected equally. First described by James Parkinson in 1817 (Box 11–1), this degenerative disease is commonly diagnosed among the elderly today. The overall incidence is 20 new cases per 100,000 population per year. The overall prevalence is 200/100,000 population but may be up to five times that level among people over age 70. Genetic, viral, and toxic causes have been implicated in small subsets of patients, but the cause of idiopathic Parkinson's disease is unknown.

Clinical Presentation

Tremor is often the symptom that brings a patient to a physician. At a first visit, a clinician will likely also observe slowness or absence of automatic movements (e.g., a decrease in facial expressions, hand gestures, arm swing) and will find increased tone in one or more extremities upon examination. The tremor of Parkinson's disease is unique. It occurs when the limb is at rest or suspended but largely disappears during intentional movements. It usually begins in one hand as a "pill rolling" motion of the thumb moving across the fingers, or as a to-and-fro movement at the wrist. Less commonly a patient will first notice a jiggling of the foot. The frequency of the tremor is 4–6 Hz. It disappears during sleep, and it can be willfully suppressed for a few moments during the early stages of the disease. The tremor is aggravated by tension and stress. With disease progression, the tremor usually appears next in the foot on the same side or in the other hand.

The cause of the tremor is thought to be a consequence of abnormal patterns of neuronal activity within basal ganglia and thalamic circuits set in motion by a deficiency of dopamine (Figure 11–1). Depth electrode recordings in patients with parkinsonian tremor show periodic bursts of neurons in the ventrolateral thalamus time-locked to the agonist-antagonist movement across a joint. Stereotaxic lesions placed here abolish the tremor and alleviate rigidity but have little effect on bradykinesia.

Slowing of movement in Parkinson's disease correlates with the loss of striatal dopamine levels. There is difficulty starting movements **(akinesia),** particularly getting out of a chair or walking, a decrease in the amplitude of movement **(hypokinesia),** and slowness of movement **(bradykinesia).** Bradykinesia and rigidity usually occur together. Both symptoms respond well to treatment with levodopa medications (see below). By contrast, not all patients develop tremor, a symptom that does not respond well to levodopa replacement therapy.

The presence of rigidity is determined by testing muscle tone. When passively moving a limb in flexion and extension across a joint, the examiner will feel an increase in resistance in both directions, called "lead pipe" rigidity. In addition, cogwheeling is characteristic

---

BOX 11–1   An Essay on the Shaking Palsy

James Parkinson (1755–1828), a practitioner of medicine, surgery, and apothecary, lived outside London in Shoreditch. He was also a humanitarian who wrote a treatise against cruel treatment of the insane and a reformer who authored pamphlets sympathetic to the social revolution in France. He founded the Geological Society and was a scholar of paleontology, having written a three-volume work, *Organic Remains of a Former World (1804–1811)*, that ran to three editions. He was 62 when he wrote his famous description of six patients with "paralysis agitans." His essay went almost unnoticed until Charcot referred to it 50 years later, and in 1912 an American resurrected the work in a publication in the Bulletin of the Johns Hopkins Hospital (23:33–45, 1912).

AN ESSAY ON THE SHAKING PALSY*

James Parkinson
London
1817

SHAKING PALSY. (Paralysis agitans.) Involuntary tremulous motion, with lessened muscular power, in parts not in action and even when supported: with a propensity to bend the trunk forward, and to pass from a walking to a running pace: the senses and intellect being uninjured.

So slight and nearly imperceptible are the inroads of this malady, and so extremely slow its progress....that the patient cannot recall the onset. The first symptoms perceived are, a slight sense of weakness with a proneness to trembling....most commonly in one of the hands or arms....in less than twelve months or more, the morbid influence is felt in some other part. After a few more months the patient is found to be less strict than usual in preserving an upright posture.

....As the disease proceeds...the hand fails to answer the dictates of the will. Walking becomes a task which cannot be performed without considerable attention....care is necessary to prevent frequent falls....The disease proceeds, difficulties increase: writing can now be hardly at all accomplished; and reading, from the tremulous motion, is accomplished with some difficulty. [Later] the propensity to lean forward becomes invincible, and the patient is forced to step on the toes and fore part of the feet....irresistibly impelled to take much quicker and shorter steps, and thereby to adopt unwillingly a running pace.

[Finally] his words are now scarcely intelligible....no longer able to feed himself...saliva is continually draining from the mouth, mixed with particles of food he is no longer able to clear from inside of the mouth.

*Reproduced, with permission, from J.M.S. Pearce. Aspects of the history of Parkinson's disease. J Neurol Neurosurg Psychiatry (Special Supplement) pp. 7–8, 1989.

---

of the resistance, a feature unique to Parkinson's disease. In the early phases of the illness, the rigidity may be subtle. Having a patient clench one fist accentuates cogwheel rigidity in the other arm, confirming the earlier finding. By contrast, in normal aging muscle tone increases symmetrically in all extremities and does not

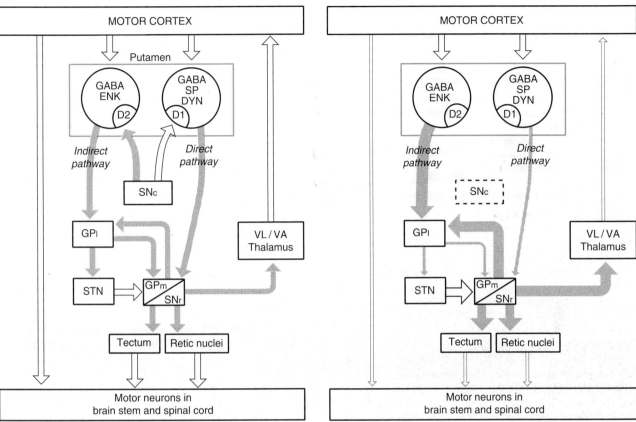

A. Normal

B. Parkinson's disease

FIGURE 11-1. This model of basal ganglia circuitry proposed by DeLong and others serves to provide testable hypotheses for understanding disease mechanisms and potential pharmacological and surgical treatments (see also Figures 3–5 and 12–3). Excitatory projections are shown by open arrows, gabaergic inhibitory pathways by solid arrows. Changes in the width of the arrows in Parkinson's disease indicate changes in activity. The dopaminergic projections from the substantia nigra, pars compacta (SNc), have their main effects on neurons in the putamen. First, dopamine is thought to *excite* a direct pathway to GPm/SNr by its action at D1 receptors on GABA/substance P/dynorphin–containing projection neurons. Increasing activity in this pathway ultimately accentuates movement. In Parkinson's disease, there would be a decrease in activity in the output from the putamen in this direct pathway. The result would be to increase inhibition on the thalamus and decrease movement. Second, dopamine is also thought to *inhibit* GABA/enkephalin–containing putamenal neurons that project to GPl by its action at D2 receptors. In Parkinson's disease, the loss of dopamine inhibition at the outset of this indirect pathway essentially disinhibits this internal loop. The result is to greatly accentuate the inhibitory activity of GPm/SNr on the thalamus. Thus, the net effect of loss of dopamine in the putamen on both pathways is to increase inhibition of thalamic projections back on the cortex. There would also be inhibition of tectospinal and reticulospinal pathways. As the cortical and brain stem motor pathways become inhibited, bradykinesia and rigidity develop. DYN, dynorphin; ENK, enkephalin; GABA, γ-aminobutyric acid; GPl, lateral globus pallidus; GPm, medial globus pallidus; SNc, substantia nigra, pars compacta; SNr, substantia nigra, pars reticularis; SP, substance P; STN, subthalamic nucleus; VL/VA, ventrolateral and ventroanterior nuclei.

have a cogwheel character. Demented patients will intermittently resist an examiner's testing of muscle tone, a paratonia called gegenhalten. This behavior is rarely confused with parkinsonian rigidity.

The combination of rigidity and bradykinesia makes complex integrative or repetitive movements particularly difficult. For example, patients will notice a change in their handwriting, in which a sentence will start off with well-formed characters that progressively deteriorate into smaller and smaller script (micrographia). Such actions as buttoning clothes, playing the piano, or opening a lock become difficult. During the examination, a patient will do poorly making repetitive rhythmic movements such as tapping a finger, hand, or foot, and with repetitive supination-pronation movements of the arms. Finding such abnormalities helps establish the diagnosis.

There are changes in facial expression and the

voice. Automatic movements are diminished or lost such that a patient gives the false appearance of sadness ("masked" face). There is a decreased frequency of blinking ("reptilian" stare). Examination of slow pursuit eye movements reveals a jerky quality comparable to cogwheeling in a limb. The voice softens, lacks emotional inflection, and demonstrates poor articulation. As the disease advances, there is difficulty initiating speech and a monotonic, mumbling dysarthria develops.

An abnormal stooped posture comes on gradually with flexion of the neck, trunk, and arms (simian posture). Since the illness usually begins on one side (hemiparkinsonism), it commonly takes 5 or more years before body posture is affected. Postural reflexes also become impaired, with an increased likelihood of falling. The gait becomes slow and short-stepped, and the patient has particular difficulty in turning and climbing steps. Festination may also occur, in which the patient takes faster and faster short steps and has difficulty stopping.

Dementia occurs in up to 40% of patients. The exact prevalence depends on the criteria used at different medical centers. In contrast to Alzheimer's disease, abnormalities of cortical function such as memory impairment, apraxia, agnosia, and aphasia are uncommon. Features of "subcortical" or "frontal" dementia are more prominent. Patients have slowed thought processes **(bradyphrenia)** and exhibit difficulty changing mental sets. There is difficulty with memory recall but not with encoding, such that patients improve their test scores with cueing. There is difficulty with visuospatial functions, such as recognizing rotated objects after a delay in presentation.

Depression occurs more often in patients with Parkinson's disease than in the general population. The diagnosis can be difficult, since a lack of facial expression and movement occurs in both conditions. Apathy, feelings of worthlessness, hopelessness, helplessness, and dysphoria distinguish the depression of Parkinson's disease. Neuronal loss in catecholamine brain stem nuclei projecting to frontal and limbic areas may underlie susceptibility to depression. Treatment with tricyclic antidepressants or specific serotonin reuptake inhibitors (SSRIs) that enhance the synaptic efficacy of catecholamines improves mood and behavior.

Changes in autonomic function are not uncommon in Parkinson's disease, probably reflecting pathological changes found in the intermediolateral cell column of the spinal cord and autonomic ganglia. Bowel problems are frequent, and most patients require treatment for constipation. In the late stages of the illness, bladder dysfunction is manifested as daytime urgency (detrusor hyperactivity) and nocturia. Orthostatic hypotension occurs in a minority of patients but is not as severe as in the Shy-Drager syndrome (see below).

Despite progressive change in motor, mental, and autonomic functions in most patients over time, other neurological systems remain uninvolved in idiopathic Parkinson's disease. Thus, there are no changes in cranial nerves, vision, sensation, or strength. The latter sometimes surprises physicians considering Parkinson's original description of shaking palsy or paralysis agitans. Whereas patients' movements are slowed and dexterity is lost, performance on tests of muscle strength remains normal. Reflexes are also preserved, and only a minority develop Babinski's sign, a finding that adds nothing *per se* to the clinical picture.

Pathology

Pathologically Parkinson's disease is defined by a loss of pigmented neurons in the substantia nigra, locus caeruleus, and dorsal motor nucleus of the vagus. With normal aging, there is a 50% loss of neurons in the substantia nigra by 70 years; symptoms of Parkinson's disease begin when there is an approximately 70% reduction (Figure 11–2). With cell loss, there is disappear-

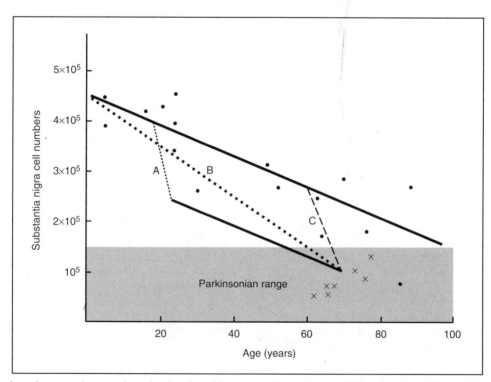

FIGURE 11–2. Number of neurons in one substantia nigra from 16 normals of increasing age (filled circles) and fitted with a linear regression line. The shaded area represents the threshold for parkinsonian symptoms. The line suggests that symptoms would be reached in normals by age 100. Seven patients are shown by crosses. Line A represents a precipitous loss by a toxin or virus followed by age-related changes. Line B suggests accelerated loss from a genetic cause. Line C represents late-life degenerative disease. (Reproduced, with permission, from P. L. McGeer, S. Itagaki, H. Akiyama, and E. G. McGeer. Comparison of neuronal loss in Parkinson's disease and aging. *In* D. B. Calne, D. Grippa, G. Comi, et al [eds.]. Parkinsonism and aging. Aging 36:25–34, 1989.)

ance of neuromelanin from the substantia nigra, an aspect of the disease that can be seen upon cutting a fresh brain at autopsy (Figure 11–3). Under microscopic examination, many remaining neurons show characteristic eosinophilic cytoplasmic inclusions called **Lewy bodies**. These granules are 3–5 μm in diameter and consist of a dense core surrounded by a halo. Under the electron microscope, they are seen to consist of aggregations of fibrils. These fibrils stain positively with antibodies to neurofilaments, tubulin, MAP 1 and 2 proteins, complement proteins, and ubiquitin, a protein involved in the nonlysosomal metabolism of cellular proteins. The degenerative process is believed to start in the ventrolateral nigra with loss of projections to the dorsolateral putamen. The destructive process is thought to begin at least 5 years prior to symptoms and continues steadily despite symptomatic treatment. With loss of nigral neurons, there is progressive loss of dopamine, the neurotransmitter for the nigrostriatal pathway, at projection sites within the putamen and other terminal fields in the ventral striatum, hypothalamus, and frontal lobe. Striatal dopamine is 80% depleted at the onset of symptoms.

Pathophysiology

the major signs and symptoms of Parkinson's disease are a consequence of the degeneration of dopaminergic neurons in the substantia nigra and their projections into the striatum. This degeneration results in an abnormal amount and pattern of neuronal firing through basal ganglia and thalamic circuits that project back to and influence premotor, supplementary motor, and primary motor cortex (see Figure 11–1). As a consequence, the onset, speed, and fine-tuning of appendicular movements are impaired. In addition, as the supplementary motor cortex projects bilaterally to midline motor systems, disruption of physiological activity in this cortical area can influence bilateral movement. Similarly, abnormal activity in nigrotectal and nigroreticular projections is thought to change the balance of activity in descending pathways to midline muscles. Mechanisms of posture and balance become abnormal.

There are several potential causes of dementia in Parkinson's disease. Some evidence indicates that pathological involvement of the frontally projecting mesolimbic dopamine system can explain the dementia. This system arises from dopaminergic neurons in the ventral tegmental area just medial to the substantia nigra. Other evidence suggests that the dementia may be due to pathology in the basal nucleus of Meynert, a cholinergic nucleus that projects diffusely to cortex. In support of this notion is the observation that patients with advanced Parkinson's disease become confused when given low doses of anticholinergic drugs. Finally, pathological analysis of some patients reveals widespread Lewy bodies throughout the cortex, whereas others have pathology consistent with Alzheimer's disease (Chapter 16).

The cause of cell death in the substantia nigra and other pigmented nuclei is unknown. Research is now focusing on mechanisms of cell death, e.g., calcium overload, glutamate toxicity, and oxidative stress. The last hypothesis receives support from several direct and indirect observations. First, biochemical analysis of brains of patients demonstrates an increase in total iron but a decrease in ferritin, the iron-binding protein, in the substantia nigra. Iron is also increased in areas of damage in other neurodegenerative diseases, but in these conditions there is also a compensatory increase in ferritin. Thus, in Parkinson's disease there is an increase in free iron in the tissue. Iron participates in the formation of reactive oxygen species that cause lipid peroxidation and damage to cell membranes. In Parkinson's disease, there is an increase in malondialdehyde, an intermediate of lipid peroxidation, and a decrease in reduced glutathione, which buffers oxygen radicals.

Second, melanin is formed by the oxidation of catecholamines. Melanin is incorporated in lipofuscin from lysosomes in pigmented brain nuclei. There may be production of free radicals or toxic quinones during formation of neuromelanin. In addition, neuromelanin may bind and thus concentrate neurotoxins such as MPTP and iron. Against the melanin hypothesis is the observation that cell loss in the substantia nigra begins in the least pigmented area.

Finally, studies of the mechanism of action of the neurotoxin MPTP have identified abnormalities in mitochondrial oxidative metabolism as a cause of oxidative stress (Box 11–2). MPP+ inhibits NAD(H)-ubiquinone oxidoreductase activity of complex I of the mitochondrial oxidative chain. This defect leads to a failure of energy supply of ATP and cell death. Assays of the substantia nigra of brains in Parkinson's disease also show a depletion of complex I, but interpretation of this finding is not straightforward. By the time of death as a result of Parkinson's disease, most neurons in the substantia nigra have been replaced by reactive and fibrous glia. Thus, a defect in complex I may indicate a defect in glia and not a primary pathophysiological event.

Evaluation and Differential Diagnosis

The clinical diagnosis of idiopathic Parkinson's disease is straightforward for a patient who presents with unilateral onset of tremor, rigidity, and bradykinesia. In this situation, there is no need to perform imaging tests or an extensive evaluation of diverse etiologies (Table 11–1). The benefit such patients receive from levodopa confirms the biochemical pathophysiology of Parkinson's disease.

In patients who have no tremor but present with bilateral rigidity, bradykinesia, and postural instability, a trial of levodopa is important to differentiate patients with Parkinson's disease from those with other degenerative diseases or conditions. Several clinical situations can cause diagnostic confusion, particularly in the elderly. First, it is important to eliminate medications that block dopamine transmission. Major tranquilizers (e.g., chlorpromazine and haloperidol) are the most common offenders. Disease states such as normal pressure hydrocephalus and multiple infarcts of subcortical structures

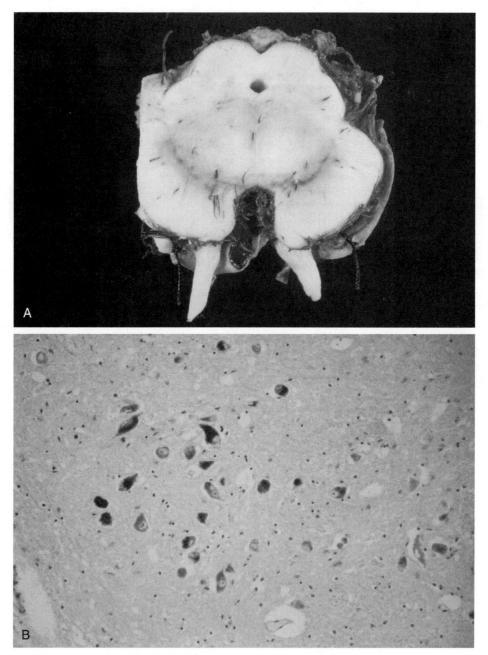

FIGURE 11–3. Neuropathology of Parkinson's disease. *A*, A fresh-cut section of a normal human brain through the midbrain reveals the dark neuromelanin pigment in the substantia nigra. *B*, Histologically there are many neurons containing neuromelanin in the normal brain.

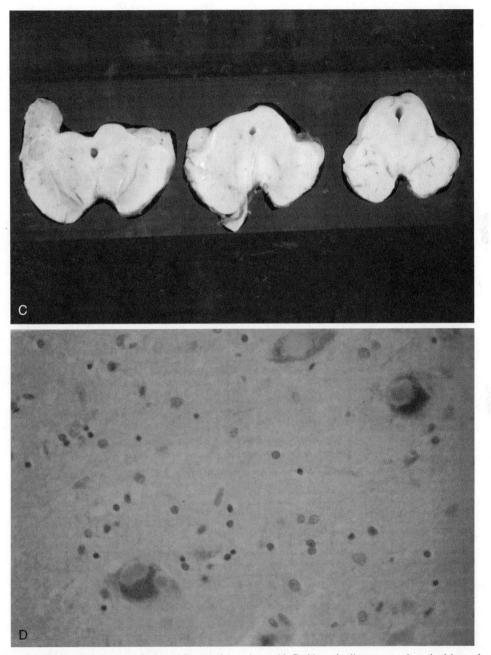

FIGURE 11-3 *Continued C,* Three sections through the midbrain of a patient with Parkinson's disease reveal marked loss of neuromelanin. *D,* Microscopic analysis shows a decrease in pigmented neurons with the presence of Lewy bodies (arrows) in several remaining neurons. These eosinophilic bodies are composed of cytoskeletal proteins and fibrils. (Photomicrographs courtesy of H. Vinters, M.D.)

BOX 11-2 MPTP Parkinsonism

In July 1982, a 42-year-old man was admitted to Santa Clara Valley Medical Center in San Jose, California, in a state of catatonic immobility. He appeared alert but was akinetic, sitting in a stooped posture with a flexed trunk. There was a fixed stare, infrequent blinking, and continuous drooling. His arm movements were exceedingly slow and there was "lead pipe" rigidity with cogwheeling in all extremities and the neck muscles. He had difficulty standing, walked slowly, and turned *en bloc*. There was no tremor, and the rest of his neurological examination was normal. The patient was given carbidopa-levodopa and improved dramatically. A week later, the patient's 30-year-old girlfriend was admitted with similar findings. Within several months, seven cases of acute parkinsonism in young adults aged 22–42 had been identified in the Santa Clara Valley.

Epidemiological investigation revealed that the affected persons had taken intravenously a "new synthetic heroin" synthesized at an illicit laboratory. Chemical and toxicological analysis of specimens indicated that the offending compound was 1-methyl-4-phenyl-1,2,3,6-tetrahydropyridine (MPTP), a by-product in the chemical synthesis of MPPP, a potent meperidine opiate analog. Subsequent studies in experimental animals determined that MPTP is selectively toxic to dopaminergic neurons in the substantia nigra. MPTP is converted by monoamine oxidase B (MAO-B) to MPP+ in glia. MPP+ is concentrated in the substantia nigra by the dopamine transporter and high-affinity binding to neuromelanin. MPP+ inhibits NAD(H)-ubiquinone oxidoreductase activity of complex I of the mitochondrial respiratory chain by a mechanism involving oxygen radicals. Nitric oxide (NO) may also play a role in destroying dopamine neurons. Subsequent degeneration of nigrostriatal projections results in a pure picture of dopamine-deficient parkinsonism.

Clinical studies of people who had taken MPTP have clarified important concepts regarding the pathophysiology of Parkinson's disease. (1) A group of asymptomatic patients were studied with PET scans and found to have a deficiency in the uptake of fluoro-dopa, indicating loss of dopamine terminals. A presymptomatic, or chemical, stage of the disease thus occurs before degenerating nigral cells reach a critical threshold. (2) Patients studied with neuropsychological tests showed a profile of deficits similar to patients with idiopathic Parkinson's disease, having abnormalities in construction, category naming, and frontal lobe functions. These deficits must therefore be a result of dopamine deficiency rather than of loss of cholinergic neurons or other pathological processes sometimes found in Parkinson's disease. (3) Patients with MPTP parkinsonism developed dyskinesias and on-off motor phenomena within months after treatment with levodopa compounds. Thus, disease severity rather than duration of levodopa treatment is the critical factor in these clinical phenomena.

The discovery of MPTP parkinsonism prompted a search for similar toxic compounds that might play a role in causing idiopathic Parkinson's disease, but none has been found. Since inhibitors of MAO-B block experimental MPTP parkinsonism, several new inhibitors are being investigated to see whether they influence disease progression in humans. Studies of the mode of action of MPTP have stimulated new research focused on abnormalities of membrane transport and oxidative metabolism as possible causative factors in human disease.

---

can cause a similar clinical picture. Characteristic abnormalities of gait and urinary incontinence distinguish the former, and pseudobulbar palsy and pyramidal tract signs are consistent features of the latter. Imaging studies are diagnostic in these situations helping to direct appropriate therapy. Toxins are rare causes of parkinsonism and usually affect other neuroanatomical systems in addition to basal ganglia. Rarely families are encountered in which members in several generations develop features of parkinsonism. Machado-Joseph disease (Chapter 12) and neuroacanthocytosis are examples. Molecular genetic studies on these families will provide further insight into basic mechanisms of neurodegeneration.

TABLE 11-1. Differential Diagnosis of Parkinsonism

Idiopathic Parkinson's Disease
Clinical: Tremor, rigidity, bradykinesia
Pharmacological: Response to levodopa
Pathological: Loss of neurons in the substantia nigra; Lewy bodies
The Multiple System Atrophies
Striatonigral degeneration
Shy-Drager syndrome (idiopathic orthostatic hypotension)
Olivopontocerebellar atrophies
Progressive Supranuclear Palsy (PSP)
Secondary Parkinsonism
Drugs: Phenothiazines (e.g., chlorpromazine); butyrophenones (e.g., haloperidol), reserpine; α-methyldopa, metoclopramide
Toxins: MPTP, manganese, carbon monoxide
Infections: Postencephalitic parkinsonism
Genetic: ? Autosomal dominant
Trauma: Dementia pugilistica
Normal pressure hydrocephalus
Vascular: Multiple infarcts

MULTIPLE SYSTEM ATROPHIES

Approximately 10% of patients who present with features of Parkinson's disease will prove on follow-up to have another type of degenerative illness. These patients are usually identified by a failure of response to levodopa. These illnesses are described in the literature under a variety of eponymic and descriptive terms (see Table 11–1) but all have in common variable neuronal loss and gliosis in subcortical structures. In contrast to Parkinson's disease, there is no preponderance of Lewy bodies in degenerating neurons. Structures commonly involved include substantia nigra, caudate, posterior putamen, lateral globus pallidus, cerebellar Purkinje cells, pontine nuclei, and the intermediolateral cell column of the spinal cord. Defects in the autonomic system in these disorders (e.g., the Shy-Drager syndrome) can cause severe postural hypotension. Studies of individual families with olivopontocerebellar atrophy have revealed different genetic defects for some of these disorders (Chapter 12).

PROGRESSIVE SUPRANUCLEAR PALSY

This neurodegenerative illness, also known as the Steele-Richardson-Olszewski syndrome, is characterized clinically by abnormal volitional eye movements. The earliest abnormality is difficulty with downward gaze, which may cause patients to stumble. Upward gaze is involved next, and volitional control of lateral gaze can also be impaired. In contrast to a loss of volitional control of saccadic eye movements, slow pursuit movements and vestibulo-ocular reflexes ("doll's eyes") are usually relatively well preserved. These clinical findings localize the lesion to the midbrain, where neuronal loss, gliosis, and neurofibrillary tangles are prominent in the pretectum, superior colliculus, and periaqueductal gray matter. The globus pallidus and pontine nuclei are also characteristically involved. Atrophy of the midbrain tegmentum can usually be appreciated on MRI scans in advanced cases. Bradykinesia, axial rigidity, dystonia, and dysarthria are prominent features. Speech and cognitive functions are slowed. The illness progresses over 5–10 years and is generally unresponsive to levodopa treatment.

Treatment

The goals of treatment in Parkinson's disease are to prevent degeneration of substantia nigra neurons and to enhance transmission at the dopamine synapse. At present, selegiline is a putative treatment for preventing degeneration. This agent blocks monoamine oxidase B (MAO-B) and has been found to prevent MPTP-induced parkinsonism in experimental animals. On the basis of the hypothesis that it might block other, yet unknown toxins, it is being tried in humans. Because it blocks the metabolism of dopamine itself, it raises endogenous levels of this neurotransmitter and thus has a symptomatic affect. Some clinicians use it as sole treatment for very mildly affected patients, since it delays the need to start levodopa.

Replacement therapy is the mainstay of treatment. In early trials of oral levodopa, 4–12 g/d of the amino acid were required to achieve a response. Since up to 75% of oral levodopa is decarboxylated peripherally, these massive amounts were required to get enough levodopa across the blood-brain barrier into the dopamine synapse (Figure 11–4). After drugs were developed to inhibit the peripheral sites of dopa decarboxylase, the oral dose was cut to less than 2 g/d, and side effects of nausea and vomiting were greatly diminished. Combinations of levodopa and carbidopa, a peripheral decarboxylase inhibitor, are used in nearly all patients (Table 11–2).

In the early phase of the illness, patients respond well to replacement therapy and can usually maintain full activity in employment and recreation for many years. The use of carbidopa-levodopa has allowed a normal life span for many. In some patients, tremor is resistant to levodopa replacement and anticholinergic medicines can be helpful as adjuvant therapy. However, in high doses they can cause confusion in elderly patients.

The management of patients in the late stages of the disease is challenging. Most patients taking levodopa experience an end-of-dose wearing-off effect or rapid fluctuations of on-off periods. These symptoms are probably due to the progressive loss of dopamine terminals with a reduction in the storage capacity for dopamine. Further increases in individual doses often cause **dyskinesias,** which are abnormal choreoathetoid or dystonic movements of the face, head, hands, or feet and represent direct dopamine stimulation. Interestingly, most patients will elect to tolerate these movements if a reduction of dose means having bradykinesia. The best approach to treating these symptoms is to change the dosing regimen to more frequent but smaller individual doses of carbidopa-levodopa. In addition, the use of dopamine agonists (e.g., pergolide) can be beneficial. Since these agents act directly on postsynaptic receptors they will be active even though the presynaptic neurons continue to degenerate.

Stereotaxic Surgery. In his original description, Parkinson noted that a patient who suffered a stroke

TABLE 11-2. Treatment of Parkinson's Disease*

Drug	Mechanism of Action	Dose (mg/d)	Common Side Effects
Early Phase of Disease			
For bradykinesia, rigidity, and tremor:			
Sustained-release carbidopa-levodopa	Replacement	400–600	Nausea, dyskinesia
Selegiline	MAO-B blocker	5–10	Nausea, lightheadedness
For persistent and prominent tremor:			
Trihexyphenidyl	Anticholinergic	2–10	Dry mouth, confusion
Amantadine	Dopamine release	200	Nausea, lightheadedness
Advanced Phase of Disease			
For rapid motor fluctuations, wearing-off, on-off phenomena:			
Carbidopa-levodopa	Replacement	200–1600 every 1–2 h	Dyskinesia, hallucinations
Pergolide	D1 and D2 agonist	1–3	Dyskinesia, hallucinations
For depression:			
Trazodone	Serotonin reuptake inhibitor	150–500	Sedation, dry mouth
Fluoxetine	Selective serotonin reuptake inhibitor	10–60	Nervousness, anxiety

*Guidelines for therapy are to start with low doses and advance slowly over days to weeks to achieve optimal response. In advanced cases, the therapeutic window between relief of motor symptoms and dyskinesias and hallucinations is narrowed.

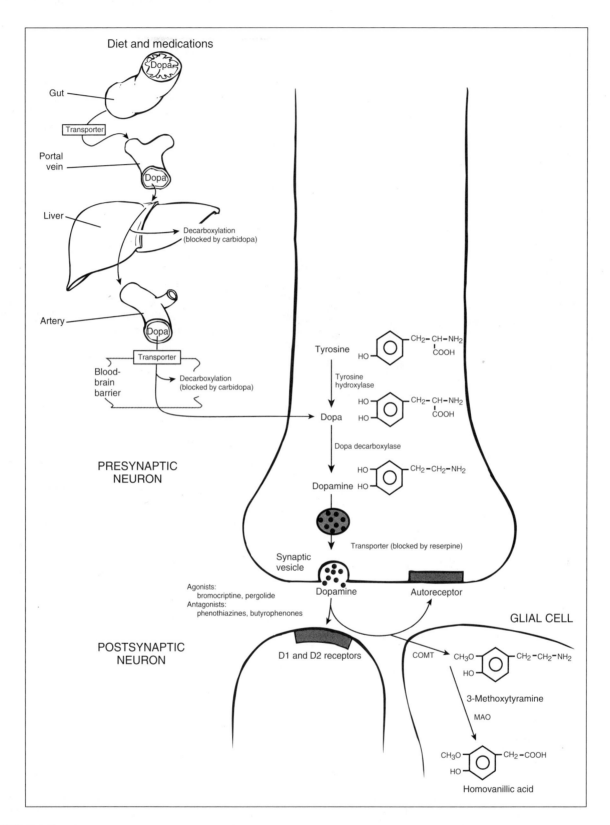

FIGURE 11–4. The dopamine synapse. The amino acid tyrosine is the main precursor of dopamine in healthy individuals. To increase synaptic dopamine, patients with Parkinson's disease are given the precursor levodopa. Dopa is absorbed from the gut and enters the systemic circulation after passage through the liver. Inhibition of peripheral decarboxylase enzymes maintains a high level of dopa in the plasma for transport across the blood-brain barrier by the neutral amino acid carrier. In the brain, dopa is decarboxylated in nerve terminals into dopamine for synaptic transmission. There are five types of dopamine receptors, with D1 and D2 being the most important in the striatum and motor circuits (see Figure 11–1). Dopamine is removed from the synapse and metabolized by catechol-*O*-methyltransferase (COMT) and/or monoamine oxidase (MAO). Drugs that block the vesicular transporter and deplete dopamine (reserpine), or block dopamine at the synaptic receptor (e.g., haloperidol) cause parkinsonism. Drugs that stimulate the receptor (e.g., bromocriptine) relieve symptoms and in high doses cause dyskinesias. Drugs that inhibit reuptake (amphetamine) or block metabolism (selegiline) increase dopamine and relieve symptoms.

had diminution of his tremor on the side of his weakness. Later, after Irving Cooper fortuitously discovered that ligature of the anterior choroidal artery in a Parkinson patient with an aneurysm abolished the patient's tremor, a variety of procedures were introduced to produce lesions in the ventrolateral thalamus. These were successful in ameliorating tremor and rigidity but did not relieve bradykinesia. More recently, lesions placed in the posteroventral globus pallidus have been found to bring relief to all symptoms. For best results these operations are done under electrophysiological guidance and MRI stereotaxic control. Graded radiofrequency stimulation is used to test the efficacy of the treatment before a permanent lesion is made. Patients with tremor or severe dyskinesias or those who become refractory to pharmacological therapy are the best candidates.

Transplantation. Adrenal-to-caudate transplantation was introduced as a means to place dopamine-producing tissue directly into the caudate. A patient's own adrenal gland was removed and sections were placed into the striatum. After several years, it was realized that any effect was short lived and operative morbidity and mortality did not justify the operation.

Transplantation of substantia nigra cells from aborted fetuses into the striatum of patients is under evaluation in controlled studies. This procedure has found more success than adrenal transplants in experimental animals with MPTP-induced parkinsonism. Transplantation of cells genetically engineered to produce high levels of dopamine and/or growth factors (e.g., GDNF; Box 10-3) provides a therapeutic effect in experimental animals.

Supportive Treatment. Physical and occupational therapy are important treatment modalities as the disease advances. All patients should practice routine daily exercise that is comfortable and enjoyable such as walking or swimming. Stretching exercises help counteract the natural tendency of the disease to cause flexed posture of the trunk and loss of flexibility in the arms and legs. Education is important for the patient and the spouse, and many are helped with psychological and social issues by joining a support group.

SUMMARY

Parkinson's disease is an idiopathic degenerative disease primarily affecting substantia nigra dopaminergic neurons. Having its onset in adult years, it becomes increasingly prevalent with aging. The loss of striatal dopamine disrupts the balance of activity in basal ganglia and thalamic circuits and causes characteristic features of bradykinesia, rigidity, resting tremor, postural instability, and gait difficulties. Stereotaxic lesions destroying the inhibitory projections from a disinhibited globus pallidus into the thalamus reduce symptoms. Replacement therapy with levodopa medicines is the mainstay of treatment and provides early and long-lasting benefit in most cases. Therapy directed at the primary cause of degeneration awaits further insight into basic pathophysiological mechanisms.

Selected Readings

Ballard, P. A., J. W. Tetrud, and J. W. Langston. Permanent human parkinsonism due to 1-methyl-4-phenyl-1,2,3,6-tetrahydropyridine (MPTP): Seven cases. Neurology 35:949–956, 1985.

Bergman, H., T. Wichmann, and M. R. DeLong. Reversal of experimental parkinsonism by lesions of the subthalamic nucleus. Science 249:1436–1438, 1990.

Calne, D. B. The free radical hypothesis in idiopathic parkinsonism: Evidence against it. Ann Neurol 32:799–803, 1992.

Cummings, J. L. The dementias of Parkinson's disease: Prevalence, characteristics, neurobiology, and comparison with dementia of the Alzheimer type. Eur Neurol 28(Suppl 1):15–23, 1988.

Cummings, J. L. Depression and Parkinson's disease: A Review. Am J Psychiatry 149:443–454, 1992.

Dexter, D. T., A. Carayon, F. Javoy-Agid, et al. Alterations in the level of iron, ferritin and other trace metals in Parkinson's disease and other neurodegenerative diseases affecting the basal ganglia. Brain 114:1953–1975, 1991.

Fahn, S., and G. Cohen. The oxidant stress hypothesis in Parkinson's disease: Evidence supporting it. Ann Neurol 32:804–812, 1992.

Laitinen, L. V., A. T. Bergenheim, and M. I. Hariz. Leksell's posteroventral pallidotomy in the treatment of Parkinson's disease. J Neurosurg 76:53–61, 1992.

Markham, C. H., and S. G. Diamond. Evidence to support early levodopa therapy in Parkinson disease. Neurology 31:125–131, 1981.

Markham, C. H. (ed.). Parkinson's disease. Clin Neurosci 1:1–68, 1993.

Parkinson Study Group. Deprenyl forestalls disability in early Parkinson's disease: A controlled clinical trial. N Engl J Med 321:1364–1371, 1989.

Tomac, A., E. Lindqvist, L.-F.H. Lin, et al. Protection and repair of the nigrostriatal dopaminergic system by GDNF in vivo. Nature 373:335–339, 1995.

CHAPTER TWELVE

HUNTINGTON'S DISEASE

AND THE

HEREDITARY ATAXIAS

HUNTINGTON'S DISEASE 139

    Introduction 139

    Clinical Presentation 139

    Genetics 139

    Pathophysiology 141

    Evaluation and Differential Diagnosis 143

    Treatment 143

THE HEREDITARY ATAXIAS 146

SUMMARY 147

HUNTINGTON'S DISEASE

Introduction

Huntington's disease is a hereditary degenerative disorder of the nervous system causing chorea (involuntary dance-like movements), psychological and behavioral abnormalities, and dementia in adults. It is the most common neurogenetic disorder presenting with degenerative disease in midlife. The condition was first described in 1872 by George Huntington from observations from his grandfather's, father's, and his own clinical practice in East Hampton, New York (Box 12–1). It is recognized worldwide with an overall prevalence of 5–10/100,000 population. The illness is inherited as an autosomal dominant disease with complete penetrance, the genetic abnormality being transmitted on chromosome 4 as an excess number of triplet repeats of CAG (see below). Owing to the late onset of symptoms, it is estimated that there are five times as many "at-risk" family members for each case.

Clinical Presentation

The mean age of onset of Huntington's disease is approximately 40 years with men and women affected equally. Approximately 6% of cases begin before age 20, and paternal inheritance is a risk factor for early onset. Cases occurring beyond age 50 are milder, progress more slowly and without prominent mental changes, and are usually diagnosed as senile chorea unless genetic testing is performed to make a definitive diagnosis. In the absence of a clear family history, the adult age of onset often means that patients have already had children before an opportunity for genetic counseling. Increased awareness of this disease and the availability of specific individual blood testing are improving this situation.

In the majority of cases, the disease becomes manifested by abnormal movements. A "nervousness" or "fidgetiness" of the hands or the face is often identified in retrospect once more overt jerky, choreic movements are recognized as clearly abnormal. At first these larger movements may be folded into mannerisms, such as continuously crossing or uncrossing the legs, adjusting one's eyeglasses, running fingers through one's hair, or clearing the throat to mask an involuntary vocalization. Over time the movements become more frequent and more abnormal. The gait takes on a dance-like quality suggesting intoxication. The voice loses normal intonation and prosody, occasionally taking on an explosive quality in speaking. Disabling, violent movements may occur such that it becomes impossible to stand or sit without falling. As the disease progresses, the quick, jerky movements become slowed with more sustained posturing called choreoathetosis. In advanced cases, there is bradykinesia, rigidity, and dystonia. Difficulties with swallowing, nutrition, and breathing eventually occur, with death coming 15–20 years after onset of first symptoms.

Juvenile onset cases often begin with bradykinesia, rigidity, and dystonia. Tremor occurs rather than chorea. Rarely patients have seizures. The rate of progression is rapid in these akinetic-rigid juvenile cases, rarely lasting more than 14 years. Up to 90% of juvenile cases inherit the defect from their father.

Approximately a third of cases begin with psychological or behavioral abnormalities, sometimes 10 years or more prior to chorea. Often there can be a change in personality, with patients becoming perfectionistic, obsessional, complaining, or irritable. Others may become apathetic and withdrawn. Still others become eccentric or impulsive or exhibit manic behavior and sexual promiscuity (as observed originally by Huntington). Occasionally a diagnosis of schizophrenia is entertained before the characteristic movement disorder appears.

Depression is common in Huntington's disease, occurring in up to a third of cases. Often changes in mood are interpreted as a situational depression, or even as an appropriate mood change considering the severity of the symptoms and the uniformly poor prognosis of the disease. However, such situational mood states are usually short lived and are not associated with the cardinal manifestations of a major depression: sustained loss of interest and energy, feelings of worthlessness and hopelessness, changes in sleep and appetite. The symptoms of depression are important to recognize, since pharmacological treatment is effective. There is an increased incidence of suicide with this disorder.

Cognitive impairment occurs as the disease advances. Patients develop difficulties in managing business and household responsibilities. Impairment in attention to tasks becomes evident with a decrease in speed and flexibility of thinking. Formal tests of cognition reveal impairment in performance skills more than in verbal skills. Mental difficulties are cumulative with time. Problems with memory impair and diminish meaningful communication. Global dementia eventually occurs. In contrast to cortical dementias, apraxia, agnosia, and aphasia are not prominent features.

The neurological examination of an adult with early Huntington's chorea reveals abnormalities of the motor system beyond the choreic movements. Abnormalities of eye movement can be appreciated as a slowness of saccades. When asked to shift the eyes quickly from one target to another, a patient will do this slowly or in small multiple steps (hypometric saccades). Occasionally a patient may involuntarily close the eyes and turn the head to accomplish the task. Slow pursuit movements may also be abnormal, being interrupted by jerky movements. Muscle tone and strength are normal, but fine dexterous movements of the hands are poorly accomplished. There is also difficulty in sustaining a tonic posture, such as protruding the tongue ("serpent's tongue") or maintaining a forceful handgrip ("milkmaid's grip"). Mental status testing may reveal difficulties with attention and concentration such as in performing serial sevens. Sensation and reflexes remain normal.

Genetics

The mutant gene in Huntington's disease was localized near the telomeric end of the short arm of chromo-

BOX 12-1   George Huntington's Disease

George Huntington (1850–1916) grew up in East Hampton, New York, and eventually returned to practice there after spending a few years in Ohio, where he presented his famous paper. In his later life, he looked back upon his boyhood and recalled his first encounters with chorea when he accompanied his father on his horse and buggy rounds.

Over fifty years ago, in riding with my father on his professional rounds, I saw my first case of 'that disorder,' which was the way in which the natives always referred to the

dread disease. It made a most enduring impression upon my boyish mind, an impression every detail of which I recall today, an impression which was the very first impulse to my choosing chorea as my virgin contribution to medical lore. We suddenly came upon two women, mother and daughter, both tall, thin, almost cadaverous, both bowing, twisting, grimacing. I stared in wonderment, almost fear. What could it mean? My father paused to speak with them and we passed on.

At age 22, George Huntington gave the classical description of hereditary chorea that now bears his name.

THE MEDICAL AND SURGICAL REPORTER

No. 789 PHILADELPHIA, APRIL 13, 1872 Vol. XXVI–No. 15.
ORIGINAL DEPARTMENTS
COMMUNICATIONS

ON CHOREA
By George Huntington
Of Pomeroy, Ohio
Essay read before the Meigs and Mason Academy of Medicine at
Middleport, Ohio, February 15, 1872

Chorea is essentially a disease of the nervous system. The name "chorea" is given the disease on account of the *dancing* propensity of those who are affected by it, and it is a very appropriate designation.... Its most marked and characteristic feature is a clonic spasm affecting the voluntary muscles. There is no loss of sense or volition attending these contractions, as there is in epilepsy; the will is there, but the power to perform is deficient, the desired movements are after a manner performed, but there seems to exist some hidden power, something that is playing tricks, as it were upon the will, and in a measure thwarting and perverting its designs; and after the will has ceased to exert its power in any given direction, taking things into its own hands, and keeping the poor victim in a continual jigger as long as he remains awake.... The disease commonly begins by slight twitchings in the muscles of the face, which gradually increase in violence and variety. The eyelids are kept winking, the brows are corrugated, and then elevated, the nose is skewered first to the one side and then to the other, and the mouth is drawn in various directions, giving the patient the most ludicrous appearance imaginable....

And now I wish to draw your attention more particularly to a form of the disease which exists, so far as I know, almost exclusively on the east end of Long Island....

The *hereditary* chorea, as I shall call it, is confined to certain and fortunately a *few* families, and has been transmitted to them, an heirloom from generations away back in the dim past.... It is attended generally by all the symptoms of common chorea, only in an aggravated degree, hardly ever manifesting itself until *adult* or *middle* life, and then coming on gradually but surely, increasing by degrees, and often occupying years in development, until the hapless sufferer is but a quivering wreck of his former self.

1. Of its hereditary nature. When either or both of the parents have shown manifestations of the disease, and more especially when these manifestations have been of a serious nature, one or more of the offspring almost invariably suffer from the disease, if they live to adult age. But if by chance these children go through life *without* it, the thread is broken and the grandchildren and great-grandchildren of the original shakers may rest assured that they are free from the original disease....

2. The tendency to insanity, and sometimes that form of insanity which leads to suicide, is marked. I know of several instances of suicide of people suffering from this form of chorea, or who belonged to families in which the disease existed. As the disease progresses the mind becomes more or less impaired, in many amounting to insanity.... At present I know of two married men, whose wives are living, and who are constantly making love to some young lady, not seeming to be aware that there is any impropriety in it. They are suffering from chorea to such an extent that they can hardly walk, and would be thought, by a stranger, to be intoxicated. They are men about 50 years of age, but never let an opportunity to flirt with a girl go past unimproved. The effect is ridiculous in the extreme.

3. Its third peculiarity is its coming on, at least as a grave disease, only in adult life. I do not know of a single case that has shown any marked signs of chorea before the age of thirty or forty years, while those who pass the fortieth year *without* symptoms of the disease, are seldom attacked.

some 4 (4p16.3) by linkage analysis in 1983. Ten years later the gene, initially termed IT15 for "interesting transcript 15," was isolated by a collaborative team of international investigators using techniques of positional cloning (Figure 12–1). The gene spans 180 kb and contains 67 exons coding for a protein called "huntingtin." The protein contains 3144 amino acids,

has a mass of 330 kDa, and does not resemble any other known protein. The abnormality within the gene was identified as an unstable, expanded trinucleotide $(CAG)n$ repeat near the 5' end of the coding region (Box 12–2). In normal chromosomes, there are 6–34 repeats with the great majority being less than 32 (mean, 18–19). In Huntington's chromosomes, there are

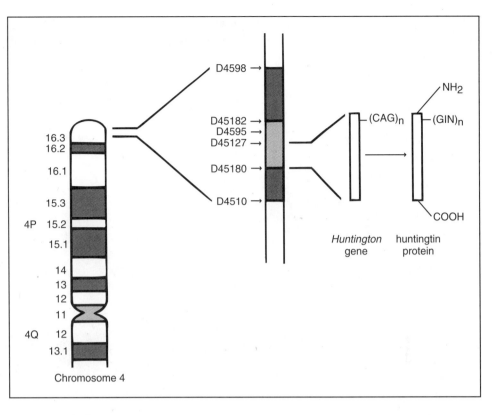

FIGURE 12-1. The Huntington's disease gene is located on the short arm of chromosome 4 near the telomeric end. Prior to its identification, markers near the gene were used to study inheritance in individual families. The 180-kb gene is shown with the triple repeat (CAG)n. Translation of this gene gives a protein of 3144 amino acids with a stretch of glutamines transcribed by the CAG code. When there are more than 39 repeats, the disease becomes manifest.

repeat lengths of 37–121 with the vast majority being greater than 40 (mean, 42–46). Asymptomatic individuals with 33–39 repeats fall in an indeterminate range with regard to diagnosis and predictability.

The number of repeats is unstable from one generation to another. Inheritance from the mother may result in an increase or decrease in 3–4 repeats. Inheritance from the father most often results in an increase in repeats, even up to a doubling of number. This reflects an increased instability of repeats during spermatogenesis. Paternal inheritance is a risk factor for juvenile onset of the disease, in which the range of repeats is very high (mean, 60). The number of repeats is one factor in determining the age of onset of symptoms; patients with greater than 50 repeats tend to present before age 30. However, there is considerable variability in age of onset, indicating the presence of other genetic or environmental factors. There is no relationship between repeat length and the type of symptoms at onset, i.e., motor versus behavioral.

Huntington mRNA is expressed at high levels in neurons throughout the nervous system. It is also expressed in systemic organs. Regional brain differences in expression of *Huntington* found with *in situ* hybridization techniques reflect differences in neuronal density, since expression per neuron is uniform. There is no increase or decrease in expression in neurons in the caudate nucleus, the site of greatest pathology in Huntington's disease, in either normal or diseased brains. Thus, the presence of expanded repeats does not interfere with the expression of *Huntington* mRNA, and there is no correlation between expression and susceptibility to degeneration. This suggests that other

factors unique to vulnerable cells interact pathophysiologically with *Huntington* or huntingtin.

The cloning of the *Huntington* gene has allowed the introduction of a highly specific PCR-based blood test for the disease. The presence of 37 or more repeats is considered diagnostic of an abnormal gene and can be used for prenatal counseling, identifying presymptomatic gene carriers within a family, and diagnosing sporadic cases. Of note, several sporadic cases have been found whose fathers had repeats in the indeterminate range, indicating that expansion of a normal number of repeats during spermatogenesis can lead to disease in offspring. The availability of this test raises ethical, legal, and psychosocial concerns. Many of these issues have received careful study since the introduction of the first linkage test. Only a fraction of at-risk individuals avail themselves of testing; others claim that they do not want to deal with the emotional and psychological consequences, they are happy not knowing, and there is no effective treatment. International committees have made recommendations concerning how diagnostic centers might counsel patients and families while protecting their autonomy and privacy (Box 12–3). In the past, supportive, nondirective counseling has been remarkably successful in reducing the gene frequency in well-identified families.

Pathophysiology

The earliest pathological change in Huntington's disease is a loss of medium-sized spiny neurons in the medial, paraventricular portion of the caudate nucleus and the dorsal putamen (Figure 12–2). These neurons

BOX 12-2 Trinucleotide Repeats in Neurological Disease

The expansion of trinucleotide repeats is recognized as a major cause of degenerative disease of the nervous system. At present, two different types of expansion have been identified (see table). Expansions of trinucleotides outside the protein coding region of the gene include the fragile X mental retardation syndromes (CGG and GCC) and myotonic dystrophy (GTC). It is thought that excessive expansions of the nucleotides interfere with expression of the gene product. For example, in the fragile X-A syndrome as the (CGG)n repeats become longer, there is less expression of the gene product (FMR-1) and the mental retardation worsens. Similarly, in myotonic dystrophy (DM) the longest expansions of (GTC)n occur in congenital cases rather than in adults. The fragile X syndromes and myotonic dystrophy are multisystem disorders affecting many organs (see Chapter 7).

Expansions of (CAG)n repeats occur within the coding region of genes in five degenerative diseases including Huntington's disease. The molecular mechanisms are unclear. The trinucleotide expansions do not seem to interfere with gene expression. For example, in Huntington's disease the gene is expressed at normal levels in the nervous system. A leading hypothesis for these disorders is that the gene products are proteins in which the abnormally long (CAG)n-coded glutamine tracts interfere with other cellular proteins of unique importance to a particular neuron. The medium-sized spiny stellate neurons in the striatum are the most vulnerable in Huntington's disease. Cerebellar Purkinje cells are particularly vulnerable in several inherited ataxias.

Expanded triplet repeats are unstable with changes in length from one generation to another. In myotonic dystrophy the greatest instability occurs between mother and child, while in the (CAG)n diseases the greatest instability occurs between father and child where there is usually an increase in repeat lengths. This phenomenon occurs during spermatogenesis and accounts for anticipation—the appearance of earlier onset of symptoms with successive generations within a family—as well as for the development of juvenile cases. There is a high correlation between the length of (CAG)n repeats and age of onset in SCA1. The longer the repeat length in adults, the greater is the likelihood of further expansion in offspring. Thus, these genetic disorders are dynamic, suggesting to some authors that the natural tendency toward expansion is increasing their incidence. In Huntington's disease, sporadic cases have been linked to an expansion of a normal, or "indeterminate," number (32–38) of repeats during spermatogenesis in the father.

Trinucleotide repeats make excellent markers for specific diagnostic testing. However, the length of the repeats cannot be used for predicting onset or severity in any one case. For example, in Huntington's disease, except for juvenile cases with the greatest number of repeats, there is a 10- to 20-year variation in age of onset for any particular repeat length. Thus, other genetic or environmental factors must play a role, and their discovery may lead to therapeutic interventions.

Trinucleotide Repeat Diseases

Disease	Locus	Repeat	Normal (Number of Repeats)	Disease (Number of Repeats)
Triplets Outside Coding Region				
FRAXA	Xq	CGG	6–50	200–>1000
FRAXE	Xq	GCC	6–25	>200
Myotonic dystrophy	19q	CTG	5–30	200–>1000
Triplets Inside Coding Region				
Huntington's disease	4p	CAG	11–34	39–120
SCA1	6p	CAG	19–36	43–81
DRPLA	12p	CAG	7–23	49–75
Machado-Joseph disease	14q	CAG	13–36	68–79
SBMA	Xq	CAG	11–34	40–62

DRPLA, dentatorubral-pallidoluysian atrophy; FRAX, fragile X a and E syndromes; SBMA, spinal and bulbar muscular atrophy; SCA1, spinocerebellar atrophy–1 (Table 12–3).

compose 80% of the cells in the striatum. They are gabaergic and project out of the striatum to the globus pallidus and substantia nigra, pars reticularis. Neurochemical markers of projection neurons are depleted in postmortem specimens of caudate, e.g., GABA, glutamate decarboxylase, enkephalins, substance P, angiotensin-converting enzyme, and cholecystokinin. The earliest pattern of cell loss identifies depletion of GABA/enkephalin projections to the lateral globus pallidus (see Figure 12–2). Loss of this projection is thought to account for the predominance of chorea in the early

phases of illness (Figure 12–3). Markers of interneurons remain relatively well preserved (e.g., somatostatin, neuropeptide Y, neurotensin, and nitric oxide synthase). As the disease progresses, severe diffuse neuronal loss and gliosis occur throughout the caudate, putamen, and globus pallidus and all projection neurons become depleted. In advanced cases, there is also variable loss of neurons in layers III, V, and VI of the frontal cortex, in the thalamus, and in the substantia nigra.

The cause of the selective vulnerability of medium-

BOX 12-3 Guidelines for the Molecular Genetics Predictive Test in Huntington's Disease*

These guidelines were developed to serve patients, at-risk individuals, clinicians, geneticists, ethical committees, and lay organizations in resolving difficulties arising from the application of the test. The recommendations reflect ethical principles based upon current knowledge and techniques in molecular genetics.

(1) All individuals who may wish to take the test should be given up-to-date, relevant information so they can make an informed, voluntary consent.

(2) The decision to take the test is solely the choice of the individual concerned. No requests from third parties—family members or otherwise—shall be considered.

(3) The participant should be encouraged to select a companion to accompany him or her throughout all stages of the testing process: the pretest stage, the taking of the test, the delivery of the results, and the posttest stage.

(4) Testing and counseling should be provided within specialized genetic counseling units knowledgeable about molecular genetic issues in HD, preferably within a university department. These centers should work in close collaboration with the lay organizations of the country.

*Adapted from J. Broholm and the committee representing the International Huntington Association and the World Federation of Neurology. Guidelines for the molecular genetic predictive test in Huntington's disease. Neurology 44:1533–1536, 1994.

sized spiny neurons is somehow related to the expression of *Huntington*. A leading hypothesis focuses on a "gain of function" due to the expression of the form of *Huntington* with the expanded allele. This hypothesis states that the gene, its mRNA, or its protein product causes a new biological function to occur rather than causing a loss of a normal function. In support of this hypothesis are the observations that a deletion of one *Huntington* allele (Wolf-Hirschhorn syndrome) does not cause Huntington's disease, and the presence of two abnormal *Huntington* genes—the homozygous condition of Huntington's disease—does not result in earlier or worse disease than does the heterozygous condition.

Attention has focused on the type of abnormality that might be conferred by excessive repeats of glutamine near the N terminus of huntingtin. A tract of polyglutamine in this protein may result in nonspecific hydrogen bonding interactions with other proteins in the cell cytoplasm where huntingtin is localized. A binding protein unique to the striatum would explain the selected vulnerability of Huntington's disease. There are also excessive CAG repeats in genes of four other inherited neurological diseases (Box 12-2) each with a different pattern of cellular degeneration. Different proteins with polyglutamine tracts may bind with proteins unique to particular neurons.

In Huntington's disease, an alternative hypothesis proposes that catabolism of huntingtin could lead to accumulation of small polyglutamine peptides. These might interact with glutamate receptors and potentiate excitotoxic cell death. Glutamate is the neurotransmitter released from corticostriate projections upon medium-sized spiny neurons. Injections of excitatory amino acids (e.g., quinolinic acid, kainic acid) into the caudate causes preferential destruction of these neurons in a pattern similar to Huntington's disease. The creation of a transgenic Huntington's disease mouse may allow testing of these hypotheses.

Evaluation and Differential Diagnosis

The clinical diagnosis of Huntington's disease is straightforward in an adult with chorea and a positive family history. A blood test identifying greater than 37 CAG repeats at the genetic locus is confirmatory in these cases and is diagnostic in the absence of a clear family history. Neuroimaging with CT or MRI often shows atrophy of the head of the caudate nucleus, but these tests are no longer indicated in routine cases.

Other causes of chorea in adults may sometimes be identified in the course of evaluating patients. **Neuroacanthocytosis** is a rare genetic disease causing chorea and mental change in young adults. A defect in plasma membranes underlies the disorder. Red blood cells form acanthocytes, an abnormality that can be used as a diagnostic test. Peripheral nerves are affected with diminution or loss of tendon reflexes, and serum levels of muscle creatine phosphokinase (CPK) can be elevated. The **inherited ataxias** are sometimes confused with Huntington's disease, since both show abnormalities of gait. However, patients with pure ataxia do not exhibit involuntary movements. Other conditions causing chorea in adults include **paroxysmal choreoathetosis, benign senile chorea, drug-induced tardive dyskinesias, basal ganglia infarction,** and **Creutzfeldt-Jakob disease** (see Chapter 16).

Treatment

At present there is no specific treatment for the genetic or degenerative processes of Huntington's disease. However, symptomatic treatment can be helpful when it is focused on specific motor or behavioral abnormalities for a limited period of time. As a general principle, it is best to try nondrug approaches to symptom management as the first step; when drugs are necessary, prescriptions should start low and go slow, monitoring for optimal response with minimal side effects (Table 12-1). Each patient's medical regimen should be evaluated regularly, since symptoms change as the illness advances.

Early in the course of the illness when chorea predominates, neuroleptics that block D2 dopamine receptors (e.g., butyrophenones) are effective in ameliorating these involuntary movements. Blocking these receptors would have the effect of increasing activity in the projection pathway from the striatum to the lateral

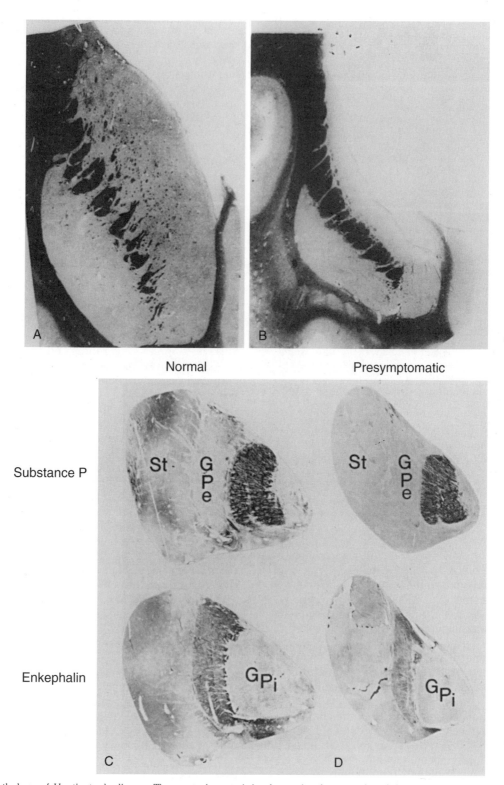

FIGURE 12-2. Pathology of Huntington's disease. The most characteristic change involves atrophy of the caudate nucleus and putamen. *A,* Normal brain. *B,* Severe atrophy from an advanced case. The earliest change involves degeneration of medium-sized spiny stellate neurons that project out of the striatum. (*A* and *B,* Reproduced, with permission, from J.-P. Vonsattell, R. H. Myers, T. J. Stevens, et al. Neuropathological classification of Huntington's disease. J Neuropathol Exp Neurol 44:559–577, 1985). *C,* A brain from a presymptomatic carrier for Huntington's disease was stained for neurotransmitter markers of these projection neurons. Neurons containing GABA and substance P that project to the medial globus pallidus are relatively preserved. *D,* Neurons containing GABA and enkephalin that project to the lateral globus pallidus (GPe) show a decrease in staining compared to control indicating early degeneration. GPi, medial globus pallidus; St, striatium. (*C* and *D,* Reproduced, with permission of Little, Brown and Company, from R. L. Albin, A. Reiner, K. D. Anderson, et al. Preferential loss of striato–external pallidal projection neurons in presymptomatic Huntington's disease. Ann Neurol 31:425–430, 1992.)

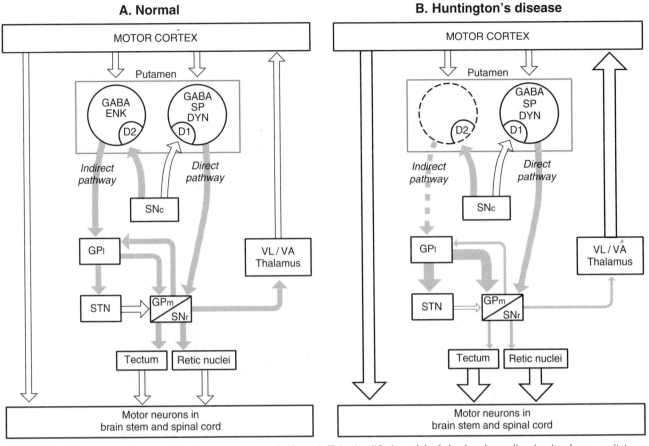

FIGURE 12–3. Functional anatomy of Huntington's chorea. *A*, Normal. This simplified model of the basal ganglia circuits shows excitatory connections in open arrows and inhibitory (gabaergic) connections in solid arrows (see Figure 3–5). *B*, In Huntington's disease, the symptom of chorea is thought to occur early in the illness owing to degeneration of striatal GABA/enkephalin neurons projecting to the lateral globus pallidus (see Figure 12–2), indicated by a thinning of the arrow. This loss of inhibitory control of the GPl results in increased firing of these inhibitory neurons and increased inhibition of the subthalamic nucleus. A diminution in firing of the subthalamic nucleus will act in concert with an augmented inhibitory drive from GPl and cause a depression of neuronal activity in GPm and SNr. The net effect is a decreased inhibition of the neurons in the motor thalamus and tectum and therefore an increased excitatory drive to cortex and spinal cord, causing excessive, asynchronous firing of anterior horn cells and chorea.

globus pallidus (Figure 12–3). However, the sedative and dysphoric side effects of these medicines limit their usefulness. Most centers use them only briefly for treating disabling chorea. As the disease progresses, choreic symptoms abate while bradykinesia and rigidity become accentuated. Neuroleptics worsen these latter symptoms and must be withdrawn.

Treatment of psychiatric symptoms of depression

with tricyclics (e.g., nortriptyline) or serotonin uptake inhibitors (e.g., fluoxetine) can be beneficial. The use of carbamazepine or valproic acid should be considered when bipolar manic-depressive symptoms occur. Finally, the short-term use of nonbenzodiazepine anxiolytics (e.g., buspirone) can help selected patients.

As the disease advances, patients develop problems with speaking and swallowing. Several guidelines

TABLE 12–1. Treatment of Symptoms of Huntington's Disease

Drug	Starting Dose	Maximal Dose	Common Side Effects
For Chorea			
Haloperidol	0.5–1.0 mg	10 mg	Sedation, dysphoria, parkinsonism
Thioridazine	10 mg	100 mg	Sedation, dysphoria, less parkinsonism
For Anxiety			
Buspirone	5 mg	30 mg	Sedation
For Depression			
Nortriptyline	10–25 mg	150 mg	Dry mouth, postural hypotension
Fluoxetine	10 mg	60 mg	Restlessness, insomnia
For Manic-Depressive Illness			
Carbamazepine	100 mg at bedtime	1200 mg	Sedation, dizziness, leukopenia
Valproic acid (systemic)	250 mg	1500 mg	Nausea, vomiting, sedation

TABLE 12-2. Common Causes of Ataxia in Adults

Acquired diseases affecting cerebellum or its pathways
    Vascular: ischemic infarction, hemorrhage
    Neoplastic: metastatic and primary tumors
    Paraneoplastic: small cell lung cancer
    Nutritional: alcoholism, thiamine deficiency
    Toxic: phenytoin use
Hereditary diseases
    Autosomal recessive (onset before age 20)
        Metabolic disorders, e.g., aminoaciduria
        Ataxia telangiectasia
        Friedreich's ataxia
    Autosomal dominant (adult onset, Table 12-3)

will help family and caregivers. Communication improves if patients are taught to speak slowly and use just the main words. The listener should repeat the idea to be certain it was sent and received correctly. Eating should be done slowly and deliberately. Considering the high caloric requirements of patients with chorea, feeding and eating require an increasing amount of time. It is important to provide some texture to the food because swallowing liquids can be particularly difficult and lead to aspiration and pneumonia.

THE HEREDITARY ATAXIAS

Patients who develop difficulty in walking in midlife present a diagnostic challenge (Table 12-2). Usually the acquired causes of ataxia can be diagnosed through history, examination, and testing. The hereditary ataxias are only beginning to be understood. The classification of these disorders by clinical features and pathological analysis alone has been inadequate. There is considerable phenotypic variability among family members with the same disease, and there is considerable overlap in symptoms and pathology between families with different genetic defects.

Molecular genetic studies have revealed some of the reasons behind these problems in nosology (Table 12-3). A single genetic defect due to the triplet repeats (CAG)n causes a range in the severity of the disease related to the range in the length of the triple repeats. For example, early age of onset, rapidity of progression, and severity of disease are associated with the longest chain of repeats. Presumably, the abnormal proteins (called ataxins) with the longest glutamine tracts disrupt neuronal metabolism the greatest amount. However, since these genes are expressed throughout the body, the pathogenetic mechanism must be related to unique biochemical features of vulnerable neurons. The vulnerable neurons lie in the cerebellar cortex, inferior olive, and basal ganglia. Neurons only marginally affected in mild cases become abnormal in severe cases. In addition, in the late stages of all of these illnesses many noncerebellar sites become damaged such that many patients develop ophthalmoplegia, dysphagia, rigidity, sensory loss, and muscle wasting.

SCA1 is the most common example of these disorders. Symptoms begin in the mid-30's with gait ataxia or dysarthria. Patients often describe having had premonitory signs for several years, such as intermittent clumsiness during sports activities or gait imbalance when under emotional stress. Over time the disease causes a full "cerebellar syndrome," with unstable posture, staggering gait, intention tremor, and dysdiadochokinesia (clumsiness of rapid, rhythmic, alternating movements). Within 5 years, patients must use canes or walkers. By 10 years, most are in wheelchairs. There are abnormalities of eye movements with nystagmus, loss of upward gaze, and slowed saccades. Behavioral and mental changes can develop, particularly of the frontal lobe type, with impaired executive decision-making functions, and emotional lability. Many patients show pyramidal and extrapyramidal signs on examination late in the disease. The disease progresses over 15–20 years with death occurring in the mid-50's. Toward the end dysphagia and respiratory failure dominate the clinical picture.

TABLE 12-3. Autosomal Dominant Cerebellar Ataxias

Name	Phenotype	Pathology	Locus
ADCA type I (SCA1)	Ataxia, dysarthria, dysphagia, ophthalmoparesis, amyotrophy, neuropathy, rigidity	Cerebellum, inferior olive, pons, spinocerebellar tract, posterior columns, cranial nerves, anterior horn cells	6p22–p23 (ataxin 1)
ADCA type I (SCA2)	Ataxia, hyporeflexia, slow saccades, rigidity	Cerebellum, inferior olive, pons, spinocerebellar tract, posterior columns	12q23–24.1
SCA3/Machado-Joseph disease	Ataxia, dysarthria, postural instability, nystagmus, eyelid retraction, facial fasciculations, distal atrophy	Cerebellar pathways, pons, spinocerebellar tract, vestibular nerve, oculomotor nerve, substantia nigra, subthalamic nucleus, anterior horn cells	14q24.3–32.1
DRPLA	Ataxia, choreoathetosis, dystonia, myoclonus, seizures, dementia	Cerebellar pathways, globus pallidus, subthalamic nucleus	12p12–ter
SCA4	Ataxia, sensory neuropathy		16q24–ter
SCA5	Ataxia, dysarthria		11, centromere
ADCA type II	Ataxia, retinal degeneration		Not mapped
Episodic ataxia 1	Brief attacks, myokymia, nonprogressive paroxysmal kinesiogenic choreoathetosis, responsive to acetazolamide		12p (potassium channel)
Episodic ataxia 2	Brief attacks, nystagmus, progressive, responsive to acetazolamide		19p

Specific genetic testing will enable specific diagnoses in the dominant inherited ataxic disorders. Following the guidelines that have been developed for Huntington's disease (Box 12–3), it will be possible to provide genetic counseling for affected families. In addition, once the molecular genetic mechanisms involved in one of the triplet repeat diseases is understood, there likely will be rapid progress in understanding all others.

SUMMARY

Huntington's disease is the most common inherited degenerative disorder in adults. Patients, typically in their 40's, develop abnormal involuntary choreic movements that become more severe over time, eventually leading to death in 15–20 years. The disease is transmitted by a gene on the short arm of chromosome 4. This gene contains excessive repeats of CAG that are coded faithfully into excessive repeats of glutamine in the transcribed protein. The abnormal protein probably binds with a protein specific for gabaergic projection neurons in the caudate and putamen and leads to the death of these cells. Treatment is symptomatic, but current experiments in understanding the molecular genetics of the disease process and protein-protein interactions promise potential therapies.

Selected Readings

Albin, R. L., A. Reiner, K. D. Anderson, et al. Preferential loss of striato–external pallidal projection neurons in presymptomatic Huntington's disease. Ann Neurol 31:425–430, 1992.

Duyao, M., et al. Trinucleotide repeat length instability and age of onset in Huntington's disease. Nature Genetics 4:387–392, 1993.

Genis, D., T. Matilla, V. Volpini, et al. Clinical, neuropathologic, and genetic studies of a large spinocerebellar ataxia type I (SCA1) kindred. Neurology 45:24–30, 1995.

Goldberg Y. P., S. E. Andrew, J. Theilman, et al. Familial predisposition to recurrent mutations causing Huntington's disease: Genetic risk to sibs of sporadic cases. J Med Genet 30:987–990, 1993.

Hardie, R. J., H. W. H. Pullon, A. E. Harding, et al. Neuroacanthocytosis. Brain 114:13–49, 1991.

Harper, P. S. (ed.). *Huntington's Disease.* London, W.B. Saunders Co., 1991.

Huntington, G. On chorea. Med Surg Reporter 26(15):317–321,1872.

Huntington, G. Recollections of Huntington's chorea as I saw it at East Hampton, Long Island, during my boyhood. J Nerv Ment Dis 37:255–257, 1910.

Huntington's Disease Collaborative Research Group. A novel gene containing a trinucleotide repeat that is expanded and unstable on Huntington's disease chromosomes. Cell 72:971–983, 1993.

La Spada, A. R., H. L. Paulson, and K. H. Fischbeck. Trinucleotide repeat expansion in neurological disease. Ann Neurol 36:814–822, 1994.

Landwehrmeyer, G.B., et al. Huntington's disease gene: Regional and cellular expression in brain of normal and affected individuals. Ann Neurol 37:218–230, 1995.

Rosenberg, R. N. Advances in the inherited ataxias. Clin Neurosci 3:1–53, 1995.

Vessie, P. R. On the transmission of Huntington's chorea for 300 years—the Bures family group. J Nerv Ment Dis 76:553–576, 1932.

Wexler, A. *Mapping Fate, a Memoir of Family, Risk, and Genetic Research.* New York, Times Books, Random House, 1995.

CHAPTER THIRTEEN

SEIZURES AND

EPILEPSY

INTRODUCTION 149

CLINICAL PRESENTATION 149

    Common Seizure Syndromes 149

    First Seizure 149

    Anoxic Seizure 150

    Febrile Seizure 150

    Common Epilepsy Syndromes 150

    Petit Mal, or Absence Epilepsy of Childhood 151

    Juvenile Myoclonic Epilepsy 151

    Grand Mal, or Generalized Tonic-Clonic Seizures 151

    Status Epilepticus 152

    Complex Partial Seizures, or Psychomotor or Temporal Lobe Epilepsy 153

PATHOPHYSIOLOGY 154

EVALUATION AND DIFFERENTIAL DIAGNOSIS 155

TREATMENT 156

SUMMARY 157

INTRODUCTION

A seizure is the expression of an abnormal, excessive discharge of neurons that causes sudden ("paroxysmal") and brief (<1–2 minutes) abnormalities of behavior. The neuronal discharges originate within abnormal circuits in the cerebral cortex or limbic system and spread downward through neuronal pathways into the brain stem, spinal cord, and muscles, causing convulsions. The clinical expression of seizures varies and includes a focal or generalized convulsion of muscle, sensory paresthesias, brief impairment of consciousness, and unconscious psychomotor automatisms. The symptoms seizures cause reflect the spread of abnormally intense discharges through local and long neuronal circuits. Clinically, seizures are classified as either **partial** or **generalized**. Partial seizures are further classified as **simple** if they do not disrupt consciousness and **complex** if they do (Table 13–1). A great many different conditions can damage the brain and cause seizures (Table 13–2). **Epilepsy** is defined as recurrent seizures of unknown etiology. Epileptic seizures are classified as different syndromes dependent on age and clinical manifestations (Table 13–3).

Seizures are common. In a person's lifetime there is a 6% chance of having a single seizure and a 3%

TABLE 13-1. Classification of Seizures

I. **Partial seizures.** These focal seizures may evolve into secondarily generalized seizures.
  A. **Simple partial seizures.** There is no impairment of consciousness. The EEG shows localized abnormalities confined to a small area of cerebral cortex, often indicating an underlying structural lesion.
    1. Focal motor seizures with convulsive jerking of a limb, side of the face, or whole side. Occasionally there is a jacksonian march or tonic extension.
    2. Focal sensory seizures with somatosensory or visual symptoms, less commonly auditory or vertiginous. Olfactory or gustatory symptoms precede complex partial seizures.
    3. Focal aphasia symptoms, often with memory impairment.
  B. **Complex partial seizures.** Impairment of consciousness occurs. The EEG shows discharges over temporal or frontal areas, and depth electrodes reveal discharges in the hippocampus and amygdala.
    1. Psychic aura only with brief alterations in perception, emotion, or memory, often with partial diminution in consciousness.
    2. Loss of consciousness with automatisms, often preceded by an aura.
II. **Generalized seizures.**
  A. **Nonconvulsive.** These occur primarily in children, with brief interruptions of consciousness. There may be brief or minor convulsive manifestations.
    1. Absence seizures (petit mal). Abrupt onset and cessation of altered consciousness with 3-Hz bilateral discharges for 5–10 seconds.
    2. Atypical absence. More heterogeneous clinical and EEG manifestations. Lennox-Gastaut syndrome.
  B. **Convulsive.** These occur at all ages and are characterized by bilateral EEG and motor manifestations from the start.
    1. Tonic-clonic (grand mal). Severe seizure: 10- to 12-Hz EEG activity, decreasing to burst discharges and postictal depression.
    2. Myoclonic. Single or repetitive asynchronous muscle jerks seen in metabolic and degenerative diseases.

TABLE 13-2. Causes of Seizures

Genetic
Primary generalized epilepsies, inborn errors of metabolism
Congenital Abnormalities
Maldevelopment of brain   — tumor
Perinatal
Anoxia, ischemia, hemorrhage
CNS Infections
Encephalitis, meningitis, abscess
Trauma
Penetrating wound, closed head injury, surgery
Neoplastic
Primary gliomas, metastatic
Vascular
Infarction, hemorrhage, arteriovenous malformations
Toxic
Alcohol or cocaine use, alcohol and sedative drug withdrawal
Metabolic
Hyponatremia, hypoglycemia, hypocalcemia
Degenerative
Alzheimer's disease, Creutzfeldt-Jakob disease

chance of having more than one. The incidence is highest at the extremes of life, being approximately 100/100,000 in the first year of life owing to congenital and perinatal insults and approaching this figure after age 70 owing to vascular and degenerative diseases. Between these extremes the incidence is approximately 25/100,000, with an overall prevalence of 0.6% in the general population. Seizures are among the most common reasons patients seek neurological care. Owing to advances in diagnosis, the availability of effective anticonvulsant medicines, and the possibility of surgery in selected cases, 70% of seizures can be effectively controlled.

CLINICAL PRESENTATION
Common Seizure Syndromes
First Seizure

Because a seizure is a *symptom* of abnormal neuronal discharge, its cause must be sought by history, examination, and laboratory testing (Table 13–4). The first step is to affirm that the "spell" was a real seizure and not a faint, TIA, migraine, or other cause of brief neurological dysfunction. A witness to the event will provide the best description of a seizure if consciousness is altered. Descriptions of facial expression, alter-

TABLE 13-3. Common Epileptic Syndromes

Focal seizure syndromes
  Benign childhood epilepsy with centrotemporal (rolandic) spikes
  Childhood epilepsia partialis continua with Rasmussen's encephalitis
  Temporal lobe epilepsy with partial complex seizures
Generalized seizure syndromes
  Benign febrile seizure
  Absence seizure (petit mal)
  Juvenile myoclonic epilepsy
  Tonic-clonic seizure (grand mal)

TABLE 13-4. Clinical Evaluation of Seizures and Epilepsy

Goals
1. Did a seizure occur?
2. Can the seizure be classified (Table 13-1)?
3. Are etiological clues present (Table 13-2)?
4. Are neurological abnormalities present?
5. Should anticonvulsants be started?

Clinical History
Description of the seizure: aura, focal or generalized ictal features, postictal behavior, time-intensity of clinical features
Differential clinical features of other spells
Frequency of seizures: time of day, asleep, on awakening
Precipitating factors: sleep deprivation, menses, alcohol or cocaine use
Developmental history: birth, febrile seizures, psychosocial development
Etiological factors (Table 13-2)
Family history of seizures

Neurological Examination
Observations for seizure: brief lapse in attention or consciousness, focal twitches, posturing
Mental status: evidence of retardation in child
Signs of focal abnormalities

Routine Laboratory Evaluation
EEG, while awake, while asleep, and during hyperventilation
MRI scan

Special Tests
EEG, sleep deprived, special electrodes, telemetry
PET or SPECT scan

ations in awareness or responsiveness, posturing, and convulsive movements of muscles and limbs are important. Seizures can last from 5 to 10 seconds (absence seizures) to several minutes (complex partial seizures) and rarely longer. They can be convulsive with strong jerking of the face or limbs, or nonconvulsive with alterations in sensation, emotion, or consciousness. A period of confusion, called postictal depression, follows prolonged seizures and can last for several minutes or even hours. Occasionally strong focal seizures of a limb will result in a period of weakness after the seizure is over, a condition called Todd's paralysis.

In patients with a single seizure, it is common to have a normal examination, EEG, and imaging study. In this situation, it is important to bear in mind that only 50% of patients who have a seizure will ever have another one. The cause of the isolated seizure in these patients can occasionally be attributed to illicit drug or alcohol use, sleep deprivation, or a combination of these factors. In many cases, no cause is found. Clinical features indicating a high likelihood of recurrent seizures and an eventual diagnosis of epilepsy include a positive family history, seizures as a child, occurrence of the seizure in the early morning hours of sleep, and abnormalities on the neurological examination. Characteristic abnormalities on the EEG will identify a portion of these patients at the time of initial workup. If no abnormalities are found, there is still a 50% chance of having another seizure within the first year. A neurologist will usually have a patient take anticonvulsant medications during this year.

Anoxic Seizure

During a simple faint, patients lose muscle power and tone and fall to the ground. The horizontal position allows an increase in return of venous blood to the heart, helping restore cardiac output and cerebral perfusion. On occasion people faint but are unable to fall, being restrained in a sitting or standing position. In this situation, cerebral hypoperfusion is more profound, and it is not uncommon for brief seizures to occur as a response to this type of insult. Commonly a brief tonic extensor convulsion occurs, or there are a few brief myoclonic jerks of the extremities. If it can be determined clinically that the faint preceded the convulsions, there is no need to evaluate the patient for other causes of seizure.

Febrile Seizure

Having a seizure during a fever is not uncommon (4%) for children between the ages of 3 months and 5 years. The peak incidence occurs between 1.5 and 2 years, usually as the fever is rising, lasts less than 5 minutes, and does not recur during the illness. The cause of fever is most often a benign viral illness or otitis media. If seizures are prolonged (>10 minutes), if they recur, or if there is suspicion of meningitis or encephalitis, a lumbar puncture must be performed. The result is normal in benign febrile convulsions. Since only a third of patients will have a second febrile seizure, and since anticonvulsants commonly cause behavioral abnormalities in children, there are no strong recommendations for treating febrile convulsions prophylactically. However, the presence of two or more risk factors for later nonfebrile convulsions prompts many pediatricians to prescribe phenobarbital or diazepam per rectum for use at the first appearance of fever. These risk factors include a positive family history of nonfebrile seizures, prolonged or complex febrile convulsion, and delayed or abnormal neurological development. There is some evidence that prolonged, intense febrile convulsions can lead to complex partial epilepsy after many years.

Common Epilepsy Syndromes

Generalized seizures affect both cerebral hemispheres simultaneously, interrupt consciousness, and cause bilateral motor manifestations. Genetics plays a role, but no specific gene has been isolated. In monozygotic twins, the concordance for childhood and adolescent syndromes of generalized epilepsy is 65%. In these identical twins, the convulsive manifestations are identical. By contrast, the concordance among dizygotic twins is 24% and the convulsive manifestations can be quite different. In families having epilepsy, some members will experience strong convulsions, others very mild manifestations such as myoclonic jerks upon awakening, and still others only an abnormality (sometimes very subtle) on the EEG. These findings seem to indicate that more than one gene is involved in creating the low threshold for seizures and clinical manifestations of the seizures in these families. Environmental factors also play a strong role.

In contrast to focal seizures, it has not been possible to discover where generalized seizures originate within the brain. Wilder Penfield, a neurosurgeon who devoted his professional life to the study of epilepsy, proposed the concept of a "centrencephalon." This hypothesis suggests that deep subcortical structures such as the intralaminar thalamic nuclei could be responsible for seizure onset and synchronization. These nuclei project widely to the cerebral hemispheres and could conceivably recruit them into synchronous action. Electrophysiological studies in cats of epilepsy caused by systemic penicillin demonstrate that cortico-thalamic "reverberating" circuits occur during generalized cortical epileptic discharges. Ethosuximide, an anticonvulsant effective in petit mal (see below), blocks this type of experimental discharge. In humans, it is likely that both orthodromic and antidromic spread of seizures tightly link cortex with thalamus during generalized convulsions, regardless of where they start.

Petit Mal, or Absence Epilepsy of Childhood

Petit mal ("little illness") is a childhood epileptic disorder occurring between ages 4 and 8 years and characterized by brief absences of less than 10 seconds' duration. A child will develop a blank stare and may blink repetitively, fumble with clothes, lick the lips, or attempt to respond. During the brief spell, the EEG shows regular 3-Hz spike-and-wave discharges (Figure 13–1). Hyperventilation and photic stimulation can often induce the discharges and seizures. With cessation of the discharges, the child returns to normal as does the EEG. A child can have many spells in a day, occasionally leading a teacher or parent to conclude that the child has a behavioral problem or continually day-dreams.

Genetic factors play a role in the cause of petit mal, but a gene has not been isolated. Some studies indicate an autosomal dominant inheritance pattern for the 3-Hz spike-and-wave EEG abnormality, although not all patients have clinical seizures. Slight variations in discharge rate may indicate different syndromes. For example, the EEG in the Lennox-Gastaut syndrome of childhood epilepsy shows 2.5-Hz discharges. This syndrome represents a heterogeneous group of disorders with diffuse cerebral abnormalities due to a variety of causes. Children have many different convulsive manifestations and exhibit mental retardation. Up to half the patients with pure petit mal can exhibit mild signs of mild retardation, and a similar number may have occasional tonic-clonic seizures. This type of epilepsy can be controlled with ethosuximide or valproic acid. The prognosis for complete remission of seizures during adolescence in children with pure petit mal is 90%.

Juvenile Myoclonic Epilepsy

Juvenile myoclonic epilepsy is the most common cause of generalized epilepsy beginning in the teenage years. A typical case begins with morning myoclonic jerks and progresses to a generalized convulsion. Sleep deprivation is a potent stimulus to morning seizures. The EEG shows 4- to 6-Hz irregular spike-and-wave discharges that are prominent frontally. A family history of myoclonic jerks and the EEG trait can often be obtained upon careful study. The genetic cause of the disorder has not been established. Both the myoclonus and the generalized seizures respond well to valproic acid. The disorder is probably lifelong.

Grand Mal, or Generalized Tonic-Clonic Seizures

A generalized convulsion is one of the most dramatic clinical events in medicine. Without warning a patient is thrown into tonic (sustained) extension as all the muscles convulse. A loud cry is often emitted as

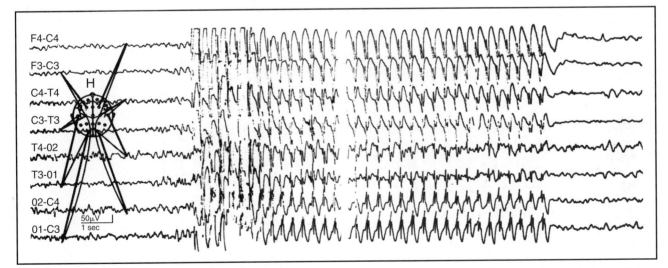

FIGURE 13–1. Absence (petit mal) seizure in a 12-year-old boy. There is abrupt onset and cessation of 3-Hz spike-and-wave discharge. During this time, the patient exhibited staring and eye blinking and was unresponsive to questions. Three seconds of the tracing are removed. (Reproduced, with permission, from E. W. Lothman and R. C. Collins. Seizures and epilepsy. *In* A. L. Pearlman and R. C. Collins [eds.]. *Neurobiology of Disease.* New York, Oxford University Press, 1990.)

forced expiration of air rushes past a closing glottis. Ventilation is interrupted and anoxia rapidly develops, turning the patient blue. Anaerobic metabolism of muscle increases several hundredfold, causing marked lactic acidosis. As the autonomic nervous system discharges, blood pressure and heart rate increase markedly, hyperglycemia occurs, excessive salivation develops, and the bladder and bowel evacuate. After approximately 30 seconds, the tonic phase gives way to the clonic phase with intermittent periods of muscle relaxation that lengthen until there is complete flaccidity, usually within 2 minutes. The EEG cannot be recorded in patients because of the violent convulsions. In paralyzed patients, the EEG shows sustained 10- to 12-Hz high amplitude discharges during the tonic phase, followed by intermittent burst discharges during the clonic phase, followed by depression (Figure 13–2). In some patients, there may be clonic-tonic phases, in others clonic-tonic-clonic. As ventilation resumes, hyperventilation develops driven by combined hypoxemia and acidosis. Consciousness returns slowly, emerging through a period of postictal encephalopathy that may last 15–30 minutes or sometimes hours. Patients may be disoriented, resist attempts at help, and even be combative in a nondirected manner during this period. Left alone they will commonly sleep for many hours, often awakening with a headache.

Grand mal seizures are a well-recognized form of clinical seizure. They can be an extended manifestation of petit mal, juvenile myoclonic epilepsy, or other generalized epileptic syndromes. They can also start with a focal seizure that becomes secondarily generalized. In many cases, the initial focal symptoms are so brief as to be unrecognized or unremembered. This is especially true of frontal lobe seizures, which gain ready access to bilateral motor pathways. In addition, generalized seizures are the most common expression of reactive seizures to drugs and alcohol, and two or more successive convulsions commonly occur in this setting. Anticonvulsants can control grand mal seizures in up to 60% of patients.

Status Epilepticus

When a second generalized convulsion follows quickly upon the first without the patient regaining consciousness, a medical emergency ensues. Without prompt treatment, recurrent generalized seizures, or status epilepticus, can lead to permanent brain damage as a result of combinations of hypoxemia, hyperthermia, and alterations in blood flow. During the time when epileptic discharges increase the neuronal metabolic rate fourfold, convulsions result in hypoxemia, acidosis, and occasionally even hypoglycemia—factors aggravating the metabolic insult to the brain. The same areas of selective vulnerability that occur after prolonged cardiac arrest are damaged by status epilepticus: layers III, V, and VI of the cortex, Sommer's sector of the hippocampus, and Purkinje cells of the cerebellum. There is experimental evidence in animals that the

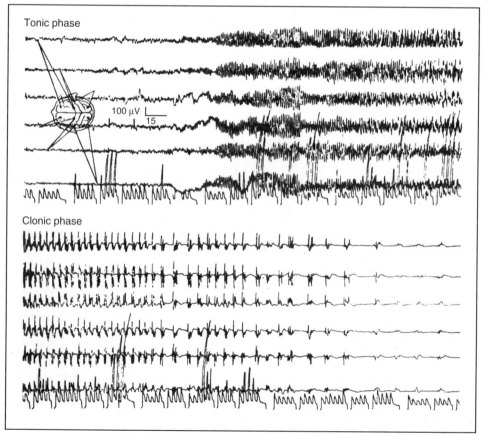

FIGURE 13–2. Generalized tonic-clonic seizure. The EEG (top six traces) shows a fast buildup of continuous high-frequency, high-amplitude discharges in all leads during the tonic phase. The discharges become discontinuous during the clonic phase, which ends in a low-amplitude depression of the electrical activity. (Reproduced, with permission, from H. Gastaut and R. Broughton. *Epileptic Seizures.* Springfield, Illinois, Charles C Thomas, 1972.)

brain damage caused by status epilepticus leads to epilepsy.

Status epilepticus occurs most commonly in patients with epilepsy who fail to take their anticonvulsant medication. Alcohol and drug intoxication and withdrawal are other common causes, followed in frequency by diffuse insults associated with encephalitis or cerebral anoxia. Status epilepticus must be controlled immediately. Patients must be given intravenous anticonvulsants and fluids and intubated to maintain the airway and control ventilation (Table 13–5).

Complex Partial Seizures, or Psychomotor or Temporal Lobe Epilepsy

Limbic system seizures cause transient abnormalities in sensation, perception, emotion, and memory and have fascinated clinicians for years. Originally called the "intellectual aura" or "dreamy state" by Hughlings Jackson (1888), psychomotor seizures by Gibbs (1948), and temporal lobe epilepsy by Penfield and colleagues (1950s), these seizures are now labeled as complex partial seizures (see Table 13–1). The earlier terms better communicate the phenomenology and pathological anatomy of the disorder. Complex partial seizures constitute approximately 40% of all seizures and usually present in the second to fourth decades. Evidence suggests these seizures represent delayed effects of birth injury, strong childhood febrile convulsions, or head trauma. Most patients respond well to anticonvulsant treatment. Surgery is beneficial in refractory patients when a clear unilateral temporal lobe focus can be found. MRI, PET scanning, and depth electrodes with telemetry are useful tools for identifying surgical patients.

Most often these seizures begin with an aura, or warning symptom that intrudes itself into the patient's consciousness. In fact, the aura is an expression of the earliest phase of the seizure. There can be sensory symptoms such as a bad smell, an unusual taste, or a rising sensation in the abdomen. The patient recognizes these sensations as distinctly unusual and not like any worldly experience. The odor is usually unpleasant but cannot be ascribed to anything in particular. The rising sensation is not like nausea or pain. The woolly vagueness of the descriptions is a characteristic feature

of internally evoked sensory, perceptual, or emotional experiences when consciousness is also affected. A patient may have a feeling of dread and show a frightful face but be unable to identify the cause. Occasionally a patient may have an evoked memory. "I saw myself as a little girl," one patient said. "I was sitting on a swing and my father was pushing me. Then it was over." This brief fragment from the past is an elaboration of a childhood event rather than a true experiential recording, since the patient could not have seen herself on the swing. Such "intellectual auras" are most common from seizures originating in the amygdala.

The aura may last 5–15 seconds and then disappear as the seizure stops. Patients describe the experience as being halfway into a dream, a "double consciousness," experiencing the evoked events but also distant from them. If the discharges continue and spread from one medial temporal lobe to the opposite side and into subcortical projections, consciousness is lost. In contrast to bilateral generalized seizures, bilateral limbic seizures do not cause muscle convulsions and usually do not cause patients to fall to the ground. Patients develop a blank stare or a frightened look, often mumble or mutter a few words, swallow repetitively, smack their lips, fumble with their clothes, or walk to a different part of their surroundings. During this time, they may react partially to environmental stimuli, but they do not respond verbally or engage in goal-directed, purposeful behavior. This automatic behavior lasts from 30 seconds to a few minutes and then changes imperceptibly to a postictal confusional state. As consciousness returns, the patient often asks what has happened but has no recollection of the events. Family or friends witnessing the events not uncommonly ascribe the behavior to stress, confusion, or psychological problems rather than a seizure. For this reason, many patients are not brought to medical attention until seizures recur and become more frequent. A significant number of patients and families first seek medical attention from psychiatrists because of the strange aspects of the behavior.

In a small number of patients, the cause of these seizures is due to a tumor, vascular malformation, or hamartoma in the medial aspect of the temporal lobe. In the majority of patients, there is sclerosis within the hippocampus (Figure 13–3), which can sometimes be

TABLE 13–5. Anticonvulsant Medications

Seizure Classification	Drug	Adult Dose [mg/kg (mg/d)]	Therapeutic Level (µg/mL)	Half-Life (h)	Toxicity
Partial seizures	Carbamazepine	15–25 (800–1600)	8–12	12	Anorexia, dizziness, leukopenia
	Phenytoin	3–8 (300–500)	10–30	24	Anorexia, ataxia, somnolence, gum hypertrophy
Generalized seizures Primary	Valproic acid	10–60 1–3 g	50–100	14	Anorexia, alopecia, weight gain, hepatotoxicity
Secondary	Carbamazepine or phenytoin				
Status epilepticus	First, lorazepam, 4–20 mg IV at a rate of 2 mg/min				
	Second, phenytoin, 1–1.5 g IV at a rate of 50 mg/min				
	Then, if necessary, phenobarbital, 1–1.5 g IV at a rate of 100 mg/min				

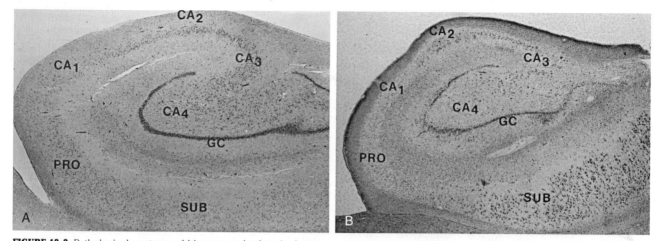

FIGURE 13–3. Pathological anatomy of hippocampal sclerosis. Autopsy specimens from a normal person *(A)* and one who had temporal lobe epilepsy and hippocampal sclerosis *(B)*. By comparing the two photomicrographs, one can appreciate loss of cells in the hilus of the dentate gyrus (labelled CA4) and subfields CA3 and CA1 of the hippocampus in *B*. There is also some thinning of the granule cell layer in this specimen. GC, granule cell; PRO, prosubiculum; SUB, subiculum. (Courtesy of G. W. Mathern, M.D.)

detected by high-resolution MRI scanning (Figure 13–4). Retrospective analysis of these patients reveals a high incidence of birth trauma, prolonged febrile convulsions, or head trauma. Although the hippocampus has long been recognized as one of the most vulnerable regions in the brain to insults of trauma and ischemia, the explanation for the long delay between insult and the development of seizures is only now becoming clear. Following strong seizures, there is damage to selected neurons with sprouting and reinnervation from adjacent neurons. Over time there is remodeling of local circuits resulting in a more excitable state.

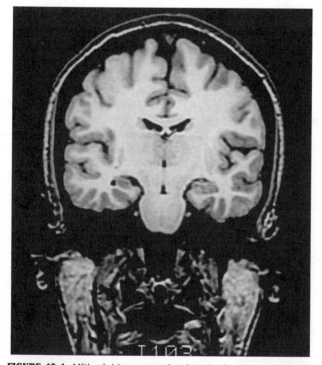

FIGURE 13–4. MRI of hippocampal sclerosis. In this patient with chronic complex partial seizures, there is characteristic sclerosis and shrinking of the left hippocampus compared with the right. (Courtesy of C. Wilson, Ph.D.)

PATHOPHYSIOLOGY

Seizures are an emergent property of neuronal circuits. As was discovered during neurosurgical operations in World War II, seizures can be induced in normal human brain. The application of penicillin directly to the cortex to prevent infection during craniotomies caused seizures. Later it was determined that the penicillin molecule blocks the receptor for the inhibitory neurotransmitter γ-aminobutyric acid (GABA). Subsequently other blockers of GABA (e.g., bicuculline), or its chloride iontophore (picrotoxin), were also found to be potent convulsants when applied to the neocortex or hippocampus of experimental animals. Conversely, pharmacological agents that potentiate gabaergic inhibition, such as the benzodiazepines and barbiturates, are potent anticonvulsants.

At the cellular level, blockade of inhibition leads to a paroxysmal depolarization shift (PDS) of the membrane potential. This results in a burst of action potentials from affected individual neurons. Research on the biochemical and biophysical events of the PDS and its transition to a full-blown seizure has revealed many basic mechanisms of seizures. One unifying hypothesis for the cause of epilepsy is the loss of inhibition within epileptic circuits. Since most insults to neurons impair their normal function, diverse conditions such as trauma, ischemia, or infection may preferentially impair and damage inhibitory interneurons or functionally isolate them from influencing other neurons. According to this hypothesis, seizures occur upon the excitation of other neurons that fire excessively owing to lack of temporal and spatial inhibitory containment.

A critical number of neurons must become synchronized into paroxysmal firing before any clinical abnormality occurs. A spike discharge on an EEG represents the synchronous firing of a small population of cortical neurons. The discharge remains contained within the cortex and does not cause symptoms (Figure 13–5). In focal motor seizures, a larger population of cortical neurons fires out of cortex and down through motor circuits to anterior horn cells in the medulla and

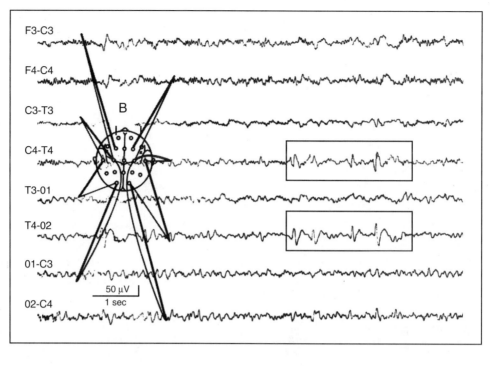

FIGURE 13–5. Interictal spikes. The sharp, high-amplitude spikes seen within the boxes are caused by synchronous paroxysmal discharges of a local population of neurons. The montage of electrodes over the skull compares the electrical activity between two points on the cortex. In this case, the montage indicates that the interictal spikes are localized to the right temporal lobe, suggesting an underlying pathological abnormality. (Reproduced, with permission, from E. W. Lothman and R. C. Collins. Seizures and epilepsy. *In* A. L. Pearlman and R. C. Collins [eds]). *Neurobiology of Disease.* New York, Oxford University Press, 1990.)

spinal cord, causing motor convulsion. A side of the face, a single digit, a limb, or an entire side of the body can be involved in the convulsion. Occasionally the convulsions will start in the hand, spread up to the shoulder and face, and then involve the leg over a 30-second period. This process involves the sequential recruitment of adjacent areas on the motor cortex into convulsive activity and is called a jacksonian march after John Hughlings Jackson, who described it in the 19th century. In other cases, a focal seizure can build in strength and spread to the other side, becoming secondarily generalized.

The projection, capture, and entrainment of neuronal circuits into abnormal epileptic discharges that recur chronically over many years are now known to involve ongoing plastic changes in circuits and synapses (Box 13–1). In patients with epilepsy, each individual seizure is nearly identical with the preceding one. This finding indicates a permanent facilitation for seizure spread within particular pathways in each patient, a phenomenon called the "conditioning effect of habitual seizures" (described by Penfield and Boldrey in 1939). Rarely it is possible to induce a focal seizure within such a pathway through sensory stimulation, a condition called reflex epilepsy. Cases are recorded in which taping a tendon induces a motor seizure of the same limb, or rarely a particular thought induces a psychomotor seizure. Photic stimulation is a well-known stimulus for absence seizures.

A change of normal anatomical pathways into highly facilitated seizure pathways can be induced in experimental animals by electrical stimulation in a paradigm called **kindling**. In a typical experiment, an electrode is placed into the limbic system of a rat (e.g., amygdala) and stimulated very briefly at a low intensity. The stimulation produces a local afterdischarge but no spread or behavioral change. After several weeks of

daily stimulation, the rat develops strong behavioral convulsions to the same stimulus. The stimulus "teaches" neuronal circuits how to become synchronized and express a seizure. The kindling hypothesis of epilepsy has gained credence through examination of the hippocampal circuits of patients operated on for intractable seizures and comparison of findings with kindled animals (Box 13–1).

EVALUATION AND DIFFERENTIAL DIAGNOSIS

The clinical evaluation of a patient suspected of having a seizure should focus on several goals. First, it is important to determine whether the clinical event under consideration represents a seizure or different type of "spell." Second, it is often possible to determine the type of seizure by its clinical phenomenology (see Table 13–1) or the presence of an epileptic syndrome (see Table 13–3). Finally, the existence of antecedent risk factors or precipitating causes should be sought. A careful history is the most important part of the evaluation, since in many cases the examination and subsequent laboratory investigation will be normal. An eyewitness description of the event represents a key piece of data, and it is always necessary to interview a family member or friend.

Upon conclusion of the history and examination, patients should have an MRI scan and routine EEG. The MRI scan aids in discovery of treatable causes of seizures such as cryptic tumors or vascular malformations. The EEG can provide supportive data and help classify a seizure disorder and direct treatment. If the EEG is normal, consideration should be given to performing a special EEG with sleep deprivation or sphenoidal leads. This approach gives a higher yield of positive abnormalities such as interictal spikes in patients with temporal lobe seizures. Since seizure discharges can be infrequent, a normal EEG does not rule out a seizure disor-

BOX 13-1 Hippocampal Sclerosis

The neuropathology of temporal lobe epilepsy is a field of intensive study because it offers the opportunity to discover the underlying cell, circuit, and molecular mechanisms of seizures in both experimental animals and humans. Over 100 years ago, two German pathologists defined the problem. Sommer proposed that hippocampal sclerosis caused seizures, while Pfleger considered that the sclerosis was the metabolic consequence of the seizures. Today it is recognized that both hypotheses were correct—seizures induce pathological changes in cells and circuits that lead to more seizures.

Patients with temporal lobe epilepsy who come to autopsy have characteristic changes in their brains called hippocampal or Ammon's horn sclerosis (Figure 13-4). The earliest lesion occurs in the hilum of the dentate gyrus with loss of mossy cells (MCs) as well as of somatostatin (SS) and neuropeptide Y (NPY)-containing-interneurons. At its fullest extent, hippocampal sclerosis includes loss of CA1 and CA3 pyramidal neurons as well, but the CA2 sector and the dentate gyrus granule cells are usually preserved. These pathological changes have been reproduced in rats by two methods. First, systemic injections of kainic acid, a rigid analog of glutamic acid, cause intense limbic system seizures. Kainic acid stimulates neurons at glutamate receptors at the synapses of the dentate gyrus mossy fibers in the dentate hilum and CA3 pyramidal layer (see figure). Second, prolonged (>12 hours) and intense electrical stimulation of the perforant pathway into the hippocampus can also damage these areas. In this event, the damage is mediated by the dentate gyrus granule cells, which are stimulated first but remain undamaged themselves.

Cytopathological studies of early lesions have given insight into epileptogenicity of the lesion. It was first proposed that there would be a loss of gabaergic interneurons in the hippocampus to explain the loss of inhibition found on electrical studies of hippocampal sclerosis. However, immunohistochemical stains revealed preservation of GABA interneurons in the dentate gyrus. Rather, there was a preferential loss of MCs and some SS and NPY interneurons as well (dotted cells in figure). The MCs are excitatory to the basket cell, a type of GABA interneuron. With removal of the MCs from the circuit, many GABA interneurons become functionally isolated, leaving the dentate gyrus granule cells relatively disinhibited.

Studies of hippocampal sclerosis have also shown sprouting of the dentate gyrus mossy fibers and other fibers within the dentate gyrus. With loss of target cells in the hilus, the granule cell axons are found to grow back into the dentate gyrus, where they reinnervate adjacent granule cells. This would provide potent feedback autoexcitation. In addition, strong stimulation of the perforant pathway into the dentate gyrus induces mossy fiber sprouting in the dentate gyrus, hilum, and CA3. Stimulus-induced mossy fiber sprouting appears to be a basic mechanism underlying the phenomenon of kindling in experimental animals and plays a role in the delayed ripening of temporal lobe seizures in humans following injury. In experimental animals, mossy fiber sprouting can be blocked by antibodies to nerve growth factors, suggesting possible new molecular genetic approaches to therapy.

Continued on opposite page

---

der. In some patients it is useful to perform telemetry, monitoring their EEG, and videotaping their behavior over several days, to determine the presence and primary site of seizure discharges. Telemetry is particularly helpful in differentiating true seizures from pseudoseizures. Special imaging with SPECT or PET scans can also be useful, particularly for localizing a seizure focus in consideration of surgery.

Several other clinical conditions cause brief spells that can be confused with seizures. In children, breath-holding spells and night terrors can usually be distinguished from seizures by observation alone or by EEG. In adults, lightheadedness and syncope are common experiences that are occasionally confused with seizures, and rarely a faint can cause a seizure (see Anoxic Seizure, above). Usually patients are standing when the faint occurs, in contrast to seizures that occur in any position. In addition, patients can usually describe the gradual alterations in sensorium that lead to a faint, whereas seizures begin abruptly without warning. Elderly patients who faint require careful cardiac evaluation including monitoring for arrhythmias. Occasionally hypoglycemia must be ruled out as a cause of a spell. Transient ischemic attacks and migraine auras are occasionally considered along with seizures as a cause of spells. In each of these conditions, the duration of symptoms is longer than the seconds or minute of a typical seizure.

TREATMENT

The goals of therapy include controlling if not eliminating seizures, avoiding toxic side effects of anticonvulsants, and maximizing the patient's educational, occupational, and social potential. The principles of treatment with anticonvulsants include (1) choosing the best drug based upon the seizure type, (2) using only one drug to achieve cessation of seizures if possible, and (3) using adequate doses commensurate with controlling seizures and avoiding toxicity. Three anticonvulsants are effective for the majority of patients (see Table 13-5). At present, of the patients who are well controlled by anticonvulsants, 48% take phenytoin, 31% carbamazepine, 13% valproic acid, and 8% other drugs.

The physician plays an important role in advising and guiding patients toward achieving a full life. Patients with epilepsy and their families require information about the causes and consequences of the disorder. Many people have a fear of epilepsy that is disproportionate to its disabling effects. The overall goal for patients should be to lead a normal life commensu-

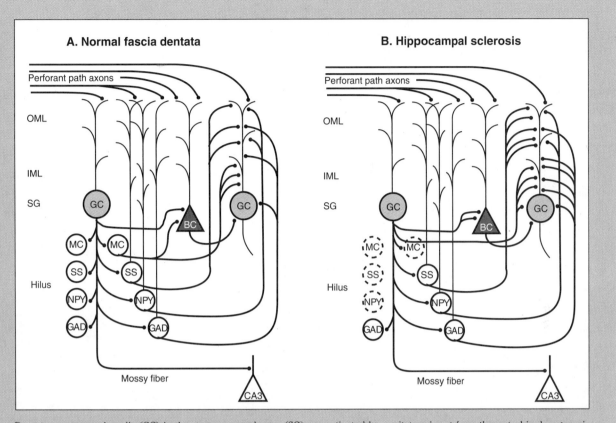

A. Normal fascia dentata

B. Hippocampal sclerosis

Dentate gyrus granule cells (GC) in the stratum granulosum (SG) are activated by excitatory input from the entorhinal cortex via the perforant pathway that ends in the outer molecular layer (OML). The granule cells send mossy fibers into CA3 of the hippocampus, giving off collaterals to basket cells (BC), mossy cells (MC), and interneurons containing somatostatin (SS), neuropeptide Y (NPY), and GABA as neurotransmitters (the latter marked GAD for the enzyme glutamic acid decarboxylase). Hippocampal sclerosis caused by prolonged febrile convulsions, status epilepticus, and perhaps other insults in humans is characterized by loss of hilus interneurons as depicted by dotted cells. As a result, the granule cells undergo sprouting and send collaterals back upon their own cells, making new excitatory synapses in the inner molecular layer (IML). This results in hyperexcitable circuits and seizures. (Reproduced, with permission, from G. W. Mathern et al. Reactive synaptogenesis and neuron densities for neuropeptide Y, somatostatin, and glutamate decarboxylase immunoreactivity in the epileptic human fascia dentata. J Neurosci 15:3990–4004, 1995.)

rate with safety for themselves and others. Education of teachers and employers is an important step in achieving these goals. The American Epilepsy Society and the International League Against Epilepsy provide useful information for the public.

Physicians and patients need to be aware of special risks associated with automobile driving. In many states, laws require physicians to report patients to the Department of Public Health if seizures cause loss of consciousness. If the Department of Motor Vehicles suspends a patient's driver's license, a successful appeal can usually be made if seizures are controlled for a period of a year or longer.

SUMMARY

Seizures are a common symptom of brain dysfunction in clinical medicine, and patients must always be evaluated for possible causes. An eyewitness description of the seizure, the clinical history and examination, and an EEG and MRI scan usually lead to the correct diagnosis and classification. There are many causes of seizures, and many of these are treatable, leading to cessation of convulsions. Research indicates that seizures change brain circuitry and potentiate the occurrence of additional seizures. Patients should be treated with anticonvulsant medications to prevent recurrent seizures, which can be physically harmful as well as disruptive of educational, social, and occupational relationships. Surgical therapy is available for some children and adults who do not respond optimally to anticonvulsants.

Selected Readings

Bone, R. C. Treatment of convulsive status epilepticus. JAMA 270:854–859, 1993.

Collins, R. C. Epilepsy: Insights into higher brain functions in humans. In *Handbook of Physiology—The Nervous System*, V, Chapter 20, pp. 811–841. Bethesda, Maryland, The American Physiological Society, 1987.

Engel, J., Jr. *Seizures and Epilepsy*. Philadelphia, F. A. Davis Co., 1989.

Lothman, E. W., and E. H. Bertram III. Epileptogenic effects of status epilepticus. Epilepsia 34(Suppl. 1):S59–S70, 1993.

Mathern, G. W., T. L. Babb, B. V. Vickrey, et al. The clinical-pathogenetic mechanisms of hippocampal neuron loss and surgical outcomes in temporal lobe epilepsy. Brain 118:105–118, 1995.

McNamara, J. O. Cellular and molecular basis of epilepsy. J Neurosci 14:3413–3425, 1994.

Sloviter, R. S. The functional organization of the hippocampal dentate gyrus and its relevance to the pathogenesis of temporal lobe epilepsy. Ann Neurol 35:640–654, 1994.

Van der Zee, C.E.E.M., K. Rashid, K. Le, et al. Intraventricular administration of antibodies to nerve growth factor retards kindling and blocks mossy fiber sprouting in adult rats. J Neurosci 15:5316–5323, 1995.

CHAPTER FOURTEEN

MULTIPLE

SCLEROSIS

INTRODUCTION 160

CLINICAL PRESENTATION 160

GENETICS 160

EPIDEMIOLOGY 163

PATHOPHYSIOLOGY 163

IMMUNOPATHOLOGY 164

EVALUATION AND DIFFERENTIAL DIAGNOSIS 167

DIAGNOSIS 169

TREATMENT 170

SUMMARY 171

INTRODUCTION

Multiple sclerosis (MS) is an immune system–mediated disease that attacks the white matter of the central nervous system and causes focal areas of demyelination. It can result in paralysis, sensory loss, and changes in mood and mentation. Although the exact cause is unknown, its autoimmune pathophysiology is well established (Table 14–1). It was first described in 1868 by Jean Martin Charcot at the Salpêtrière hospital in Paris who drew attention to the *sclerose en placques* as the pathological correlate of patients' symptoms. The disease can begin between the ages of 10 and 60 years but most commonly causes the first clinical abnormalities in young adults between the ages of 20 and 40. It affects women more than men in a ratio of approximately 1.5 to 1. The first attack often reaches its peak within hours to days and subsides in 2–6 weeks, but the subsequent clinical course is highly variable (Box 14–1).

CLINICAL PRESENTATION

The first attack of multiple sclerosis can cause limb weakness (40%), sensory symptoms (20–33%), optic neuritis (25%), brain stem symptoms and signs (10–15%), or combinations of these. Occasionally MS begins as transverse myelitis with weakness of the legs, decrease in sensation below a dermatomal level, and urinary retention. Mild sensory symptoms that last only a few days can be dismissed by a patient or even a physician and only recognized in retrospect as the first attack.

With advancing years, more complex symptoms can develop including alterations in mood with depression and the development of mild dementia. These symptoms are thought to reflect cumulative widespread involvement of hemispheric white matter. Loss of sexual function and problems with bladder and bowel control can develop early with impairment of descending spinal cord pathways, or later as a result of widespread hemispheric involvement.

Approximately 15% of patients will have a benign course following the first episode with relatively few clinical attacks and little or no disability (Figure 14–1). Sixty percent will experience a relapsing and remitting course with recurring symptoms and signs separated in space and time. Many patients experience a high re-

lapse rate early in the course of the disease with one or more attacks per year. Approximately 10 years after onset, half of these patients will begin to experience incomplete recovery from each attack and enter a chronic progressive phase of the disease. Another 15% of all MS patients have a slowly progressive course from the onset, often beginning with spinal cord involvement.

In 1955, Kurtzke developed a disability status scale for patients as a measure of the individual pace of the natural history of the disease and as a tool for judging the efficacy of new treatments in slowing or stopping its progression (Table 14–2). This scale had 10 steps for measuring change and was later expanded to 19 steps for clinical research protocols. Studies of large numbers of patients offer some general guidelines. By 15 years after onset, approximately 50% of the patients will have reached step 6, requiring a cane or other assistance to walk. Less than 20% will have reached step 7, requiring a wheelchair, and less than 5% will have died. Life expectancy at 25 years is approximately 75% of normal. These milestones apply to large populations and so cannot predict the course of a particular patient at the time of onset. Nevertheless, a more favorable course is suggested if the onset is prior to age 40, with a low attack rate of relapses and remissions in the first 5 years, and with predominately visual or sensory symptoms. Onset after age 40 with a predominance of motor signs, a high attack rate, or a progressive course are unfavorable prognostic variables.

GENETICS

A large population-based study of the incidence of MS among twins was conducted throughout the Canadian nationwide system of MS clinics in 1980–1990. The concordance rate for dizygotic twins was found to be 2–5%. This is higher than the cumulative lifetime risk of 0.02–0.1% for MS in the general population, and higher than figures for first-degree relatives of MS patients at 1–2%. Monozygotic twins were found to have concordance rates between 25% and 38% depending on the age of the patients and the use of MRI criteria for

TABLE 14–1. Evidence for Autoimmunity in Multiple Sclerosis*

Immunopathology of the plaque
Similarities to experimental allergic encephalomyelitis (EAE) in animals
Similarities to post–rabies vaccination encephalomyelitis in humans
IFN-γ causes clinical worsening in patients
Treatment with IFN-β decreases clinical worsening in patients
Immunological abnormalities
Immunogenetic background

*Data from R. Martin, H. F. McFarland, and D. E. McFarlin. Immunologic aspects of demyelinating diseases. Annu Rev Immunol 10:153–187, 1992.

TABLE 14–2. The Disability Status Scale (DSS) in Multiple Sclerosis*

0. Normal neurological examination
1. No dysfunction, minimal signs (Babinski sign, tremor, nystagmus, etc.)
2. Minimal dysfunction (slight weakness, ataxia, visuomotor disturbance)
3. Moderate dysfunction (mono- or hemiparesis, ataxia, prominent sensory, eye, bladder symptoms)
4. Relatively severe dysfunction, but up and about 12 h/d, performs normal activities of living
5. Unable to work; able to walk several blocks unaided
6. Assistance required for walking
7. Restricted to wheelchair; able to transfer
8. Restricted to bed; able to use arms
9. Totally helpless, bedridden
10. Death due to multiple sclerosis

*Data from J. Kurtzke. A new scale for evaluating disability in multiple sclerosis. Neurology 5:580–583, 1955.

BOX 14-1   A Clinical History of MS

A 37-year-old woman sought medical attention for numbness and difficulty in walking. She was referred to a neurologist by her family physician. She had been well until 6 days previously when she awoke with numbness on the left side of her face. Feeling especially tired and having no appointments, she returned to sleep for another 3 hours. When she reawakened in midmorning the numbness was more dense and additionally included the right arm and hand. Arising from bed, she discovered considerable difficulty with balance although she was able to shower, dress, and prepare breakfast. Believing this condition to be a mild ear infection following an upper respiratory infection, she decided not to seek medical attention but to "let it run its course" instead. Over the next 3 days she became worse.

Neurological consultation on day 6 found a pleasant but concerned woman who was in no acute distress. While walking into the examination suite, her gait was wide based and unsteady and she occasionally used her arms to counterbalance unexpected lurches away from her center of gravity. She joked upon greeting the neurologist, "you probably think I've been drinking!"

She gave a clear history during the interview without any evidence of difficulty with language, articulation, cognition, or memory. Her own observations consisted of numbness of the left face and right arm and hand, inability to close her left eye, double vision on looking to the left, and difficulty in walking for reasons of imbalance. The symptoms had progressed in the first 2–3 days but then stabilized. There had been no headache or facial pain, fever, or stiff neck.

Her past history was of interest for her having had an episode of difficulty with vision in her left eye at age 19 while a college student. The campus physician assured her it was a case of "neuritis" and that it would resolve in 2 weeks, which it did. No investigations were performed at that time. There was no other pertinent history to suggest prior neurological illness, cardiovascular disease, systemic lupus erythematosus, or infection. There was no history of neurological illness in the family.

The neurological examination confirmed the evidence of dysfunction of the left side of the brain stem. There was decreased appreciation of light cotton touch and pinprick on the left side of the face, a depressed corneal reflex (cranial nerve V), and decreased movement of the left facial muscles upon command with incomplete eye closure (cranial nerve VII). Left lateral gaze was incomplete with poor abduction of the left eye (cranial nerve VI). There was a slight decrease in appreciation of touch, movement, and pinprick on the right hand and forearm (crossed ascending sensory pathways). Strength was preserved throughout all extremities to resistive testing. Coordinative movements were slightly impaired in the right upper and lower extremities compared to the left side and she was unable to perform a tandem walk without falling to either side (pontocerebellar pathways). The knee and ankle reflexes on the right side were more active than on the left, and there was a right Babinski sign (left descending pyramidal tract for the right extremities).

The clinical evidence indicated a subacute 3-day process in the left lateral brain stem with ipsilateral and crossed signs. The diagnostic possibilities included infection (brain stem encephalitis), vascular disease (lupus vasculitis), and multiple sclerosis. The prior episode of transient visual loss favored a diagnosis of MS with lesions separated in space and time. After discussion, she agreed to proceed with an MRI scan and lumbar puncture. The MRI scan revealed multiple lesions in hemispheric and brain stem white matter. The former were located around the ventricles as well as above and perpendicular to the corpus callosum. There were several brain stem lesions in the midbrain and pons. The pontine lesion was enhanced with gadolinium. The lumbar puncture did not reveal any white cells, and the total protein was normal at 40 mg/dL. There was an increase in CSF IgG, and there were oligoclonal bands on gel electrophoresis. The clinical and laboratory data provided clear evidence for a diagnosis of definite multiple sclerosis.

Over the next 3 months, the symptoms and signs of brain stem dysfunction slowly resolved without treatment. She returned to her work in an art studio after 2 months. For the next 3 years, she was not bothered in her daily activities except for occasional recurring feelings of fatigue lasting for several days or a week at a time. During these episodes, she felt she had difficulty concentrating on her work and that her walking became somewhat worse. On each occasion, she returned to a fuller sense of well being after the episode. These vague spells possibly represented exacerbations in hemispheric white matter, but they were not investigated or treated.

Her annual visit at age 41 occurred 22 years after her initial optic neuritis and 4 years after her major relapse with brain stem involvement. She had not had any more dramatic exacerbations, but her overall neurological function had deteriorated slightly. She observed that her mental skills were not as sharp as they had been although there was nothing she could point to in particular. Simple mental status testing revealed slowness and uncertainty in mathematical calculations and spelling. Her mood was normal. There was a titubating tremor of her head and body while sitting, and her gait was both mildly ataxic and stiff. There were increased tone and reflexes in her legs with bilateral Babinski signs. Her walking was slow and mildly unsteady and she chose to use a cane. She had obtained a disability pass for parking her car and had moved into an apartment with central air conditioning to avoid hot weather. She continued to work steadily as an artist and had participated in several group shows. She was active socially but had noticed a decrease in her sexual feelings.

Comment. This history represents a typical case of multiple sclerosis, beginning at age 19 with a bout of optic neuritis, then relapsing clinically at age 37 with a brain stem lesion. Evaluation at that time indicated far more evidence for disease on the MRI scan than was appreciated clinically or that had caused any clear abnormalities in her personal history to that time. On the disability status scale (Table 14–2), this patient would be ranked at step 3. After her diagnosis, she read widely about MS and discussed clinical trials as well as new therapies with her neurologist but concluded she would maintain close contact and wait for the ultimate "breakthrough."

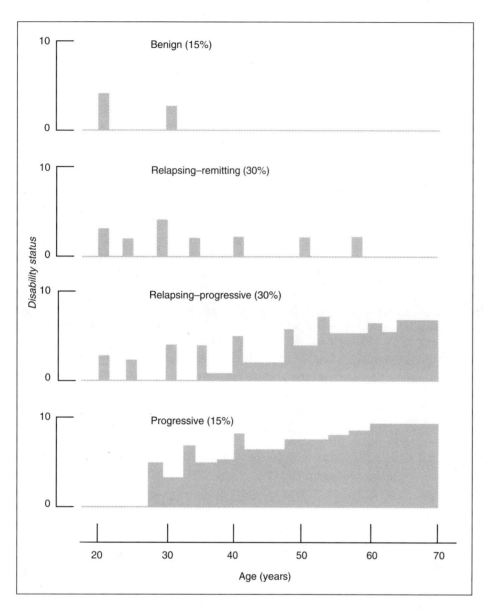

FIGURE 14-1. The clinical profile of MS can be quite variable over time. At one extreme, a patient may have one or two attacks only, a pattern called benign MS. At the other extreme, a patient may experience relentless progression of disability without remission. The clinical profile depends on plaque formation in critical functional systems. Since small plaques can also occur in hemispheric white matter without causing overt symptoms, the true biological pace of the illness is best measured by serial MRI scans.

inclusion. While these data indicate a strong genetic component as an etiological factor for MS, they also indicate the importance of environmental factors, since the majority of monozygotic pairs of twins are discordant. The differences between the concordance rates for monozygotic versus dizygotic twins indicate that two or more genes are involved rather than a single autosomal dominant or recessive gene.

Investigators have been interested in a variety of candidate genes in MS including those for immunoglobulins, the T-cell receptor, myelin basic protein, and the HLA (human leukocyte antigen) class II molecules. The only consistent finding has been an increased frequency of the Dw2 HLA haplotype in patients with MS compared with controls. The finding is more robust in families of northern European descent than outside of Europe and is more robust in multiplex families with many affected members than in families with isolated MS cases. In high-incidence families, the increased incidence of the Dw2 haplotype can be two to three times that of control populations.

The HLA genetic locus is on the short arm of chromosome 6. The class I genes are located telometrically, and the class II genes are closer to the centromere (Figure 14–2). There are three major loci for the coding of the α- and β-chains of the class II molecules, called DP, DQ, and DR. The genes located here are among the most polymorphic genes known in humans. For example, there are at least 71 known DR β-chain alleles, 21 DQ β-chain alleles, and 10 for the DQ α-chain site. Macrophages express class II molecules on their surface, which is important for the presentation of antigen to T lymphocytes. The extreme genetic polymorphism among these surface proteins probably reflects the success of different evolutionary strategies among different families for combating infection. The Dw2 haplotype in MS is known as DR15,DQ6 by serological nomenclature and as DRB1*1501,DQA1*0102,DQB1*0602 in genomic nomenclature.

The influence of this genetic locus on MS is uncertain. It is not required for developing the illness, nor is it sufficient. The Dw2 haplotype is also increased in

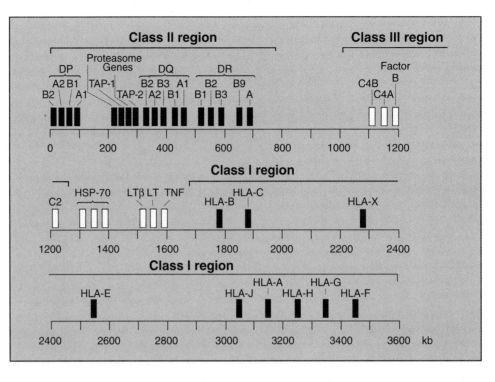

FIGURE 14-2. The HLA locus is found on the short arm of chromosome 6 where many different genic sites are associated with the immune response in addition to the class I and class II regions. C2, C4A, and B and factor B are complement proteins. HSP-70 is a heat-shock protein. Lymphotoxin (LT), lymphotoxin-β (LTβ), and tumor necrosis factor (TNF) are cytokine genes. TAP, transporter antigen processing. (Reproduced, with permission, from A. K. Abbas, A. H. Lichtman, and J. S. Pober. *Cellular and Molecular Immunology*, 2nd ed. Philadelphia, W.B. Saunders Co., 1994.)

narcolepsy, which is not an immune-mediated condition. While its presence clearly plays a role, some investigators suggest that its influence may be only 10% among all MS patients, leaving open the search for other genetic as well as environmental factors.

EPIDEMIOLOGY

The distribution of multiple sclerosis throughout the world varies widely. The prevalence of the disease is higher in temperate zones compared with equatorial zones. In addition, in racially homogeneous populations such as Australia and New Zealand, the prevalence of MS increases with increasing latitude. For example, the prevalence in Waikato, North Island, New Zealand, is 27.9/100,000, whereas in Otago, South Island, it is 79.4. The prevalence is higher in the northern part of the United States, generally 60–70, compared with the southern states, 10–30. The highest rates are found in Sweden (130), northern Scotland (144), and the Shetland (170) and Orkney (224) islands. Curiously, there is evidence for an increased prevalence in Rochester, Minnesota, increasing over the last 70 years from 46 in 1915, to 108 in 1978, to 173 in 1985. It is not clear whether this finding represents a true increase in incidence or improved diagnostic techniques and case ascertainment.

The interpretation of prevalence data is not straightforward and cannot be used to support simple theories of infectious or genetic causes of MS. For instance, the latitudinal distribution of cases cannot be explained by the distribution of an infectious agent, since there are many exceptions among different populations. For example, the prevalence of MS among Asians is much lower than among other populations living at the same latitude. In Japan the prevalence is 1–4 cases per 100,000, approximately 10% of the prevalence of populations at similar latitudes in the United States and Europe. The prevalence of MS among Eskimos is low despite their northern latitude. Conversely, the high incidence of MS in Rochester, Minnesota, compared with other sites at a similar latitude may reflect the predominant Scandinavian origin of the population instead of, or in addition to, local environmental factors.

Some epidemiological studies have suggested that migrating populations will carry the incidence of MS from their region of origin if they move after the age of 15 but will adopt the incidence of the new region if they move in childhood. These data from studies of people who have emigrated from Britain to South Africa or Israel after World War II suggest an environmental influence such as infection with a latent virus prior to the age of puberty. However, these studies have been criticized on methodological grounds for drawing inferences from small sample sizes and for failing to account for ethnic and genetic variables among the migrants. Epidemiological studies have provided fascinating data for analysis, but the complexity of potential environmental and genetic factors makes it difficult to reach secure conclusions regarding etiology at present.

PATHOPHYSIOLOGY

The symptoms and signs of MS reflect abnormalities in central myelinated pathways. During an acute phase of an attack, a focal area of inflammation develops with disruption of the blood-brain barrier and edema causing local conduction block of impulses

**TABLE 14–3. Abnormalities of Functional Pathways
in Multiple Sclerosis**

Functional Pathway	Signs and Symptoms
Pyramidal system	Spastic weakness: mono-, hemi-, or paraparesis; Babinski sign
Cerebellar pathways	Gait ataxia; intention tremor
Brain stem pathways	Dysarthria, dysphagia, diplopia, nystagmus; facial weakness, sensory loss; crossed sensory or motor signs
Sensory systems	Loss of touch, vibration, position sense; pain in face, hand, foot, truncal band; tingling paresthesias
Visual system	Central scotoma, blindness; hemianopia
Bladder and bowel	Hesitancy, urgency, frequency, retention; incontinence
Cerebral white matter	Alterations in mood and mentation

along fiber pathways. Negative symptoms result. With time, there is a resolution of the acute phase in which the recovery of function coincides with the removal of harmful inflammatory cytokines and edema. Demyelination is an active component of the lesion, but axons are largely spared. Destruction and removal of the myelin sheath result in the loss of the fast saltatory conduction of impulses. In addition, the denuded axon undergoes changes in the distribution of sodium and potassium channels, resulting in a loss of conduction efficiency and failure of propagation. These demyelinated axons are particularly sensitive to increased temperature (fever, high ambient temperature) and changes in calcium and other electrolyte levels, which can cause temporary fluctuations in the expression of symptoms.

Early in the course of the disease, the attacks typically present as a simple loss of function such as monocular blindness (optic neuritis), weakness, numbness, ataxia, or diplopia depending on the pathway affected (Table 14–3). Positive symptoms can also occur, especially as the disease progresses. These can become manifest as simple tingling paresthesias in the face, hand, or foot or as a band sensation around a thoracic dermatome, or they can be quite dramatic such as the occurrence of paroxysmal facial pain similar to trigeminal neuralgia, tonic extensor spasms of the legs, or Lhermitte's sign. These brief, positive symptoms are thought to reflect abnormal initiation and local ephaptic spread of discharges among demyelinated axons in sensory or motor pathways. Lhermitte's sign occurs as a feeling of "electric" discharge down the back and into the legs upon flexion of the neck. It probably reflects local stretching of the spinal cord and the posterior columns causing generation of discharges from a local lesion. It is common but not specific for MS and occurs in the presence of other causes of local damage such as cervical spondylosis.

IMMUNOPATHOLOGY

The precise immunological steps that occur during an acute attack of MS and the development and evolu-

tion of the demyelinated brain lesion are not fully known. Nevertheless, in the last several years advances in molecular immunology applied both to the study of acute plaques from human brains and to animal models of MS in inbred strains of rodents (experimental allergic encephalomyelitis [EAE], Box 14–2) have allowed development of a coherent story that permits testing new hypotheses relevant to etiology and treatment.

The first abnormality that occurs is the attachment of sensitized lymphocytes to postcapillary venules in white matter. It is not clear what initiates this event. It is now appreciated that lymphocytes can move in and out of the brain without causing damage, perhaps in some type of monitoring activity or "immune surveillance." In experimental animals, when lymphocytes are sensitized to brain tissue antigens they enter the brain and stay. In addition, sensitized lymphocytes can initiate a series of events that cause the up-regulation of adhesion molecules on vascular endothelium leading to the attraction and intraparenchymal migration of additional blood cells. It is important to recognize that a few lymphocytes sensitized to brain antigens can initiate the full cascade of cellular and humoral events associated with inflammation and host defense (Figure 14–3). In contrast to MS, during infections of the brain this inflammatory response attacks and clears foreign pathogens and does not lead to demyelination, even when the myelin membrane becomes damaged and exposed. A basic goal of research is to discover what steps are involved in the initiation and perpetuation of autoimmune demyelination in MS.

There have been many hypotheses concerning the cause of MS. Viruses have long been attractive candidates, since several cause demyelination in humans. The JC papovavirus causes demyelination by destroying oligodendrocytes in a disease called progressive multifocal leukoencephalopathy (PML). This latent viral infection occurs in immunosuppressed patients such as those with cancer of the reticuloendothelial system or AIDS. The pathological features of PML do not resemble those of MS.

Postinfectious encephalomyelitis is an immune-mediated demyelinating illness that follows viral infections. It is most common following measles in children under 2 years of age, ~1/1000 cases. The pathological lesions show perivascular lymphocytes and focal demyelination. Lymphocytes show activation against myelin proteins. Surviving patients often have permanent deficits. The pathological features resemble those of MS, but there is no relapsing-remitting course following this monophasic illness. The association of measles with MS remains intriguing, since a majority of MS patients have an increased titer of measles antibody (among others) in their CSF compared with controls.

Whereas there is currently no evidence for a specific viral cause of MS, it is clear that incidental viral infections in patients with MS can be associated with worsening. Approximately one-third of patients will relapse following an upper respiratory infection. Environmental factors such as viral or other infections probably stimulate an abnormal immune response in MS patients as part of a nonspecific activation of host defense

BOX 14-2   Experimental Allergic Encephalomyelitis

Experimental allergic encephalomyelitis (EAE) is an autoimmune disease of white matter that can be induced in mice, rats, guinea pigs, and primates. Immunization of these animals with myelin basic protein (MBP), myelin-associated glycoprotein (MAG), myelin-oligodendrocyte protein (MOG), or proteolipid protein (PLP) in complete Freund's adjuvant causes an encephalitis of brain and spinal cord resulting in paralysis. MBP has been studied extensively. The illness is monophasic in some inbred strains of rodents and relapsing-remitting in others. Pathologically there is perivenular infiltration of lymphocytes and macrophages with demyelination. The disease can be transferred to naive animals via lymphocytes but not serum. The T-cell lymphocytes conferring disease are specific for MBP, and they are CD4+ and belong to the IL-2– and IFN-γ–producing subset of T helper cells (Th$_1$; Figure 14-3). For reasons of the similarity between the clinical, pathological, and immune features of EAE and MS, there is great interest in exploring the molecular mechanisms and potential treatments of EAE.

It is not clear why immunization of experimental animals with autologous myelin produces autoimmunity. One suggestion is that T cells sensitive to myelin proteins were not deleted during thymic maturation. Transgenic mice engineered to express MBP-specific T-cell receptor escape clonal deletion during development. It is now known that lymphoid tissue expresses an isomer of myelin basic protein in the periphery, raising the possibility that sensitization and activation occur outside the nervous system but become secondarily magnified in brain white matter.

Different animal strains show different selective vulnerability to various epitopes of MBP. For example, in PL/J mice the nine N-terminal amino acids are encephalogenic only if the terminal amino acid is acetylated. Treatment with a nonacetylated peptide blocks the disease. Alanine substitution at position 4 enhances binding of the peptide to the class II MHC molecules, and alanine substitution at position 3 abolishes recognition of the peptide by MBP-sensitized T cells. Treatment of animals with an alanine-substituted peptide at the 3 and 4 positions at the time of adoptive transfer of EAE by peptide-specific T-cell clones blocks the development of disease. Thus, in these inbred strains where there is relatively limited heterogeneity of expression of class II MHC molecules and T-cell receptor molecules, it is possible to rationally engineer specific peptides for immunotherapy. In this case, the synthetic peptide presumably binds tightly to the MHC locus of antigen-presenting cells but blocks recognition by CD4+ lymphocytes. Following this lead, peptides have been synthesized with random sequences of four amino acids common in MBP—alanine, glutamate, lysine, and tyrosine. A mixture of such peptides (MW 14,000–23,000) is called copolymer 1 (Cop 1). This strategy recognizes the complex heterogeneity of class II MHC molecules in outbred species like humans. In this outbred setting, it would not be likely that a single highly specific peptide would block all possible trimolecular interactions. Evidence indicates that Cop 1 may also act through the antigen-specific production of suppressor T cells. Clinical trials with Cop 1 indicate that it can suppress the number and severity of relapses.

Other studies in PL mice have found some limited expression of T-cell receptor molecules during EAE, specifically an increase in the expression of V-β 8.2 and V-α 4.3. Treatment of animals with a monoclonal antibody to deplete V-β 8.2+ T cells prevents development of the disease and reverses neurological dysfunction in animals with the disease. The use of antibodies or immunization strategies to deplete CD4+ T cells in humans is under investigation.

EAE can also be blocked or ameliorated by two other immune therapies. First, inbred LE rats can be made tolerant to MBP by feeding them large amounts of the protein. This effect may be related to an MBP epitope different from the encephalogenetic site, and CD8+ T cells may be involved. Second, TGF-β is a cytokine released by T cells that has a pronounced antiinflammatory role inhibiting macrophages and cytotoxic T cells. Small amounts can block EAE in both rats and mice. In humans, separate clinical trials are directed at testing the efficacy of both oral myelin and injections of TGF-β.

---

mechanisms. Of note, transgenic mice with T-cell receptors recognizing myelin will not develop autoimmune demyelination if they are raised in a germ-free environment.

Another hypothesis for the cause of MS focuses on the possibility of abnormal immune regulation. Considerable effort is directed at determining whether patients are abnormally sensitized to specific brain antigens, particularly those associated with proteins of the myelin sheath—myelin basic protein (MBP), myelin-associated glycoprotein (MAG), myelin-oligodendrocyte protein (MOG), and proteolipid protein (PLP) (Box 14-2). Isomers of MBP are synthesized in lymphoid tissue, raising the possibility that the sensitization of lymphocytes may occur initially outside the CNS. One isomer contains an exon that is expressed only during early myelination and remyelination. Autoimmune attack on this form of MBP could play a role in reactivated and chronic lesions. Although it may not be part of the initial attack of MS, this isomer and other antigenic sites may become involved through a process of epitope spreading as the disease advances.

The immune response of identical twins concordant and discordant for MS has been studied to determine whether the affected twin has abnormal cellular immunity compared with the unaffected twin. These studies provide the best type of control for the genetic diversity found among patients selected at large. No important differences were found among twin cases and controls in studies of peripheral blood for the frequency of MBP-sensitized lymphocytes, epitope specificity, or HLA restriction. Other studies focus on whether T lymphocytes in MS lesions are restricted in regard to which V α- or β-chain of the T-cell receptor is used. These studies, similar to those which explore the linkage between HLA genes and disease susceptibility, add evidence to immunogenetic factors playing a role in the etiology of MS.

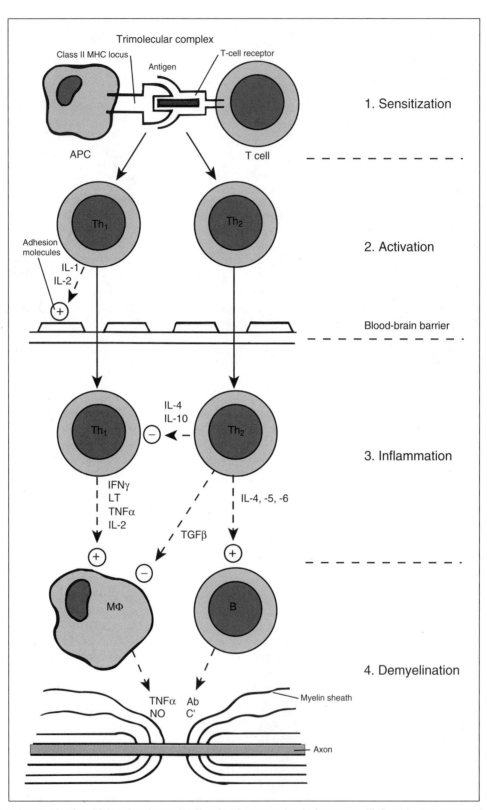

FIGURE 14–3. The pathogenesis of multiple sclerosis can be thought of as occurring in four steps. (1) Sensitization occurs when a CD4+ class II MHC antigen-presenting cell (APC) presents an antigen to a T lymphocyte. The exact antigen in MS is unknown, but proteins from the myelin sheath are the most potent antigens for inducing experimental allergic encephalomyelitis in animals (see Box 14–2). (2) Activation involves the proliferation of sensitized T cells. Both sensitization and activation may begin in the periphery, but they become magnified within the brain owing to stimulation of other lymphocytes and glial cells by lymphokines (dashed lines). (3) Inflammation is mediated by Th₁ cells and macrophages (MΦ), which cause breakdown in the blood-brain barrier and tissue edema. The inflammatory edema blocks nerve conduction, resulting in symptoms. The factors involved in the inflammatory stage are not specific for MS. (4) Demyelination is mediated by TNFα, nitric oxide (NO), antibodies (Ab) from B cells, and complement (C′).

Once activated lymphocytes cross the vascular endothelium and enter the white matter, they initiate a cellular inflammatory process. Studies on experimental allergic encephalomyelitis and fresh plaques in humans indicate that macrophages with the class II major histocompatibility complex (class II MHC) play a prominent role. Through presentation of antigen to CD4+ T cells, they initiate the expression of potent cytokines that recruit and stimulate additional lymphocytes (see Figure 14–3). Some of these factors, such as the interleukins IL-1 and IL-2, serve mainly to up-regulate adhesion molecules and stimulate other lymphocytes. Other factors secreted by T helper cells such as LT (lymphotoxin), TNF-α (tumor necrosis factor alpha), and IFN-γ (gamma interferon) can cause tissue damage and stimulate the expression of class II molecules on astrocytes and microglia. These potent factors have been found in human lesions and CSF. An acute lesion is characterized by lytic dissolution of the myelin membrane with phagocytosis of myelin debris by macrophages. The production of nitric oxide is an important part of this destructive process. Immunoglobulin may play a role in attaching the myelin fragments to the macrophage membrane.

The acute lesion usually persists for several weeks with resolution often beginning by one month. Cytokines such as IL-10 and TGF-β (transforming growth factor beta), which inhibit inflammatory processes, may play a role in stopping the attack. At this point, macrophages no longer stain positive for myelin debris but show a foamy sudanophilic cytoplasm representing partially digested lipids. This recovering lesion also shows evidence of remyelination with axons exhibiting thin, short segments of myelin membrane (Figure 14–4). There is reasonable speculation that, if this lesion does not experience a second wave of inflammation, the thinly remyelinated plaque will survive as a shadow plaque, allowing some, albeit slower, conduction of impulses through this zone. The ability of some plaques to remyelinate is of great interest with regard to potential therapies. Some evidence indicates that oligodendrocytes can survive a single acute attack; other evidence shows that they subsequently proliferate or differentiate from precursor cells. The identification of cytokines or growth factors that play a role in oligodendrocyte function is under investigation.

Brains of patients with a long history of MS show many chronic plaques that are white and hard to the touch on gross inspection. Histologically these plaques have centers that are devoid of myelin. Reactive macrophages are replaced by fibrillary astrocytes and gliosis. The peripheral rim of the plaque may show abortive attempts at remyelination. These plaques may be the result of several recurring attacks in the same place, as is now appreciated from studying serial MRI scans in patients (Figure 14–5).

EVALUATION AND DIFFERENTIAL DIAGNOSIS

MRI is a potent tool in the diagnosis and clinical study of MS. In contrast to CT, MRI results in prominent demonstration of even small lesions in the white matter in brain, spinal cord, and optic nerve. Multifocal lesions

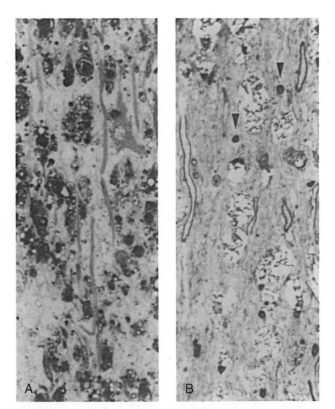

FIGURE 14–4. Pathological evolution of the MS plaque. In *A*, a recently active plaque, axons are naked and stain darkly, glial fibers are sparse, cells with round nuclei (mostly oligodendrocytes) are difficult to identify, and macrophages are filled with toluidine blue–positive myelin particles. By contrast, in *B*, from a remyelinating shadow plaque from the same patient, the conspicuous watery compartment evident in *A* is occupied by glial fibers, oligodendrocytes have appeared (arrowheads), toluidine blue–positive myelin sheaths are present on axons that now stain palely, and macrophages are filled with unstained lipids ($\times$340 before 21% reduction). (Reproduced, with permission of Little, Brown and Company, from J. W. Prineas, R. O. Barnard, E. E. Kwon, et al. Multiple sclerosis: Remyelination of nascent lesions. Ann Neurol 33:137–151, 1993.)

are seen in MS but can also be found in systemic lupus erythematosus, Behçet's syndrome, sarcoidosis, Sjögren's syndrome, and leuko-arteriolar sclerosis in the elderly. The MS lesions follow the distribution of plaques found in pathological studies with a predominance in the hemispheric white matter, particularly in periventricular zones. In addition, the use of gadolinium-enhanced scans allows detection of new lesions where there is breakdown of the blood-brain barrier during acute inflammation. Because many of these are small (<10 mm) and located in deep cortical white matter, they do not always produce overt symptoms. In clinically sensitive white matter pathways such as the optic nerve, the duration of gadolinium enhancement correlates with the development of clinical abnormalities, and the onset of recovery usually begins with the end of gadolinium enhancement. Serial monthly scans of patients have revealed new lesions or expanding lesions at rates 5–10 times the attack rates for new clinical symptoms (see Figure 14–5). These imaging data confirm autopsy studies in patients that demonstrate more lesions pathologically than were appreciated clin-

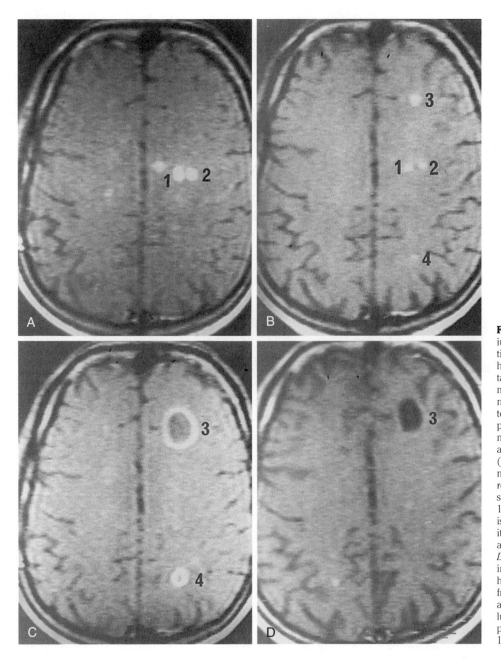

FIGURE 14–5. Serial monthly gadolinium-enhanced MRI scans in a patient with MS. These views of the hemispheres show how small attacks can come and go on a monthly basis. These lesions might not have caused any overt symptoms. *A,* Two enhancing lesions are present in the right parietal white matter. *B,* A month later, lesions 1 and 2 are smaller and a new lesion (3) has appeared in frontal white matter. Enhancement of lesion 4 represents reactivation of a previous lesion. *C,* Another month later, lesions 1 and 2 no longer enhance, lesion 3 is larger with ring enhancement at its expanding edge, and lesion 4 is also bigger with ring enhancement. *D,* At 4 months, lesion 3 is smaller in size and lesion 4 no longer enhances. (Adapted, with permission, from W. I. McDonald, D. H. Miller, and D. Barnes. The pathological evolution of multiple sclerosis. Neuropathol Appl Neurobiol 18:319–334, 1992.)

ically, as well as postmortem studies showing typical plaques in persons unsuspected of having MS during life. In patients with MS, careful quantitative measurements of these enhancing lesions on serial scans have yielded a correlation between increased frequency and area and clinical worsening (Figure 14–6).

The evidence from MRI scanning has changed traditional concepts about the natural history of the illness. Whereas patients might be divided clinically into relapsing-remitting and chronic-progressive categories, serial imaging indicates that the disease is more active on a continuous basis than can be appreciated from analysis of symptoms and signs alone. The differences among patients clinically reflect differences both in the pace of the disease and, more importantly, the likelihood that any particular lesion will affect a clinically sensitive pathway. For example, a patient with a small new lesion

in the brain stem will have overt symptoms indicating progression on clinical scales, whereas another patient might have several new larger lesions in the hemisphere indicating more aggressive disease but the progression could go undetected clinically. Clinical trials now use MRI analysis as well as clinical scales to judge progression and treatment efficacy.

Evoked potential studies can be useful in MS but they are neither as sensitive nor as comprehensive as MRI scans in identifying new lesions. The technique involves repetitive stimulation of a sensory pathway while measuring the speed and amplitude of the response as it arrives at the cortex. Somatosensory, auditory, or visual pathways can be studied. The visual evoked response (VER) is most commonly tested in patients suspected of having MS. Patients sit comfortably in front of a monitor that flashes on and off,

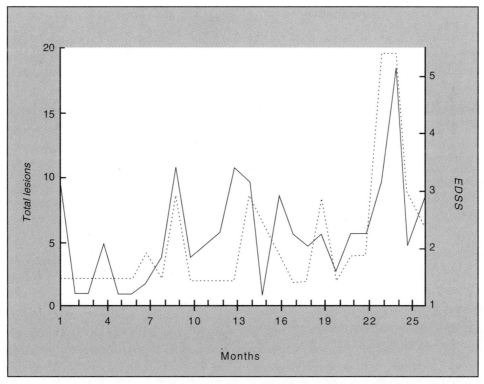

FIGURE 14–6. Correlation of changes in the number of total gadolinium-enhanced lesions (solid line) with changes in a patient's clinical activity (broken line) as measured by the expanded disability status scale (EDSS). (Adapted, with permission of Little, Brown and Company, from M. E. Smith, L. A. Stone, P. S. Albert, et al. Clinical worsening in multiple sclerosis is associated with increased frequency and area of gadopentetate dimeglumine–enhancing magnetic resonance imaging lesions. Ann Neurol 33:480–489, 1993.)

repetitively stimulating the visual system. The arrival of the cortical evoked peak is measured through occipital EEG leads and summed over time. In patients with previous optic neuritis, there will be prolongation of the latency of the cortical peak compared with normative data and compared with the patient's uninvolved eye. This finding reflects the slowness of conduction through demyelinated pathways in which saltatory conduction is lost, or through remyelinated zones where the internode distance is shortened. The test is not specific for MS, since other types of visual pathway lesions (tumor, stroke, etc.) can also produce slowing.

Cerebrospinal fluid analysis is an important component of clinical evaluation in patients suspected of having MS, particularly when the history and examination are equivocal and MRI is inconclusive. The abnormalities found in the spinal fluid in MS reflect *de novo* synthesis of immunoglobulin in the brain associated with immune-mediated illness. There is an elevated level of immunoglobulin G (IgG) and the presence of oligoclonal bands on gel electrophoresis. These findings clearly indicate the presence of an immune or infectious condition and would eliminate considerations of vascular, degenerative, and other disease processes from the differential diagnosis. These findings are not specific for MS but also can occur in viral infections, Lyme disease, sarcoidosis, and neurosyphilis. In many of these other conditions, the increase in immunoglobulin synthesis reflects antibodies directed against a specific organism or antigen. Cell counts in CSF are usually negative or only slightly elevated with

a preponderance of lymphocytes. A cell count >30 should raise suspicion of an illness other than MS.

DIAGNOSIS

The diagnosis of MS rests upon the clinical history, examination, and laboratory studies. There is no specific diagnostic test. In 1983, clinical investigators studying potential new therapies developed diagnostic criteria for *definite* and *probable* MS (Table 14–4) in order to assure patient homogeneity in different studies. These definitions reflect the need to determine two separate attacks at two separate anatomical sites in CNS white matter. Each attack must last longer than 24 hours, and the attacks must be separated by a month. For example, a 35-year-old patient may present with spastic weakness of the lower extremities that indicates a spinal cord lesion. If the evaluation also reveals evidence of a prior occurrence of optic neuritis, then there would be two white matter lesions separated in space and time indicative of clinically definite MS. Without clinical evidence of a prior episode, laboratory evidence of another lesion by MRI or evoked potentials along with an abnormal CSF immunoglobulin would satisfy the criteria for laboratory-supported definite MS.

Diagnostic criteria are important for individual patient evaluations and consultations as well as for clinical trials. Patients seeking a firm diagnosis can be told whether or not they fulfill diagnostic criteria for definite or probable MS at any given time. This is important for their own personal and professional plans, for consider-

TABLE 14-4. Diagnostic Classification of Multiple Sclerosis*

Clinically definite MS
  Two attacks and clinical evidence of two separate lesions *or*
  Two attacks, clinical evidence of one lesion, and laboratory evidence of another lesion
Laboratory-supported definite MS
  Two attacks, either clinical or laboratory evidence of one lesion, and CSF IgG or oligoclonal bands *or*
  One attack, clinical evidence of two separate lesions, and CSF IgG or oligoclonal bands *or*
  One attack, clinical evidence of one lesion and laboratory evidence of another, and CSF IgG or oligoclonal bands
Clinically probable MS
  Two attacks and clinical evidence of one lesion *or*
  One attack and clinical evidence of two separate lesions *or*
  One attack, clinical evidence of one lesion, and laboratory evidence of another
Laboratory-supported probable MS
  Two attacks and CSF IgG or oligoclonal bands
Note: The two attacks must involve different parts of the nervous system, must be separated by 1 month, and must each have lasted at least 24 hours.

*Data from C. M. Poser, D. W. Paty, L. Scheinberg, et al. New diagnostic criteria for research protocols. Ann Neurol 13:227–231, 1983.

ations of consultation regarding further symptoms, and for decisions regarding available or experimental therapy. Securing a diagnosis can end doubt and allow patient and family to focus on education, therapy, and support.

TREATMENT

At present there is no known cure for MS. Therapy is directed at immunosuppression, relief from disabling physical and emotional symptoms, and physical and occupational rehabilitation (Table 14–5).

Immunosuppression is the primary form of treatment for MS and includes use of broad-spectrum agents as well as some that are highly selective for specific components of the immune response. Treatment strategies are similar to those for other idiopathic autoimmune diseases such as lupus erythematosus. Since in relapsing-remitting diseases there is always the possibility of spontaneous improvement, the efficacy of any treatment must be proved by carefully controlled clinical trials.

Broad-spectrum Immunosuppression. ACTH and glucocorticoids have been used in MS since the 1950s. A double-blind control trial of ACTH showed its effectiveness in increasing the speed of recovery from an exacerbation but it had no significant effect on the degree of recovery or on long-term outcome. Corticosteroid preparations have not proved effective in preventing relapses or slowing the course of disease. In patients with optic neuritis, the use of prednisone was associated with an increase in relapses, whereas intravenous methylprednisolone was not. Many neurologists use steroids to hasten a patient's recovery from an acute attack, commonly prescribing 3–5 days of intravenous methylprednisolone followed by 7–10 days of oral prednisone. Glucocorticoids have a great variety of immunosuppressive actions, including inhibiting the

secretion of TNF-α, IL-2, IL-6, and INF-γ. Long-term daily use of high-dose steroids is associated with significant side effects, including weight gain, diabetes, hypertension, osteoporosis, compression fracture, gastrointestinal complications, and psychological disturbances and should not be prescribed for MS (see Table 14–5).

A variety of antinucleotides have been tried or are under investigation. These include inhibitors of nucleic acid synthesis (azathioprine), antifolates (methotrexate), and alkylating agents (cyclophosphamide and chlorambucil). These wide-spectrum agents can be associated with considerable toxicity, and none has proved of significant value. Cyclosporine has been tried, since it interferes with cytokine secretion, and 2-chlorodeoxyadenosine (cladribine) is under investigation since it is a lymphotoxin. Results are uncertain at present.

Selective Immunosuppression. The first agent to prove beneficial in MS was IFNB (β-interferon). In a double-blind, placebo-controlled trial of two doses, IFNB was given subcutaneously every other day for 2 years. Results indicated a decrease in the frequency and severity of clinical relapses as well as a decrease in the total area of lesions on MRI. A dose effect was apparent. In a 6-week study of a cohort of these patients there was also a decrease in the appearance of new, recurrent, and enlarging lesions on MRI in treated patients compared with controls. Despite these positive results there was little difference in the clinical disability among the patient groups, perhaps owing to the insensitivity of the disability status scale or the short duration of the study.

IFNB is thought to work in part by inhibiting the production of IFN-γ by activated lymphocytes. While IFN-γ has toxic effects on the blood-brain barrier and myelin and stimulates the expression of the MHC on macrophages and astrocytes, IFNB is also thought to

TABLE 14-5. Treatment of Multiple Sclerosis

Immunosuppression

Acute Attack	Methylprednisolone, 1 g IV daily for 3–5 days, followed by oral prednisone, 60 mg tapering over 2 weeks. Speeds recovery.
Prophylaxis	IFNB, 8 million international units subcutaneously every other day. Lessens attacks by ~30%. Side effects include injection site pain, flu-like illness, headache.
	Copolymer 1, 20 mg subcutaneously daily. Lessens attacks by ~30%. Side effects include chest tightness.

Symptomatic Treatment

Spasticity	Diazepam, 5–50 mg/d
	Baclofen, 10–80 mg/d
	Clonidine, 0.2–0.6 mg/d
	Dantrolene, 25–100 mg/d
Incontinence	Propantheline, 7.5–15 mg/d
	Oxybutynin, 5–15 mg/d
Fatigue	Amantadine, 100–200 mg/d
Tremor	Clonazepam, 0.5–2 mg/d
	Propranolol, 40–160 mg/d
	Primidone, 500–1500 mg/d
Paroxysmal pain	Carbamazepine, 400–1600 mg/d

block the release of LT and TNF-α from activated monocytes. The positive results of this clinical research will be followed up to learn whether other factors can be used to improve these results, since even treated patients eventually had attacks and some deteriorated.

Copolymer 1 has been found efficacious in clinical trials. This agent is a mixture of short peptides (Box 14–2) that collectively block the antigen-binding site for myelin basic protein within the trimolecular complex. As with IFNB, patients are taught to give themselves injections. It has decreased the frequency and severity of relapses at about the same order of magnitude as IFNB.

Several strategies are being developed or trials are in progress that are directed against MHC class II cells presenting antigen to CD4+ T cells. These include using antibody against the MHC class II locus and antibodies against specific components of the T-cell receptor. Agents that block lymphocyte adhesion and migration through the blood-brain barrier are under consideration, as are drugs or antibodies that block the secretion or effect of harmful cytokines. Trials with TGF-β, an inhibitor of inflammation, are under way.

Symptomatic treatment is an important component of lifelong disease management. Many drugs are effective against spasticity, incontinence, paroxysmal pain, and fatigue (see Table 14–5). Fever should be evaluated promptly, since patients with spastic bladders are prone to urinary tract infections (UTIs) and kidney damage. Prophylactic treatment for UTIs should be considered in patients with recurrent infections.

Patients should be encouraged to lead as active a life as possible. Exercise is important for maintaining strength, flexibility, and a sense of well-being. Exercise in a cool swimming pool can be particularly helpful. Physicians should provide guidance on the institution and use of orthotics, canes, walkers, and wheelchairs as appropriate. Health care providers work with patients to assure that advancing physical disability does not automatically signal an end to gainful employment or pleasurable activities in society.

SUMMARY

Multiple sclerosis is a devastating disease that attacks young adults and can lead to paralysis, sensory loss, and changes in mood and mentation. Brain imaging studies indicate that the disease is far more active than can be appreciated from clinical observations alone. Although the cause is unknown, evidence indicates that both genetic and environmental factors interact with the immune system and lead to an autoimmune demyelination (see Table 14–1). Studies of the molecular immunology of reactive T cells, macrophages, and their cytokines in EAE and MS have led to specific types of therapy. β-Interferon and copolymer 1 are biological agents that decrease the pace of the disease. Many other potential immune therapies are under investigation. Long-term disease management helps patients maintain full and productive lives.

Selected Readings

Governman, J., A. Woods, L. Larson, et al. Transgenic mice that express a myelin basic protein-specific receptor develop spontaneous autoimmunity. Cell 72:551–560, 1993.

The IFNB Multiple Sclerosis Study Group. Interferon β-1b is effective in relapsing-remitting multiple sclerosis. 1. Clinical trials of a multicenter, randomized, double-blind, placebo-controlled trial. Neurology 43:655–661, 1993.

Kurtzke, J. F. Rating neurologic impairment in multiple sclerosis: An expanded disability status scale (EDSS). Neurology 33:1444–1452, 1983.

Martin, R., R. Voskhul, M. Flerlage, et al. Myelin basic protein-specific T-cell responses in identical twins discordant or concordant for multiple sclerosis. Ann Neurol 34:524–535, 1993.

McDonald, W. I., D. H. Miller, and D. Barnes. The pathological evolution of multiple sclerosis. Neuropathol Appl Neurobiol 18:319–334, 1992.

Paty, D. W., D.K.B. Li, the MS/MRI Study Group, and the IFNB Multiple Sclerosis Study Group. Interferon β-1b is effective in relapsing-remitting multiple sclerosis. 2. MRI analysis results of a multicenter, randomized, double-blind, placebo-controlled trial. Neurology 43:662–667, 1993.

Poser, C M., D. W. Paty, L. Scheinberg, et al. New diagnostic criteria for multiple sclerosis: Guidelines for research protocols. Ann Neurol 13:227–231, 1983.

Prineas, J. W., R. O. Barnard, E. E. Kwon, et al. Multiple sclerosis: Remyelination of nascent lesions. Ann Neurol 33:137–151, 1993.

Sadovnik, A. D., and G. C. Ebers. Epidemiology of multiple sclerosis: A critical overview. Can J Neurol Sci 20:17–29, 1993.

Silberberg, D. H. (ed.). Multiple sclerosis: Approaches to management. Ann Neurol 36 (Suppl.), 1994.

Smith, M. E., L. A. Stone, P. S. Albert, et al. Clinical worsening in multiple sclerosis is associated with increased frequency and area of gadopentetate dimeglumine–enhancing magnetic resonance imaging lesions. Ann Neurol 33:480–489, 1993.

Voskuhl, R. R., R. Martin, and H. F. McFarland. A functional basis for the association of HLA class II genes and susceptibility to multiple sclerosis: Cellular immune responses to myelin basic protein in a multiplex family. J Neuroimmunol 42:199–208, 1993.

Youl, B. D., G. Turano, D. H. Miller, et al. The pathophysiology of acute optic neuritis: An association of gadolinium leakage with clinical and electrophysiological deficits. Brain 114:2437–2450, 1991.

CHAPTER FIFTEEN

CEREBROVASCULAR

DISEASE

INTRODUCTION **173**

ISCHEMIC STROKE **173**

   Clinical Presentation **173**

   Risk Factors **176**

   Pathophysiology **177**

   Evaluation and Differential Diagnosis **180**

   Treatment **180**

INTRACRANIAL HEMORRHAGE **181**

   Primary (Hypertensive) Intraparenchymal Hemorrhage **181**

   Saccular "Berry" Aneurysms **182**

   Vascular Malformations **182**

SUMMARY **182**

INTRODUCTION

Stroke is the third leading cause of mortality in the United States, accounting for approximately 150,000 deaths annually. It is also a major cause of morbidity, with 3,000,000 stroke survivors living at any one time. It is the most common diagnosis for admission to extended care facilities and nursing homes, and approximately 25 billion dollars is spent on stroke each year. Stroke has been recognized clinically since ancient times when the Greeks called it *apoplexy*—being struck suddenly and violently. Sudden clinical impairment occurs with the three major causes of stroke—thrombosis, embolus, and hemorrhage. The acute onset of a focal neurological deficit is the hallmark of cerebrovascular disease at any age, but the incidence increases steadily with advancing years: at age 50 approximately 100/100,000 population but 1000/100,000 by age 75. With the advent of new neuroimaging techniques for brain, blood vessels, and blood flow have come improvements in diagnosis and management. Medical and surgical control of risk factors is preventing stroke for many, and new interventional treatments during the acute ischemic process promise reversal of brain infarction.

ISCHEMIC STROKE

Occlusion of a blood vessel to the brain with subsequent ischemic infarction accounts for 80% of stroke cases, with intracerebral hemorrhage (10–15%) and subarachnoid hemorrhage from an aneurysm (5–10%) accounting for the remainder. Approximately 40% of ischemic strokes are due to atherosclerotic thrombosis of a large vessel, 25% are from small vessel occlusions with "lacunar" infarcts, 25% are cardioembolic, and the remainder result from less common conditions such as arteritis, infections, or inherited conditions. Men are affected 1.5–2 times more often than women. In the United States, stroke incidence and mortality are higher among blacks than whites. The incidence varies only slightly around the world, being higher in China and Japan for intracerebral hemorrhage.

Clinical Presentation

Stroke can often be classified from the history alone by one of three causes—thrombosis, embolus, or hemorrhage (Table 15–1). The examination and laboratory investigation will secure the etiological diagnosis. Similarly, the history should provide clues about whether the symptoms lie within either the anterior or the posterior circulation (Figure 15–1). Finally, in many cases it will be possible to determine the exact neurovascular syndrome (Table 15–2). In some circumstances, this exercise begins in a physician's office several days after the event has occurred. Even then a workup can be completed within 24–48 hours and lead to decisions regarding anticoagulation, vascular surgery, or other treatments. In other circumstances, the workup will begin within minutes to a few hours of the onset of symptoms in an emergency room. Here rapid diagnostic evaluation may lead either to intraarterial thrombolysis of an occlusion or to arteriography and

TABLE 15-1. Clinical Features in the Diagnosis of Stroke

Cause	Clinical Features
Thrombosis (60%)	Preceding TIAs are often stereotyped episodes. Strokes commonly occur during sleep or upon awakening. Stuttering progression to full deficit occurs over minutes to hours. Subcortical pure motor or pure sensory "lacunar" strokes are common with hypertension.
Cardiac embolus (20%)	Preceding TIAs reflect different vascular distributions. Strokes commonly occur while awake and active, reaching a maximal deficit within minutes of onset. Cortical deficits are common. Cardiac arrhythmia, valvular disease, or recent myocardial infarction often present.
Hemorrhage (20%)	Bleed occurs without warning while awake and active. The deficit progresses over 15–30 minutes. Hypertension present. Headache, vomiting, stiff neck (subarachnoid blood), stupor, and coma can occur quickly.

aneurysm surgery. The clinical exercise in both settings is the same in terms of determining anatomical localization, neurovascular localization, and etiology.

Occlusion of a cerebral vessel causes focal symptoms within seconds to minutes. The timing and severity of symptoms reflect the size of the particular vessel, the neuroanatomical volume of perfusion, the duration of ischemia, and the adequacy of collateral flow. If the occlusion is brief or incomplete, then blood flow may be reduced below the ischemic level of 20 mL/100 g/min but not to the level of infarction, 12 mL/100 g/min. In this situation, symptoms may be mild and evanescent and sometimes so slight that they are dismissed by a patient. For example, transient weakness, numbness, and visual obscuration are not uncommonly found as unheeded warning signs on taking a history from a patient with a completed stroke. If the occlusion is intermittent, there may be a stuttering pattern of symptoms over days, weeks, or longer that eventually results in a permanent stroke.

It is important for physicians to keep these variables in mind when taking a history. In addition, since stroke can damage a patient's capacity to observe, recall, and report symptoms, it is important to note the patient's language and cognitive skills at the outset of the evaluation. A corroborative history should be obtained from a relative or friend in these circumstances. In addition, stroke of the nondominant hemisphere impairs awareness of the body such that symptoms are often overlooked (neglect) or even denied (anosognosia). For example, loss of a visual field is commonly unappreciated unless it interferes with reading or complex visual processing. Finally, since ischemic stroke is usually painless, transient deficits can fail to activate behavioral arousal and can even mute adaptive responses.

Weakness. The acute onset of focal weakness is the most common symptom of stroke. It can signal ischemia of an entire hemisphere from a large vessel, or subcortical ischemia from a small arteriole penetrating the internal capsule or brain stem. Determining

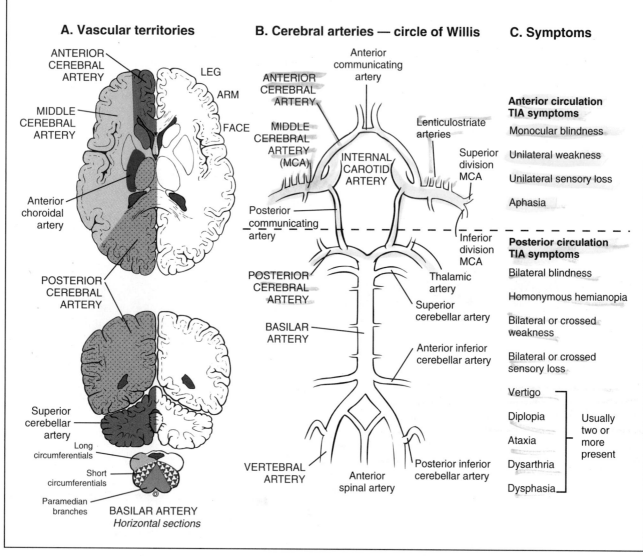

A. Vascular territories

ANTERIOR CEREBRAL ARTERY

LEG

ARM

FACE

MIDDLE CEREBRAL ARTERY

Anterior choroidal artery

POSTERIOR CEREBRAL ARTERY

Superior cerebellar artery

Long circumferentials

Short circumferentials

Paramedian branches

BASILAR ARTERY
Horizontal sections

B. Cerebral arteries — circle of Willis

Anterior communicating artery

ANTERIOR CEREBRAL ARTERY

Lenticulostriate arteries

MIDDLE CEREBRAL ARTERY (MCA)

Superior division MCA

INTERNAL CAROTID ARTERY

Posterior communicating artery

Inferior division MCA

POSTERIOR CEREBRAL ARTERY

Thalamic artery

Superior cerebellar artery

BASILAR ARTERY

Anterior inferior cerebellar artery

VERTEBRAL ARTERY

Anterior spinal artery

Posterior inferior cerebellar artery

C. Symptoms

Anterior circulation TIA symptoms

Monocular blindness

Unilateral weakness

Unilateral sensory loss

Aphasia

Posterior circulation TIA symptoms

Bilateral blindness

Homonymous hemianopia

Bilateral or crossed weakness

Bilateral or crossed sensory loss

Vertigo

Diplopia

Ataxia

Dysarthria

Dysphasia

Usually two or more present

FIGURE 15–1. Functional anatomy of the cerebral circulation.

the site of the damage leads quickly to identifying a neurovascular syndrome (see Table 15–2 and Figure 15–1) and the probable causes that require therapy. The site is best determined by noting the pattern of weakness as well as the presence or absence of other neurological symptoms or signs.

When weakness is accompanied by aphasia, the dominant left hemisphere is involved. Similarly, the additional presence of a hemianopia, cortical-type sensory loss, agnosia, or seizures indicates hemispheric dysfunction. This situation is common with cardioemboli, which frequently travel into the cortical branches of the anterior, middle, and posterior cerebral arteries. Weakness that is greater in the face and arm than in the leg suggests ischemia in the distribution of the middle cerebral artery. However, the cause of the ischemia here could be a local thrombus, stenosis at the extracranial origin of the internal carotid artery, an embolus from the carotid artery (artery-to-artery embolus), or an embolus from the heart. Weakness that is

greater in the leg than in the arm or face is consistent with ischemia in the distribution of the anterior cerebral artery. This pattern of deficit reflects the blood supply to the medial convexity of the hemisphere that contains the motor cortex for the leg and foot. When weakness is accompanied by cranial nerve symptoms or signs on the side opposite to the weakness, a posterior circulation brain stem stroke is evident. Pure motor weakness, without any cognitive, sensory, or cranial nerve dysfunction, occurs most often from occlusion of a small vessel in the internal capsule, cerebral peduncle, or pons, commonly in the setting of hypertension and diabetes. Since the motor system extends from the cortex to the spinal cord, ischemia from most vessels will cause weakness or awkwardness of motor performance.

Visual Impairment. Loss of vision in one eye alarms patients and usually leads them to seek medical evaluation. Physicians should attempt to determine whether the visual symptom is unilateral or bilateral,

TABLE 15–2. Common Neurovascular Syndromes

Cerebral Artery	Symptoms
Internal Carotid Artery	Highly variable because of collateral flow around the circle of Willis No symptoms to complete anterior circulation syndrome
Anterior Cerebral Artery	
Unilateral	Weakness and sensory loss in leg Transient expressive aphasia
Corpus callosum	Apraxia of left hand
Bilateral	Abulia, gait apraxia and weakness, incontinence
Anterior Choroidal Artery	
Unilateral	Pure motor weakness, monoplegia, hemiplegia
Middle Cerebral Artery	
Complete occlusion	Contralateral hemiplegia, sensory loss, and gaze palsy Global aphasia (left hemisphere) Contralateral hemispatial neglect (right hemisphere)
Superior division	Weakness and sensory loss of face and arm greater than that of leg Contralateral gaze palsy Broca's aphasia (left frontal) Spatial neglect, constructional apraxia (right parietal)
Inferior division	Superior quadrant or hemianopic visual loss Wernicke's aphasia (left planum temporale) Spatial neglect, constructional apraxia (right parietal)
Posterior Cerebral Artery	
Thalamic arteries	Contralateral sensory loss, thalamic syndrome
Unilateral cortical	Contralateral hemianopia Alexia without agraphia (left hemisphere)
Bilateral cortical	Bilateral "cortical" blindness Color blindness, prosopagnosia
Vertebrobasilar Arteries	
Basilar artery	Highly variable depending on collateral flow Asymptomatic (rare), mild hemiparesis, complete quadriparesis with gaze palsy (locked-in syndrome)
Long circumferentials (superior cerebellar, anterior inferior cerebellar, posterior inferior cerebellar)	Ipsilateral ataxia Eye skew, nystagmus, gaze palsy Contralateral sensory loss Dysphagia, dysarthria, vertigo, nausea, vomiting Ipsilateral Horner's syndrome
Paramedian branches	Contralateral weakness, isolated or with ataxia Ipsilateral cranial nerve palsies III, VI, VII, XII

monocular or hemianopic, and if there are positive visual phenomena as well as negative symptoms. Some patients will cover one eye during a spell of visual loss and thus discover the presence of monocular loss as opposed to hemianopic loss. The sensation of a "shade" or a "curtain" coming down suggests ischemia in a branch of a retinal vessel. Often this is evidence of atherosclerosis in the internal carotid artery or its ophthalmic branch just above the intracranial carotid siphon. Artery-to-artery emboli cause transient blindness, a clinical syndrome called **amaurosis fugax.** If contralateral weakness or other hemispheric signs accompany monocular blindness, embolic disease of the internal carotid artery is likely. As with retinal ischemia, the hemianopic symptoms of unilateral occipital ischemia reach completion within a minute and persist for variable periods of time. Rarely, emboli from the basilar artery travel to both occipital arteries and bilateral visual loss occurs. In this condition, patients exhibit a pupillary response to light but have no conscious visual perception and cannot recognize objects, faces, or colors.

Sensory Loss. Numbness most often occurs with weakness, but many patients confuse the two. When a patient's subjective awareness of numbness is present, the objective findings can be subtle, such as extinction of one area during double simultaneous stimulation, rather than overt loss of light touch or pinprick sensation. Paresthesias help localize the abnormality and indicate abnormal electrophysiological activity in ischemic sensory pathways. Sensory loss of all modalities along with spontaneous pain and paresthesias maximal in the arm are characteristic of a stroke in the thalamus (thalamic syndrome). The penetrating vessels coming off the posterior cerebral artery are implicated, and often there is choreoathetosis and intention tremor due to ischemia of adjacent extrapyramidal and cerebellar projection pathways. Bilateral perioral numbness is characteristic of brain stem ischemia and involvement of crossing trigeminal sensory pathways.

Language and Speech. Dysphasia must be distinguished from dysarthria. Difficulty with word finding is a characteristic complaint of frontal ischemia of the dominant hemisphere. Patients usually have weakness of the face and hand owing to involvement of the neighboring motor cortex. Their speech will be short and effortful, conveying much frustration. This nonfluent Broca's aphasia is a common stroke syndrome. Most patients can distinguish this difficulty from dysarthria—the slurred speech of too much alcohol. Dysarthria usually signals abnormalities in motor pathways in the brain stem or cerebellum subserving the tongue, pharynx, and larynx.

In contrast to the frustration of patients with Broca's aphasia, patients suffering ischemia of the dominant hemisphere's temporoparietal cortex seemingly are unaware of their language difficulties. These patients have Wernicke's aphasia and speak in long, fluent, melodious sentences mostly devoid of nouns and containing little meaning. They have great difficulty in understanding language. Family or friends may describe the symptoms as a transient spell of confusion.

Risk Factors

Careful control of risk factors has lowered the incidence and mortality rate for stroke over the last five decades. In particular, control of **hypertension** is recognized as the most important factor in stroke prevention (Table 15–3). Elevation of either systolic (>140 mm Hg) or diastolic (>90 mm Hg) pressure increases risk for stroke of all types: large vessel atherosclerotic thrombosis, small vessel lacunar disease, and intracranial hemorrhage. Hypertension is also identified as a cause of arteriolar sclerosis of hemispheric white matter vessels (leukoariosis) that leads to a type of vascular dementia (Chapter 16). Chronic hypertension causes

TABLE 15–3. Risk Factors for Stroke

Common Risk Factors

Transient ischemic attack
Recent stroke
Hypertension
Cigarette smoking
Cardiac disease
   Arrhythmias
   Valvular disease
   Myocardial infarction
   Cardiomyopathies
   Congenital heart disease
Diabetes mellitus

Uncommon Risk Factors

Inflammatory disorders
   Lupus erythematosus
   Giant cell arteritis
   Syphilis
Fibromuscular dysplasia
Hematological disorders
   Polycythemia vera
   Sickle cell disease
Coagulation disorders
Drug abuse

Possible Risk Factors

Increased fibrinogen
Oral contraceptives
Hyperlipidemia
Obesity
Physical inactivity
Alcohol
Pregnancy

small aneurysms or weakening of vessel walls that bleed into the basal ganglia, thalamus, pons, and cerebellum, and it also plays a role in subarachnoid hemorrhage from large saccular aneurysms on vessels around the circle of Willis. In addition, hypertension damages the heart, which can lead to embolic strokes of the brain.

Cigarette smoking accentuates both intracranial and extracranial atherosclerosis. Cessation of smoking will decrease accumulated risk of stroke. **Alcohol consumption** is not related to ischemic stroke but may be a factor in hemorrhage. **Diabetes** increases risk for stroke for both large and small vessel disease. The combination of diabetes and hypertension is particularly pathogenetic for small vessel disease. There is suggestive evidence that hyperglycemia in diabetics at the time of stroke may result in more severe infarction than will occur with normal levels of glucose. Experiments in animals show that tissue with high levels of glucose or glycogen produces more lactic acidosis under ischemic conditions, resulting in greater damage.

Heart disease is a major risk factor for embolic infarction of the brain. Atrial fibrillation, valvular heart disease, cardiomyopathies, and congenital heart disease all require consideration for long-term anticoagulation to reduce the risk of cerebral embolus. Atrial fibrillation carries a 5% risk of stroke per year, approximately 10 times normal. It may be the major cause of stroke in women over age 75. Treatment with warfarin reduces risk by approximately 70%. In addition, since atherosclerosis affects both cardiac and cerebral vessels, many patients who present with stroke have ischemic heart disease as well. Myocardial infarction is the leading cause of death in stroke survivors. While there is relatively good correlation between abnormalities of blood lipids and of lipoproteins and coronary artery disease, the correlation is not so strong for stroke. Several studies have unexpectedly found a correlation between *low* serum cholesterol and cerebral hemorrhage.

Carotid stenosis is a risk factor for stroke, a condition that can occasionally be identified by finding a bruit upon auscultation of the neck on routine physical examination. Imaging studies should be performed to evaluate the severity of any atherosclerotic lesion (Figure 15–2A). In patients with brain ischemia, stenosis of greater than 70% is found in up to 20% of cases. Randomized studies have indicated the importance of surgery when asymptomatic stenosis is greater than 70%. Medical therapy alone results in a 2-year, 26% incidence of ipsilateral stroke. Endarterectomy reduces this percentage to 9%. The presence of ulceration in all degrees of stenosis worsens the prognosis and favors need for operation.

Transient ischemic attack (TIA) was originally defined clinically as a focal neurological deficit that disappeared in 24 hours. Imaging studies now indicate that up to 20% of TIAs cause persistent signs of infarction. Nevertheless, the clinical event itself indicates a 5% likelihood of a subsequent completed stroke within a year. Stroke is also a strong indicator of subsequent stroke, with 4–8% of patients suffering a second infarction within 30 *days* and 14% within 2 years. Treatment of TIA and stroke patients with antiplatelet agents

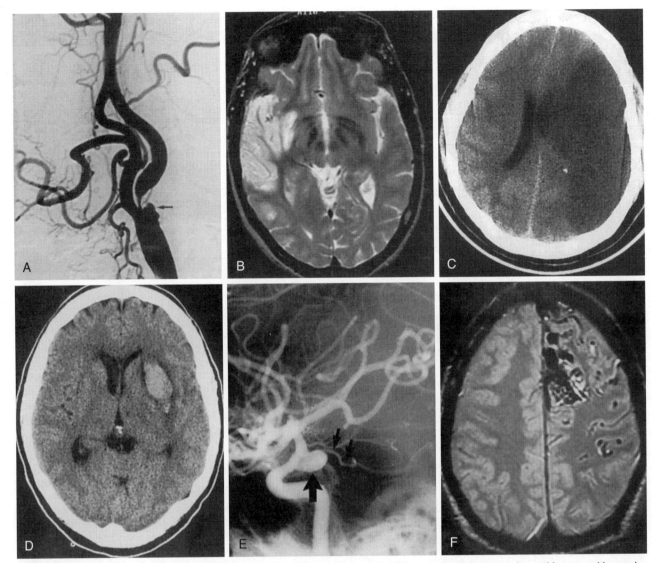

FIGURE 15–2. Neuroimaging of stroke. *A*, Angiogram of the carotid artery showing 90% stenosis of the internal carotid artery with an ulcer (arrow). *B*, T2-weighted MRI scan showing acute infarction in the distribution of the right middle cerebral artery. The increase in signal intensity is due to early vasogenic edema. There is no mass effect. *C*, CT scan of a left middle cerebral artery infarction after 3 days showing massive vasogenic edema and mass effect compressing the lateral ventricle. *D*, CT scan of an acute hemorrhage into the left putamen with compression of the lateral ventricle. *E*, Angiogram of the carotid artery showing an aneurysm (large arrow) at the origin of the posterior communicating artery (small arrows). *F*, MRI showing a right hemisphere arteriovenous malformation. The dark profiles are flow voids from enlarged feeding arteries and draining veins. (Reproduced, with permission, from S. T. Willing. *Atlas of Neuroradiology.* Philadelphia, W.B. Saunders Co., 1995.)

(aspirin or ticlopidine) reduce this risk by up to 25%. These facts emphasize the importance of carefully evaluating all patients with even mild transient focal neurological dysfunction for treatable risk factors (see Table 15–3). Stroke prevention is an important responsibility for all physicians.

Pathophysiology

Stroke is not a disease of neurons, nor is it a "cerebrovascular accident." It is the natural outcome of disease processes affecting the heart and blood vessels of the brain. The greatest impact on the natural history of stroke will therefore come from understanding and treating atherosclerosis and aggravating risk factors, as discussed above. Once an ischemic process starts in the brain, however, a series of unique events

are initiated within nervous tissue that lead to neuronal death and infarction (Box 15–1).

The maintenance of normal levels of cerebral blood flow is the key factor in preventing tissue damage. Whole-brain blood flow is approximately 50 mL/100 g/min. Blood flow to gray matter is 80 mL/100 g/min, whereas in white matter tracts it is much lower, approximately 20 mL/100 g/min. Autoregulation is the process whereby whole-brain blood flow is kept constant despite fluctuations in systemic blood pressure. In normal individuals, mean arterial pressure can be experimentally changed from 60 to 150 mm Hg without changing cerebral blood flow because vessels will automatically dilate and constrict to changes in pressure within this range. When mean pressure falls below 60 mm Hg, humans develop global symptoms leading to syncope, e.g., lightheadedness, dim vision, and loss of

BOX 15-1   The Biochemistry of Brain Ischemia and Infarction

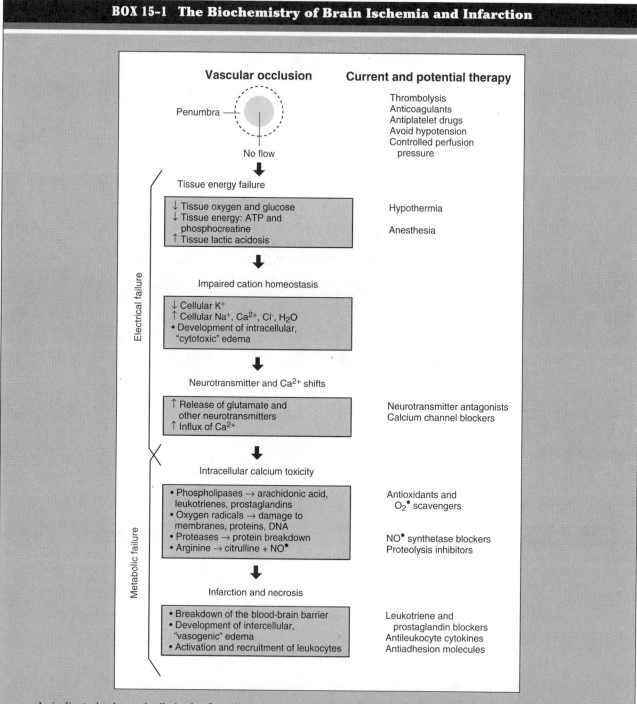

As indicated schematically in the flow diagram, when ischemia results in a drop in tissue energy levels, membrane pumps are unable to maintain ion homeostasis. Intracellular edema develops in the dendrites and axon terminals, leading to transmission or "electrical" failure. Subsequently there is a massive release of neurotransmitters into the extracellular space. The excitatory amino acids are particularly toxic because they stimulate glutamate receptors, which leads to further influxes of calcium through voltage-dependent channels. "Metabolic" failure begins when a marked rise in intracellular calcium causes excessive and chaotic activation of kinases, proteases,

phospholipases, and other enzymes. Activation of one of these metabolic pathways leads to peroxidation of lipid membranes with the production of toxic levels of arachidonic acid, prostaglandins, leukotrienes, and free radicals. Levels of neuronal nitric oxide (NO) also increase and add to the destructive process.

The exact time point for irreversible damage and the specific biochemical steps involved in neuronal death probably differ for different neurons. Hippocampal CA1 neurons with high levels of glutamate N-methyl-D-aspartate (NMDA) receptors are particularly vulnerable, while dentate gyrus granule cells with high levels of calcium-binding

Continued on opposite page

proteins are relatively resistant. Following the initial period of ischemia, delayed biochemical processes can occur over several days. There is induction of the protooncogenes c-*fos* and c-*jun*, whose protein products act as transcriptional regulators of other genes. In some cells, there is also production of heat shock proteins, which signal a cell's response to injury. At present, it is not known whether these molecular events help protect against damage or signify vulnerable neurons destined for elimination. In tissue that recovers from ischemia, there is restoration of energy levels, reestablishment of ion gradients and neurotransmitter compartments, removal of tissue lactate, and

eventual recovery of protein synthesis. In tissue that goes on to infarction, these steps remain incomplete. The delay in injury and final cellular death can last from 3 to 72 hours in the hippocampus in some experimental animals, indicating a time period when reperfusion and cytoprotective therapy could be useful.

The final phase of infarction begins within 24 hours and is characterized by breakdown in the blood-brain barrier. Endogenous factors (leukotrienes) and leukocyte cytokines probably act synergistically in causing this damage. Brain tissue loses its protection against extravasation of blood plasma, and intercellular edema develops.

consciousness. Above 150 mm Hg, vessels undergo spasm and autoregulation is lost. This extreme condition can lead to hypertensive encephalopathy, a clinical syndrome characterized by fluctuating focal neurological signs, encephalopathy, papilledema, and seizures.

At the local level, brain blood flow is intimately linked to tissue needs and regulated by metabolism. For example, the increase in physiological activity caused by opening and closing a hand is associated with an increase in neuronal firing in several discrete motor hand areas in primary and secondary motor cortex and supplemental motor cortex. This results in increased consumption of oxygen and glucose and a transient, small (5–15%) increase in regional blood flow in these areas. The augmentation in local blood flow increases the delivery of metabolic substrates as well as removes metabolic products such as lactic acid and carbon dioxide. Experimentally, local lowering of tissue pH associated with an increase in metabolism has been identified as one factor that causes vasodilation and a local increase in blood volume. An increase in endothelial nitric oxide has been found to mediate the vasodilation associated with hypercapnia, brain stimulation, and release of excitatory amino acids.

When blood flow begins to fall, the brain maintains homeostasis by increasing the extraction of oxygen and glucose from capillary blood. This compensatory mechanism is effective at flow levels of approximately 20 mL/100 g/min. Below this level, the supply of nutrients is insufficient to maintain tissue energy stores, particularly phosphocreatine and ATP, and membrane ion pumps fail. Dendrites and axon terminals are particularly vulnerable, since energy expenditure here is associated with maintaining cation homeostasis and membrane charge. With a fall in energy, intracellular potassium leaks out, while sodium, calcium, and chloride enter. There is a shift of water from extracellular to intracellular space with *intracellular* edema (see Box 15–1). This water shift can be detected by diffusion-weighted MRI in the early phases of stroke in humans. With intracellular edema, dendrites swell, neurotransmission is interrupted, and neurological symptoms develop. At this point, there is "electrical failure." With a decrease in whole-brain blood flow, as in cardiac arrest, the electroencephalogram will become slowed and suppressed as the patient becomes comatose. If there is a

fall in regional blood flow, focal signs and symptoms develop.

Electrical failure is reversible, but the length of time the brain can sustain ischemia without becoming permanently damaged is dependent on many factors. A general rule of thumb is that after 5–10 minutes of total cessation of cerebral blood flow, "metabolic failure" results and neuronal death occurs. These guidelines hold for cardiac arrest. In this condition, particular areas of brain exhibit selective vulnerability, including Sommer's sector of the hippocampus (CA1 and the subiculum); layers 3, 5, and 6 of the cerebral cortex; and Purkinje cells of the cerebellum. Survivors of prolonged cardiac arrest commonly have difficulties reflecting tissue destruction in these areas such as memory loss, cognitive impairment, and ataxia.

Local ischemia of the brain will be most intense at the core of the territory supplied by the occluded vessel, while the surrounding tissue may remain relatively well perfused or even "luxury perfused" by collateral flow from neighboring vessels. The tissue surrounding the central zone has been called the "ischemic penumbra," a term that is now best thought of as having time and intensity variables as well as a spatial domain. In essence, the degree of infarction depends on the severity and duration of blood flow reduction in a particular area. A rule of thumb for stroke is that an hour of total occlusion will lead to a central core area of infarction. However, the size of the infarction is a dynamic process and therefore open to therapeutic interventions that might either reopen occluded vessels or interrupt the cascade of metabolic events that lead from ischemia to infarction over subsequent hours and days. New therapies for stroke are aimed at emergency treatment that addresses these issues (Box 15–1).

The development of brain infarction involves breakdown of the blood-brain barrier. Exudation of blood plasma into the brain causes extracellular edema and swelling. In humans, the mass effect of edema reaches its peak in approximately 3 days as seen on CT and MRI scans (Figure 15–2*B* and *C*). Blood neutrophils subsequently enter the zone of infarction and together with macrophages, microglia, and activated astrocytes begin the process of converting a necrotic lesion into a gliotic scar. This process requires several months. The area destroyed removes a component of brain function that cannot be recovered. However, through rehabilitation this function can be compensated for by developing new strategies and functions using other brain areas.

Evaluation and Differential Diagnosis

The history and physical examination should lead to a high probability that a patient's symptoms are the result of vascular disease. There may be evidence of risk factors in the history or on the examination. However, the acute onset of focal neurological symptoms should suggest vascular disease at any age even in the absence of risk factors. Lying and standing blood pressures should be taken as part of the evaluation for hypertension. Careful auscultation of the heart should be performed for arrhythmias and murmurs, and of the neck for bruits. Absence of a peripheral pulse will give evidence of peripheral atherosclerotic vascular disease. Funduscopic examination can reveal evidence of hypertension, diabetes, and carotid emboli.

The transient neurological symptoms that occur with classical migraine (Chapter 4) can be confused with those of a TIA. However, there are usually positive phenomena such as a scintillating scotoma with migraine. Characteristically these scotomata move across the visual field from central to peripheral vision, the march taking approximately 20 minutes. The visual aura is followed by unilateral headache, often with nausea and vomiting. In the elderly, a scotoma can occur as an isolated event, called a migraine equivalent. If a patient with vague visual complaints has not had previous migraines, a family history, or characteristic clinical features, the patient cannot be presumed to have had a migraine as the cause of the transient visual symptoms and must be evaluated for vascular disease.

Occasionally the symptoms of a seizure can be confused with those of a TIA. If the convulsive phase is not witnessed, the loss of function seen during the postictal phase of the seizure will appear no different from that of a resolving ischemic event. However, it must be noted that a focal seizure can also be the first sign of a cortical stroke, especially in the elderly. Finally, epileptic discharges from within the zone of language should be a consideration in the differential diagnosis of aphasia, since focal seizures here can cause transient disruption of language in a pattern similar to transient ischemia.

Other brief or isolated symptoms may indicate vascular disease, but other possibilities must be kept in mind. These include vertigo due to labyrinthine dysfunction, tinnitus due to middle ear disease, diplopia due to a myasthenic or nerve problem, and ataxia or dysarthria due to metabolic or degenerative disease of the cerebellum and its pathways. Generalized neurological symptoms such as confusion, lightheadedness, dizziness, and generalized weakness most often do *not* indicate cerebrovascular disease. Clinical evaluation in these circumstances should be directed toward disorders that interrupt or interfere with substrate supply to the whole brain. These disorders include cardiac arrhythmias, anemia, hypoglycemia, and end-stage pulmonary, renal, or liver disease.

The laboratory evaluation includes blood analysis and imaging (Table 15–4). In the emergency setting, the CT scan is the preferred test for detecting hemorrhage owing to speed and sensitivity to the blood signal. In all other settings, the MRI scan is more sensitive to subtle pathological changes and provides higher resolution (see Figure 15–2). If carotid artery disease is suspected, ultrasound should be performed to evaluate stenosis, plaques, or occlusion. Additional studies with MR angiography or invasive dye angiography depend on the practice at different centers. An ECG and chest x-ray are routine. If cardiac emboli are suspected, ultrasound is performed to determine the presence of an intracardiac thrombus (Table 15–5).

Treatment

Treatment of ischemic cerebrovascular disease has three phases. First, preventive treatment includes identification and control of risk factors, the use of antithrombotic therapy, and carotid endarterectomy in selected cases (Table 15–6). Regular neurological follow-up and evaluation are an important component of preventive therapy. Control of hypertension and diabetes, cessa-

TABLE 15–4. Evaluation of the Patient with TIA or Stroke

History

Define each episode of symptoms
Determine anterior versus posterior circulation (Figure 15–1)
Determine time versus intensity profiles
Identify risk factors (Table 15–1)
Explore differential features of migraine and seizures
Estimate etiological classification (Table 15–2)

Examination

Complete neurological examination
Funduscopic examination
Cardiac examination
Auscultation for cervical bruits
Palpation of cranial and peripheral pulses

Routine Blood Tests

Complete blood count (CBC)
Platelet count
Erythrocyte sedimentation rate (ESR)
Prothrombin time (PT)
Partial thromboplastin time (PTT)
Glucose

Additional Blood Tests

VDRL
ANA
Cholesterol and lipids

Routine Imaging Tests

Chest x-ray
CT scan (in emergencies)
MRI scan

Additional Imaging Tests

Carotid duplex ultrasound
Echocardiography
Cerebral angiography
MR angiography

TABLE 15-5. Common Causes of Cardiac Emboli

Atrial fibrillation
    Clot in left atrium or left atrial appendage
Recent myocardial infarction
    Hypodynamic left ventricular wall
Valvular heart disease
    Rheumatic heart disease
    Nonbacterial thrombotic endocarditis (systemic cancer)
    Bacterial endocarditis (intravenous drug abuse)
    Prosthetic valve
Dilated cardiomyopathy
    Hypodynamic left ventricular wall
Congenital heart disease
    Right-to-left shunt
Cardiac tumor
    Left atrial myxoma

tion of smoking, and the use of antiplatelet or warfarin anticoagulation have reduced the incidence of stroke.

Second, acute TIA and evolving stroke are emergencies in which decisions are made in response to emerging data and the evolution of the clinical profile. Patients should be sent to an emergency room, where attention is first directed to evaluation and control of breathing and cardiac function. Hypertension should not be treated unless it is greater than 220/120 mm Hg on several repeat measurements. If chronic hypertension has been present, it is a mistake to lower pressure acutely, since the brain has adapted to a high perfusion pressure to overcome the high resistance of rigid vessels. Autoregulation is lost. Lowering pressure even to normal levels could cause further ischemia. The hypertension should be treated by gradually lowering it over several weeks, allowing time for collateral circulation to develop around an infarct as well as for vessels to adapt to more normal levels of pressure.

A neurological examination is performed, an intravenous line established, and a CT scan performed to determine whether bleeding has occurred. In large vessel ischemic stroke, it may be efficacious to perform immediate angiography and intraarterial clot lysis. In a progressing deficit, the use of heparin should be evaluated. The presence of arrhythmia and cardiac emboli also warrant consideration of rapid anticoagulation to prevent recurrent emboli.

Finally, treatment of the patient with a completed stroke involves the use of antithrombotic therapy to prevent further stroke and consideration of vascular

surgery in appropriate cases. Attention must be directed to the common complications of acute stroke, especially in bedridden elderly: hypoventilation and pneumonia, deep vein thrombosis and pulmonary emboli, urinary tract infection, and skin ulcers. Instituting physical therapy within several days of a completed stroke helps prevent these complications, helps prevent joint stiffness and contractures, and engages the patient in the process of regaining functional use of the body.

INTRACRANIAL HEMORRHAGE
Primary (Hypertensive) Intraparenchymal Hemorrhage

Hemorrhage accounts for approximately 20% of all strokes, with the incidence of intraparenchymal bleeding twice as common as that of subarachnoid bleeding (Table 15–7). Hypertension is the most important cause of intraparenchymal bleeding and probably also plays a role in the eventual rupture of vascular malformations such as saccular aneurysms and arteriovenous malformations (AVMs), although many malformations bleed in the absence of hypertension.

Hypertension is known to cause damage to long and deep penetrating arteries. Arteriole walls become thinned, showing lipohyalinosis and fibrinoid necrosis. Microaneurysms develop, and extravasation of red blood cells occurs. First described by Charcot and Bouchard in 1868, these microaneurysms are thought to break open and cause hypertensive hemorrhages. The primary sites of occurrence of intraparenchymal hemorrhage reflect the sites of deep penetrating vessels and the greater density of microaneurysms. These include the lenticulostriate arteries from the middle cerebral artery into the putamen (approximately 50% of cases), the penetrating arteries into the thalamus from the posterior cerebral artery, long arteries into the hemispheric white matter, and arteries into the cerebellum and pons.

Hemorrhage into the putamen and adjacent internal capsule produces contralateral hemiparesis and eye deviation (Figure 15–2D). As the hematoma develops, it grows medially and inferiorly, pushing against the reticular activating system in the thalamus and midbrain, causing stupor and coma. Symptoms can develop rapidly over 15–30 minutes. Hemorrhage into the pons produces coma immediately. The pupils become pinpoint owing to destruction of the descending sympa-

TABLE 15-6. Treatment for TIA and Ischemic Stroke

Clinical Situation	Recommendation	Comment
TIA or early stroke (first 6 hours)	Evaluate, perform CT, give intraarterial thrombolytic and/or cytoprotective agents	Under clinical study
TIA or stroke	Control risk factors, give ASA 325 mg/d or ticlopidine 250 mg twice a day	Use both drugs, or add warfarin if symptoms recur
Carotid stenosis		
>75% Asymptomatic	Perform endarterectomy	
<75% Asymptomatic	Give ASA 325 mg/d or perform endarterectomy	Under clinical study
Symptomatic	Perform endarterectomy	
Atrial fibrillation	Give warfarin INR 2–3	Give ASA 325 mg/d if warfarin not tolerated
Cardiac embolus	Give heparin acutely, warfarin	Contraindicated in large strokes

TABLE 15-7. Common Causes of Intracranial Hemorrhage

Chronic hypertension
    Putamen, hemisphere, thalamus, pons, cerebellum
Saccular "berry" aneurysm
    Subarachnoid space—anterior circle of Willis
Vascular malformations
    AVMs, cavernous malformations
Trauma
Tumor
    Metastatic melanoma, embryonal tumors, choriocarcinoma
    Acute myelogenous leukemia
    Glioblastoma
Drug abuse
    Cocaine
Hemorrhagic conditions
    Idiopathic thrombocytopenic purpura, thrombotic
        thrombocytopenic purpura, hemophilia, anticoagulation
Amyloid angiopathy

thetic pathways in the pons. Death usually occurs within hours. Cerebellar hemorrhages usually present with acute headache, dizziness, vomiting, and inability to walk. Eyes become deviated away from the side of the cerebellar hemorrhage owing to compression of the lateral parapontine gaze center. Large cerebellar hemorrhages can expand and compress the brain stem or obstruct CSF flow, leading to coma over several hours. Early diagnosis, imaging studies, and surgery for cerebellar hemorrhages before deep coma develops can be lifesaving. Surgery is only rarely indicated for other intraparenchymal hemorrhages.

Hemorrhage into the hemispheric white matter, lobar hemorrhage, is associated with hypertension in half the cases. Other patients will have amyloid angiopathy, a hereditary condition that leads to hemorrhage in the elderly. "Occult" vascular malformations and tumors are also causes of lobar hemorrhages. These etiologies should be considered when intraparenchymal bleeding occurs in the absence of hypertension.

Saccular ("Berry") Aneurysms

Cerebral aneurysms are the result of developmental weakness of the walls of arteries around the circle of Willis. They occur most commonly on the anterior communicating artery (Figure 15–2E), on the internal carotid artery at the origin of the posterior communicating artery or the middle cerebral artery, or at the first bifurcation of the middle cerebral artery. They are usually asymptomatic until they rupture, although large posterior communicating aneurysms can cause a third nerve palsy with a dilated pupil by compressing cranial nerve III. Rupture of a saccular aneurysm characteristically causes severe headache, nuchal rigidity, hypertension, fever, bilateral decerebrate motor signs, stupor, and coma.

The clinical diagnosis of subarachnoid hemorrhage is substantiated by finding blood on a CT scan or lumbar puncture. This finding should lead directly to angiography in most cases. Early repair of the aneu-

rysm is important for prevention of rebleeding. In addition, subarachnoid blood causes vasospasm, which can secondarily lead to cerebral ischemia. Vasospasm can be treated with calcium channel blockers (nimodipine) and occasionally angioplasty. If hypoperfusion develops, cerebral perfusion pressure should be maintained with volume expansion and intravenous dopamine. Patients are best managed in neurointensive care units where intracranial pressure, EEG, and blood flow can be regularly monitored. With aggressive therapy, the eventual outcome is good.

Vascular Malformations

Arteriovenous malformations (AVMs) are developmental abnormalities of the cerebral vasculature (Figure 15–2F). They can be quite small and go undetected until a brain MRI scan is performed or until autopsy. Alternatively they can be quite large and symptomatic, detected shortly after birth. The most common clinical presentation occurs between 10 and 30 years of age with a gradually declining incidence into late adult life. Approximately one-third of patients will have a bleed and develop headache and focal neurological deficits. Large bleeds can lead progressively to coma and death. Another third of patients will present with seizures, and an additional third of cases will be discovered during evaluation of severe or recurrent headache. Since the incidence of bleeding is approximately 3–5% per year, surgery should be considered for AVMs. New intravascular techniques have been developed for obliterating AVMs.

Cavernous and venous malformations are usually small and detected in symptomatic patients by MRI scans. A central, dark "flow void" is seen within a lesion. When these lesions bleed or cause seizures, they can be treated with focused proton or gamma irradiation.

SUMMARY

Stroke is one of the most common causes of morbidity and mortality worldwide. By treatment of hypertension, use of antithrombotic agents, control of diabetes, cessation of smoking, and careful management of carotid artery and heart disease, physicians can greatly reduce the incidence of stroke. The clinical presentation of ischemic stroke can be quite variable, but each patient must be evaluated as soon as possible. The prompt performance of intraarterial thrombolysis in select cases and antithrombotic therapy in most cases can prevent brain damage in the emergency situation. New neuroprotective agents may interrupt the pathophysiology of tissue infarction. In cases of hemorrhagic stroke, the determination of aneurysmal bleeding should lead to prompt surgery, which together with the treatment of vasospasm promises good recovery for many patients.

Selected Readings

Caplan, R. C. *Stroke, A Clinical Approach,* 2nd ed. Boston, Butterworth-Heinemann, 1993.

Dobkin, B. (ed.). Management of the patient with stroke. Neurology 45 (suppl 1):S5–S35, 1995.

Feigin, V. L., D. O. Wiebers, and J. P. Whisnant. Update on stroke risk factors. J Stroke Cerebrovasc Dis 4:207–215, 1994.

Fisher, M., and J. Bogousslavsky (eds.). *Current Review of Cerebrovascular Disease.* Philadelphia, Current Medicine, 1993.

Hachinski, V., and J. W. Norris (eds.). Cerebrovascular disease. Curr Opin Neurol 7:3–60, 1994.

Hossmann, K.-A. Viability thresholds and the penumbra of focal ischemia. Ann Neurol 36:557–565, 1994.

McDowell, F. H. and Consensus Panel Members. Stroke: The first six hours—Emergency evaluation and treatment. Stroke 4:3–12, 1993.

Pulsinelli, W. A. (ed.). Cerebrovascular disease. Curr Opin Neurol 8:3–68, 1995.

CHAPTER SIXTEEN

ALZHEIMER'S DISEASE

AND THE

PRIMARY DEMENTIAS

ALZHEIMER'S DISEASE **185**

   Introduction **185**

   Clinical Presentation **185**

   Risk Factors **186**

   Pathophysiology **188**

   Evaluation and Differential Diagnosis **190**

   Treatment **192**

PRIMARY DEMENTIAS **192**

   Frontal Lobe Dementia **192**

   Subcortical Dementias **193**

   Lewy Body Dementias **193**

   Prion Diseases **193**

SUMMARY **194**

ALZHEIMER'S DISEASE

Introduction

Dementing illnesses are among the most common causes of morbidity and mortality in the elderly. Approximately 5% of persons between ages 65 and 70 years have dementia, with this figure doubling every 5 years to >45% above age 85. Alzheimer's disease accounts for 50–70% of the cases of dementia with a third of all people over age 85 affected by this disease alone. It is the fourth leading cause of death in the United States. The annual cost of care for a patient is $47,000 in 1990 dollars. The direct cost of all dementias is 20 billion dollars, with an additional 38 billion dollars of calculated indirect costs. The lifetime risk for developing Alzheimer's disease for the general population is 15–25%, but much higher for those with risk factors (see below). When Alois Alzheimer first described the disease and its pathological basis in a 51-year-old woman (Box 16–1), it was thought that he had described a *pre*senile illness and that senility was a natural process of aging or the result of "hardening of the arteries." It is now known that the characteristic pathological process of Alzheimer's disease increases with aging, while vascular disease, trauma, and other causes of dementia account for less than half the cases.

Clinical Presentation

Alzheimer's disease begins insidiously, progresses relentlessly, and runs its course over 5–10 years, robbing the mind of its history and purpose. The exact time of onset is difficult to determine. Patients or family commonly attribute early, subtle changes in cognitive behavior to reaction to stress, adjustment to retirement, or even normal aging. Most often the first difficulty is forgetfulness. Patients have problems recalling little used proper names or low-frequency words. In contrast to "benign forgetfulness of aging," patients with Alzheimer's disease are often unaware of their difficulty, talk around it, or deny it. With time, patients will misplace possessions, forget appointments, and fail

---

BOX 16–1 About a Peculiar Disease of the Cerebral Cortex by Alois Alzheimer

Alois Alzheimer (1864–1915) was a clinician and a neuropathologist working in Germany at the turn of the century. He was a colleague of many pioneering anatomists responsible for defining the histological boundaries of the human brain: Oscar Vogt, Korbibian Brodmann, Franz Nissl, and Auguste Forel. It was Emil Kraeplin, a founder of psychiatry, who championed the work of Alzheimer and provided him with a laboratory. Alzheimer made important contributions in correlating clinical neuropsychiatric illness with neuropathology in the general paresis of syphilis, atherosclerosis, and senile dementia. His classical description of the disease that bears his name comprised but a 2-page report.

ALLGEMEINE ZEITSCHRIFT FÜR PSYCHIATRIE UND PSYCHISCH-GERICHTLICHE MEDIZIN

64:146–148, 1907
Über eine eigenartige Erkrankung der Hirnrinde*

Case Presentation

The first noticeable symptom of illness shown by this 51-year-old woman was suspiciousness of her husband. Soon, a rapidly increasing memory impairment became evident; she could no longer orient herself in her own dwelling, dragged objects here and there and hid them, and at times, believing that people were out to murder her, started to scream loudly.... She is completely disoriented to time and place.... At times she is totally delirious, drags her bedding around, calls for her husband or daughter, and seems to have auditory hallucinations. Often she screams for many hours in a horrible voice.... Only through constantly repeated efforts was it possible to eventually establish some limited information.

Clinical Evaluation

Her ability to encode information is most severely disturbed. If one shows her objects, she usually names them correctly. Immediately thereafter, however, she has forgotten everything. In reading, she confuses lines, reads by spelling, or with senseless intonation. When writing, she repeats single syllables many times, omits others and gets stuck altogether very quickly. When speaking, she frequently uses phrases indicating perplexity or embarrassment, or single paraphasic expressions (milk pourer instead of cup); some-

times one observes that she is completely at a loss for words....

...general imbecility keeps progressing. The 4½-year illness ended in death. Terminally, the patient was totally dulled, lying in bed with legs drawn up, incontinent, and despite all care, developed decubiti.

Autopsy

The autopsy reveals a consistently atrophic brain. Preparations stained with Bielschowsky's silver method reveal peculiar changes of the neurofibrils. Inside an otherwise apparently still normal cell, first one or more fibrils stand out prominently because of their unusual thickness and unusual ability to take up stain. Later on, there are many such fibrils lying next to each other, all changed in the same way. These are eventually seen clustering together in thick bundles which gradually emerge at the surface of the cell.... About one-quarter to one-third of all ganglion cells in the cortex show such changes, and numerous ganglion cells, especially in the upper cell layers, have altogether disappeared.

Scattered over the entire cortex, and especially numerous in the upper layers, there are miliary foci distinguishable by the deposit in the cerebral cortex of a peculiar substance which can be recognized without stain and is, in fact, very refractory to staining....

---

*Translation reproduced, with permission, from L. Jarvic and H. Greenson. Alzheimer's Disease and Related Disorders 1:7–8, 1987.

to register items in a conversation, asking for the same information over and over again. During the early phase of the illness, the patient's personality will remain intact with preservation of social skills such that problems with memory may be unappreciated by colleagues or family. Only later are errors in business and family affairs discovered.

Early in the illness, patients show their greatest functional problems with learning new material and recalling recent memories. They spend longer amounts of time at mental tasks and accomplish less. Mental fatigue becomes apparent, causing frustration in some patients but indifference in others. In contrast to difficulty with new memories, recall of remote memories seems well preserved. Clinicians commonly observe that patients can remember events of their own childhood but not their grandchildren's names. However, investigators point out that items of personal history are over-rehearsed and formal tests of distant events reveal difficulties with past memory in patients as well. In normal aging, the speed and detail of recollections decline; however, cues and prompting reveal that recognition of events is well preserved. This finding is easily appreciated during the neurological examination when short-term memory is tested. Patients with Alzheimer's disease will have difficulty recalling three unrelated test items, such as a "ball," "sweater," and "train." When they are prompted with a list of possibilities, their performance will barely improve, indicating difficulty with registration and encoding as well as with recall.

Patients undergo a characteristic dissolution of language functions. This appears first as difficulty with word finding and eventually results in speech that is impoverished of nouns. Patients will exhibit difficulty generating word lists, such as names of animals or words beginning with a particular letter, as well as with confrontational naming of objects. Syntax, the grammatical structure of language, remains relatively preserved. For example, a patient asked to name the "collar" of a physician's white coat might reply, "that's the part that goes around the thing you're wearing." This type of language might be interpreted as a difficulty with memory for words rather than a difficulty with language *per se*. The localization of anomic aphasia in early Alzheimer's disease cannot be resolved anatomically or physiologically. In contrast to language production, language comprehension is well preserved. A patient asked to point to the collar of a physician's coat will perform this act correctly. However, as global dementia progresses, language comprehension also fails, and patients show confusion or even indifference to multiple-step commands and eventually to simple commands. Semantic paraphasias (calling a spoon a fork), phonemic paraphasias (calling a spoon a sploom), and neologisms will appear in speech and go uncorrected. Eventually, fluency and grammar become curtailed and disrupted as patients become stuck in meaningless perseverations, simply repeat what they hear (echolalia), or become mute.

In a minority of patients, abnormalities with language are prominent early, suggesting a focal dominant hemisphere process. The discovery of other cognitive deficits on detailed neuropsychological testing aids in the diagnosis of a more diffuse, global process. Similarly, a minority of patients may present first with prominent deficits of visuospatial functions, properties predominantly localized in the nondominant hemisphere. Eventually, all patients show visuospatial deficits. There will be progressive difficulty with drawing familiar objects on command, such as a house or a face. Details drop away as the drawings become simplified and distorted (Figure 16–1). Copying three-dimensional and then two-dimensional objects and designs becomes impaired. Determining the right and left sides of the examiner, or copying different hand positions and movements, will be difficult. Early in the course of the disease, patients may become lost in unfamiliar surroundings. In the final stages, there will be difficulty in dressing and in recognizing and using common objects, such as opening a lock with a key, folding a letter and putting it in an envelope, or using eating utensils properly. Disruption of well-learned manual behaviors or gestures is called apraxia and is common in Alzheimer's disease.

In the final stage of the illness, the patient requires total care for dressing, eating, and personal hygiene. Features of parkinsonism may become evident with rigidity and difficulty with posture and gait. Myoclonus and seizures can develop. Difficulty with eating and swallowing accelerate debility and can lead to aspiration and pneumonia, a common cause of death.

In the early and even middle stages of Alzheimer's disease, the loss of cortical functions predominates: amnesia, aphasia, apraxia, and agnosia. While there is relative preservation of simple processes of movement, strength, sensation, vision, and hearing, the integration of these functions into complex thought and behavior is disrupted. Eventually the patient's personality is affected. There is a change in temperament, with some becoming irritable and even agitated and others apathetic and placid. Overt symptoms of depression may become apparent early in the illness. Delusions are not uncommon and are often directed at a spouse's fidelity (see Box 16–1). Rarely, patients may believe that a spouse or a relative is an impostor. These behavioral symptoms are important to recognize and treat promptly for the patient's as well as the caretaker's comfort and safety.

Risk Factors

Risk factors for developing Alzheimer's disease include **older age, family history,** and **head trauma**. There is a progressive increase in the prevalence of Alzheimer's with advancing years. It was once speculated that the illness represented accelerated aging, since autopsies of brains of nondemented elderly commonly demonstrated some pathological evidence of the Alzheimer process. There are increasing numbers of amyloid plaques in the brain with aging, but detailed neurochemical studies reveal that only certain types are pathological. In addition, it is now recognized that genetic factors play a prominent role in forming

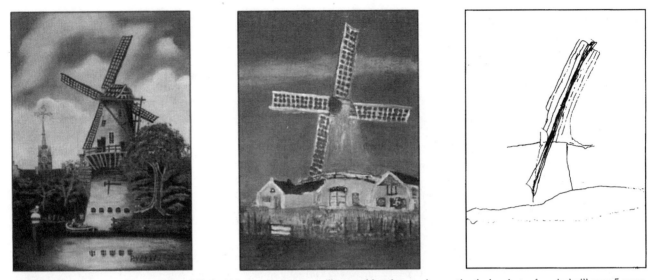

FIGURE 16–1. Deterioration in cognitive skills in Alzheimer's disease as illustrated by changes in a patient's drawings of a windmill over 5 years. There is progressive simplification, loss of detail, and overall geometric distortion. (Reproduced, with permission, from J. L. Cummings. Probable Alzheimer's disease in an artist. JAMA 258:2731–2734, 1987. Copyright 1987 American Medical Association.)

pathological lesions in late- as well as early-onset Alzheimer's disease.

Genetic linkage for developing Alzheimer's disease has been found on chromosomes 1, 14, 19, and 21 (Table 16–1). The gene on the long arm of chromosome 14 accounts for most early-onset familial cases. Patients commonly present before age 50 and experience an accelerated course of dementia with increased muscle tone, seizures, and myoclonus. The gene codes for a membrane protein with seven transmembrane regions typical of channels or receptors, although its exact function is currently unknown. Members of different families with Alzheimer's disease have been found to have different missense mutations in the protein.

The locus on chromosome 19 codes for apolipoprotein and is a major risk factor determinant for autosomal-dominant, late-onset disease; it plays a role in sporadic cases as well. There are three alleles for the gene—E2, E3, and E4—which differ by one or two amino acids. ApoE4 is the pathogenetic allele. Systemically, these proteins transport cholesterol in the blood. In the brain, they are secreted by astrocytes and are thought to play a role in reparative processes along with other acute-phase reactants—complement and α_1-antichymotrypsin. All three molecules are found deposited within neuritic plaques in Alzheimer's disease. If a person carries one copy of E4 (20% of the population),

there is a two- to fourfold increased risk for Alzheimer's. If a person is homozygous for the allele, E4/E4 (2–3% of the population), the risk is increased 5–15 times. It is estimated that 25–40% of all Alzheimer's is related to ApoE4. The exact pathogenetic mechanism of this protein may relate to its interaction with other proteins in forming amyloid (Box 16–2).

Genetic linkage to chromosome 21 is the gene that codes for the β-amyloid precursor protein (APP), a membrane glycoprotein in neurons. This protein contains a fragment of variable length that accounts for the amyloid staining in the neuritic plaques of Alzheimer's disease. This fragment, called β-amyloid (Aβ), is a family of peptides 39–44 amino acids long found within and extending beyond the transmembrane region of APP (see Box 16–2). In Alzheimer's disease, the peptides form β-pleated sheets in the extracellular space and stain positive for Congo red and thioflavine, features that define amyloid. The genetic abnormalities associated with Alzheimer's disease cause amino acid substitutions in regions of APP outside the Aβ region. This finding indicates that alterations in the metabolism and breakdown of APP are associated with rapid accumulation of amyloid deposits and early Alzheimer's disease. The most common abnormality, accounting for 10% of early-onset familial Alzheimer's cases, is an amino acid substitution at APP717 (valine to isoleucine,

TABLE 16–1. Genes Associated with Alzheimer's Disease

Gene	Chromosome	Onset	Percentage	Protein
Disease Gene				
FAD 1	21	45–65	1%	Amyloid precursor protein
FAD 2	14	30–50	5–10%	S182 Membrane protein
FAD 3	1	30–50	2–3%	STM2 Membrane protein
Risk Gene				
Acquired	19	>60	40–50%	Lipoprotein ApoE4

BOX 16-2 The Amyloid Hypothesis of Alzheimer's Disease

A leading hypothesis of the pathogenesis of Alzheimer's disease states that the formation of β-amyloid (Aβ) from the membrane amyloid precursor protein (APP) is the primary abnormal event in the disease process. Upon formation, Aβ fibrils condense in the extracellular space, disrupting fine neurites and synapses, activating astrocytes and microglia, ultimately leading to neuronal death.

APP is a glycoprotein that spans the plasma membrane and acts as a cell surface receptor (see Figure, *opposite*). Its short internal carboxyl portion anchors the protein to the cytoskeleton or acts in signal transduction (or both). It is found mainly in the nervous system but also exists in platelets and lymphocytes. Up to 18 exons participate in coding different isoforms comprising 695, 714, 751, or 770 amino acids. APP695 is the dominant human CNS isoform, although the relative percentage of longer isoforms may increase with aging. The control of transcription and splicing events for the relative production of different APP isoforms is unknown.

The Aβ domain of APP is 39–43 amino acids long and lies partly within and partly extracellular to the plasma membrane. Aβ40 is the form normally found in CSF, but Aβ42 is the predominant form in Alzheimer's plaques. Aβ39 predominates in vascular amyloid. Two points are noteworthy regarding these Aβ peptides. First, they represent genetic coding from apposed portions of exons 16 and 17 and thus are not derived by alternative splicing. Second, the favored proteolytic pathway for APP breakdown and turnover is enzymatic cleavage at a point *within* Aβ. Thus, Aβ formation is thought to represent accentuated metabolism of a minor proteolytic pathway of APP

with cleavage sites on either side of Aβ. In familial Alzheimer's disease, genetic substitutions within APP may lead to amino acid sequences or protein conformational changes that block normal proteolysis and favor Aβ formation. Since these genetic diseases account for less than 1% of Alzheimer's disease, other mechanisms must play a role in altered APP metabolism in the majority of cases.

Loose or diffuse amyloid plaques are found in brains of nondemented elderly as well as brains of people with Down syndrome (trisomy 21). The latter condition may represent an example of increased substrate for Aβ formation by a mass action effect, since there are three copies of APP gene. These plaques are relatively simple and do not contain reactive proteins or form dense condensations around neurites and synaptic endings.

Aβ peptides spontaneously associate into β-sheets forming fibrils *in vitro*. The rate of fibril formation is greatly accelerated by α1-antichymotrypsin and ApoE, two proteins released by reactive glia in the brain in Alzheimer's disease. ApoE4 is more potent than the other ApoE isoforms, consistent with its being the greatest risk factor for Alzheimer's disease. Fibrillary plaques in Alzheimer's disease contain these reactive proteins, condense around dystrophic neurites and synaptic endings, and are associated with activated glia and microglia. The pathogenesis of neuritic senile plaques may be simply related to the number of diffuse senile plaques. With advancing age, diffuse plaques accumulate before the appearance of neuritic plaques. Alternatively, there may be factors that accelerate the formation of the elaborated neuritic plaque such as genetic abnormalities in membrane proteins S182 and STM2.

Continued on opposite page

glycine, or phenylalanine), just two amino acids removed from the Aβ portion of APP (see Box 16–2). A substitution at APP695 (glutamine for glutamic acid) causes a familial disease characterized by excess deposition of Aβ in vessel walls, leading to cerebral hemorrhage (hereditary cerebral hemorrhage with amyloidosis–Dutch type, HCHWA-D).

Head trauma may also be a factor in Alzheimer's disease, increasing the risk up to twofold in some studies. The degree of trauma must be moderately severe, causing loss of consciousness or hospitalization. It is suggested that head trauma may initiate secretion of ApoE and acute-phase reactants, which accelerate the formation of amyloid and neuritic plaques.

Estrogen may provide a protective effect against Alzheimer's disease. Women taking estrogen replacement medications after menopause have a lower incidence of the disease compared with other women. A decline in estrogen production within the brain with aging may play a role in pathogenesis.

Lack of formal education is also a relative risk factor; persons with no schooling have a twofold greater risk than those with 6–8 years of education. Interpretation of this finding probably involves the greater development and functional reserve of cognitive skills in the educated.

Pathophysiology

The identification of several genetic and epigenetic factors in the cause of Alzheimer's disease likely indicates that there are several different diseases with a similar phenotypic expression. Nevertheless, it has not been possible to define these separate diseases on clinical or pathological grounds. Since the first description of Alzheimer, the clinical disease has been defined on the basis of neuronal loss, gliosis, and two pathological criteria that are found in all genotypes: intraneuronal neurofibrillary tangles and extracellular β-amyloid-rich senile plaques. The former is related to the metabolism of cytoskeletal proteins called τ (tau). The latter is related to the metabolism of the membrane protein APP. It is possible that different disease processes affect metabolism of these proteins by different mechanisms but lead to a similar pathological and clinical picture.

Neurofibrillary tangles are intracellular deposits of paired helical filaments formed by an abnormal excessive phosphorylation of τ proteins. These proteins (six isoforms) normally bind to microtubules and stabilize them in a polymerized state in the neuron's cytoskeleton. In Alzheimer's disease, they become separated from microtubules, undergo abnormal phosphorylation, and associate into paired helical filaments

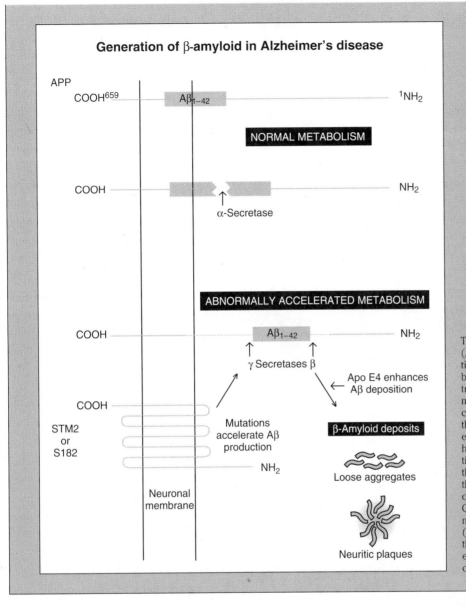

Generation of β-amyloid in Alzheimer's disease

NORMAL METABOLISM

α-Secretase

ABNORMALLY ACCELERATED METABOLISM

γ Secretases β

Apo E4 enhances Aβ deposition

Mutations accelerate Aβ production

β-Amyloid deposits

Loose aggregates

Neuritic plaques

Neuronal membrane

The amyloid precursor protein (APP) contains the amyloid peptide partly within the transmembrane portion and partly in the extracellular domain. The major metabolic pathway involves α-secretase splitting the β-peptide, thereby preventing formation of extracellular deposits. In Alzheimer's disease, there is acceleration of a minor metabolic pathway that cleaves the β-peptide on either side, thus allowing formation of amyloid deposits in the tissue. Genetic mutations in APP, or in the membrane protein STM2 or S182 (Table 16–1), seem to accelerate this metabolic pathway. The presence of ApoE4 enhances amyloid deposition.

(PHFts). Neurofibrillary tangles are found principally in large pyramidal cells of the hippocampus and neocortex. Involvement of neurons in layers II and III of the cerebral cortex is particularly intense. Involvement of these cells disrupts the association pathways from one cortical area to another, probably accounting for deficits in higher cognitive functions. Tangles are also prominent in the entorhinal cortex, where they disrupt neocortical projections into hippocampus, probably accounting for problems with memory and learning. PHFts also form neuropil threads, which are fine fibrillary structures seen in dendrites with silver staining. The progressive accumulation of intraneuronal neurofilaments leads to neuronal degeneration and cell death. Occasionally neurofibrillary tangles are seen as the only remnant of a cell body. More commonly, PHFts are found in dystrophic neurites in association with senile plaques.

Senile plaques are composed of aggregations of Aβ fibrils. These aggregations can exist loosely in the

neuropil as diffuse senile plaques. They are commonly found in brains of nondemented elderly persons and are not considered of pathological significance unless they are in excessive numbers or are accompanied by other pathological changes. However, Aβ fibrils can also become condensed into radial arrays associated with neuritic processes—swollen terminals and abnormal synaptic boutons (Figure 16–2). These are called neuritic senile plaques and are characteristic of Alzheimer's disease. In addition to amyloid, they contain τ, ApoE, complement, and α₁-antichymotrypsin. These are localized to the cerebral gray matter. The pathogenesis of these abnormal structures is unclear. Some evidence suggests that there are separate processes for the generation of Aβ and PHFts, while recent studies have found that the τ proteins bind with a conformation-dependent domain of APP714-723. One unifying hypothesis submits that phosphorylated τ proteins disrupt neurites and cause excessive secretion of APP amyloidogenic peptides. These proteins become

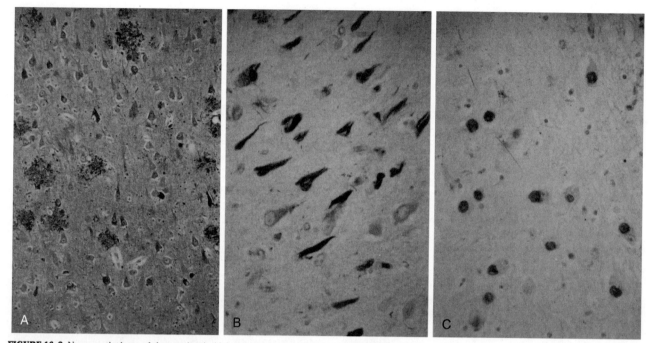

FIGURE 16-2. Neuropathology of dementia. *A,* Alzheimer's disease. Section of hippocampus showing abundant senile plaques and neurofibrillary tangles. *B,* Alzheimer's disease showing intracellular neurofibrillary tangles. Gallyas technique. *C,* Pick's disease. Section from the frontal lobe showing intracellular inclusions. (Courtesy of H. Vinters, M.D.)

concentrated in the extracellular space as the neuritic senile plaque. The amyloid hypothesis holds that the primary abnormality is the metabolism of APP into Aβ (Box 16–2).

The severity of dementia in Alzheimer's disease correlates only weakly with the quantity of neuritic senile plaques and neurofibrillary tangles. These gross structures represent final products of processes that disrupt neuronal function more widely. Immunohistochemical stains for synaptic proteins indicate progressive loss of synapses in Alzheimer's disease. The magnitude of synaptic loss correlates well with the degree of dementia. Particular synapses may be depleted early, such as in hippocampus. Destruction of neurons in the nucleus basalis in the basal forebrain causes a progressive loss of widely projecting cholinergic neurons to the cortex. In addition to depletion of cortical levels of acetylcholine, there is also loss of somatostatin. Therapeutic strategies have been devised to improve cholinergic and somatostatin neurotransmission in Alzheimer's disease.

Evaluation and Differential Diagnosis

A diagnosis of dementia requires the presence of a decline in memory and cognitive functions that impairs daily activities. In contrast to patients with delirium or encephalopathy, demented patients retain a normal level of consciousness. The clinical approach to a specific diagnosis follows the steps for history taking, examination, and laboratory testing (Table 16–2). The list of possible causes is long but easily evaluated clinically within a few days (Table 16–3). The discovery of a treatable or reversible illness requires a comprehensive approach.

The clinical diagnosis of *probable* Alzheimer's disease rests upon finding progressive deterioration of memory and cognitive functions in the absence of other brain or systemic disease that could account for the findings (Table 16–4). Lacking a specific laboratory test, a diagnosis of *definite* Alzheimer's disease requires a brain biopsy that reveals significant numbers of neuritic senile plaques and neurofibrillary tangles. Practitioners can make a diagnosis of probable or possible Alz-

TABLE 16-2. Clinical Approach to Dementia

History (points of emphasis)
    Patient's history, with confirmation from a collateral source
    Familial cases
    Current medical conditions
    Medicines
Physical examination
    Mental status testing and Mini-Mental State Examination
        Memory
        Language
        Reasoning and judgment
        Visual or spatial skills
        Personality and social skills
    Hearing and vision
    Stance and gait
    Focal neurological signs
Laboratory tests
    Blood: CBC, ESR, chemistry panel, thyroid test, vitamin B_{12} level
    Chest x-ray
    ECG
    Imaging: CT or MRI
Supplementary tests if indicated
    VDRL and HIV
    EEG
    Lumbar puncture
    Neuropsychometric testing

TABLE 16-3. Differential Diagnosis of Dementia (Common or Treatable Causes)

Primary degenerative conditions
   Cortical
      Alzheimer's disease
      Pick's disease
   Subcortical
      Parkinson's disease
      Huntington's disease
      Multiple system atrophies
      Progressive supranuclear palsy
Vascular disease
   Multi-infarct dementia
   Lacunar state
   Binswanger's disease
   Postcardiac arrest
Traumatic injury
   Subdural hematoma
   Dementia pugilistica (boxer's dementia)
Infectious disease
   AIDS
   Syphilis
Nutritional and metabolic conditions
   Hypothyroidism
   Vitamin B_{12} deficiency
   Alcoholism
Neoplastic disease
   Frontal lobe tumors
   Disseminated metastasis
Hydrocephalus

heimer's disease by clinical examination and laboratory testing alone (see Table 16–2). The important steps include careful documentation of memory and cognitive performance on a standardized test such as the Mini-Mental State Examination (Box 6–4), repeat evaluations over time that reveal deterioration, and elimination of other possible causes. The diagnosis is supported by a positive family history and the finding of atrophy as the only abnormality on a CT or MRI scan.

Normal aging can cause mental changes that superficially resemble Alzheimer's disease. There is a decrease in reaction time and a decline in tests of memory and problem solving. Memory for names is the most fragile, but in contrast to Alzheimer's disease,

TABLE 16-4. Criteria for Diagnosis of Alzheimer's Disease

Definite
  Clinical criteria for probable Alzheimer's disease
  Biopsy or autopsy showing plaques and tangles
Probable
  Progressive worsening of memory
  Deficits in at least one other cognitive area
  No disturbance of consciousness
  Onset between 40 and 90 years of age (usually after 65)
  Absence of other brain or systemic disorders that could explain
    deficits
Possible
  Dementia syndrome with variation in onset, features, or course
    atypical of Alzheimer's disease, but in the absence of other
    causes of dementia
  Presence of a second causative or contributing process (e.g.,
    vascular disease) thought not to be the major cause of the
    dementia

immediate memory for short lists and logically associated materials (working memory) is preserved. Language and abstract thinking are also relatively well preserved. The elderly commonly develop problems with vision and hearing that can accentuate cognitive problems. In addition, advancing age brings an increased prevalence of cardiac, pulmonary, digestive, and musculoskeletal disease. These illnesses and their treatment can adversely affect mental functions. Persons over age 65 commonly take five or more medicines daily, which alone or in combination often prove to be the cause of cognitive impairment. Careful evaluation of concurrent illness and medication use is of great importance in the workup for possible dementia.

Depression can occur as an early manifestation of Alzheimer's disease or appear independently in the elderly. In the latter situation, it is not uncommon to find features of dementia along with primary mood depression and difficulty with memory, problem solving, and learning tasks. These deficits probably reflect primary problems with sustained attention and speed of processing. They clear with the treatment of depression. However, the presence of apraxia, visuospatial disorder, or aphasia should alert the examiner to the probability that the depression is a feature of a more widespread dementing illness. The depressive symptoms may respond to treatment, but the cognitive deficits will remain.

Vascular disease is a common cause of dementia in the elderly, being second only to Alzheimer's disease. In addition, many patients with Alzheimer's have concomitant vascular disease that adds to the dementia. Three types of vascular syndromes are recognized. First, **multiinfarct dementia** is the result of multiple strokes that progressively destroy more and more functioning brain. A careful history reveals abrupt onset of symptoms and stepwise progression reflecting multiple vascular events. The examination often demonstrates focal neurological signs such as asymmetric spastic weakness, hemisensory loss, or a characteristic aphasia. Imaging studies reveal multiple areas of small or large brain infarction.

The **lacunar state (état lacunaire)** is the name given to the clinical picture that results from multiple strokes of subcortical structures, particularly basal ganglia, thalamus, and pons. Pseudobulbar palsy is often present, with slow dysarthric speech and emotional incontinence. Responses to questions are particularly slow and often incomplete. Language is often abbreviated or telegraphic, although understandable, whereas in Alzheimer's disease, language can be quite effusive but devoid of meaning. The neurological examination reveals abnormalities in the motor system with increased tone, slowed awkward movements, and abnormal reflexes.

Binswanger's disease, once thought to be a rare vascular disease of hemispheric white matter, is now recognized more commonly in the elderly by means of CT and MRI scans. T2-weighted MRI scans (Chapter 2) are particularly sensitive for detecting ischemia or infarction from occlusion of deep penetrating vessels into the white matter and periventricular zone

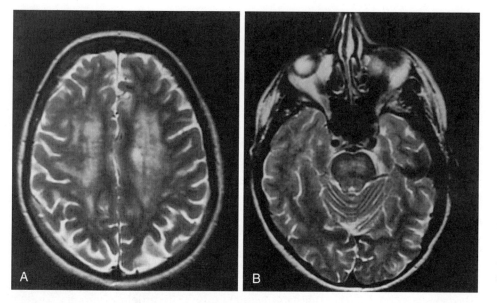

FIGURE 16–3. MRI scan of a patient with vascular dementia showing changes consistent with a diagnosis of Binswanger's disease. This 82-year-old man had a slow, glue-footed gait in addition to slowed thinking, forgetfulness, and deterioration in behavior and speech. *A,* There are hyperintense coalescent lesions deep in the cortical white matter, particularly around the ventricles. *B,* Lesions can also be seen in subcortical sites in the midbrain and pons.

(Figure 16–3). The progressive accumulation and co-alescence of lesions disrupt corticocortical connections, impairing cognitive functions and leading to dementia. Often there are no characteristic clinical features of the Binswanger's vascular dementia that can be reliably used to distinguish it from Alzheimer's disease. The history of a stroke-like episode, the presence of stroke risk factors, or the finding of focal weakness on examination will provide suggestive evidence. Imaging studies are essential in identifying the presence of occult white matter vascular disease.

Treatment

At present there is no primary treatment for Alzheimer's disease. Owing to recent advances in understanding the biochemical pathways for β-amyloid, new therapies will be targeted on blocking its formation or enhancing its normal degradation.

Symptomatic therapies directed at improving cholinergic neurotransmission in Alzheimer's disease have been under investigation for many years. The "cholinergic hypothesis" of dementia rests upon several observations. First, there is damage to cholinergic nuclei in the basal forebrain (basal nucleus, nucleus of the diagonal band, septal nuclei) with depletion of acetyl choline in the cortex and hippocampus. Second, pharmacological blockade by scopolamine of central cholinergic synapses in healthy volunteers causes a memory deficit similar to that found in Alzheimer's disease. Third, the scopolamine-induced memory deficit can be reversed by physostigmine, an acetylcholinesterase inhibitor. Clinical trials of physostigmine or tacrine, another central acetylcholinesterase inhibitor, have not resulted in consistent or sustained improvement in memory in Alzheimer's disease, although there is a psychotropic or alerting affect. At best, a third of patients taking tacrine will show a modest improvement in memory for 6–12 months.

When vascular disease is found as the underlying cause of dementia or in combination with Alzheimer's disease, it is important to guide therapy toward treatment of risk factors for stroke: hypertension, diabetes, hyperlipidemia, and heart disease (see Chapter 15). Although successful treatment of these factors should stabilize the disease process, clinical studies indicate that the overall prognosis for survival with vascular dementia is the same as for Alzheimer's disease.

Patients with dementia are benefited by treatment of symptoms of depression and agitation. Participation in scheduled, routine daily activities in the home or in community centers is also helpful for patients in the early stages of the illness. These activities also provide relief for family caretakers.

Patients and families should be told the diagnosis of Alzheimer's disease as early as possible, although care should be taken to minimize the psychological stress that comes with the diagnosis. Failure to counsel and educate patients and families during the illness can increase stress and discomfort. Many find joining a support group particularly helpful. Patients need to attend to financial and legal affairs early in the illness. They should be told not to drive. In some states, laws require physicians to report cases to the Public Health Service for possible revocation of the driver's license. With advancing disability, plans for institutional or permanent home care should be considered.

PRIMARY DEMENTIAS
Frontal Lobe Dementia

Diseases of the frontal lobes cause a characteristic dementia that is different from Alzheimer's disease. The illnesses are uncommon. Pick's disease is a degenerative process characterized pathologically by fibrillary inclusion bodies in neurons of the frontal and temporal lobes. Dementia of the frontal lobe type (DFT) is the name given to a disease process lacking specific pathology other than neuronal loss and gliosis. Rarely, a structural process affecting both frontal lobes, such as a parasagittal or basilar meningioma, can cause frontal dementia.

Patients' first symptoms of frontal lobe dementia reflect a change in personality rather than a change in memory or specific cortical functions. Apathy and indifference develop along with disinhibition from social standards. They may make inappropriate comments or gestures, often of a sexual kind, seemingly unaware or unconcerned with the effects or consequences on themselves or others. They develop rigid behavior, a characteristic that is appreciated in cognitive function tests where there is difficulty in changing mental sets. The Wisconsin Card Sorting Test is sensitive to this type of frontal lobe dysfunction. With advancing disease, problems with word finding develop, manifested on direct testing as difficulty in generating lists of animals, or words beginning with a specific letter. Speech becomes curtailed. Features of the Klüver-Bucy syndrome may emerge, in which patients excessively explore objects by touching them or putting them in their mouth.

The diagnosis of frontal lobe dementias is aided by neuroimaging. CT and MRI scans can demonstrate atrophy of the frontal and anterior temporal lobes in advanced cases. In earlier stages, PET or SPECT scans will reveal a decrease in blood flow and metabolism in the frontal lobes that precedes the development of overt atrophy. By contrast, in early Alzheimer's disease there is hypometabolism in the parietal lobes.

Subcortical Dementias

Changes in cognition and behavior commonly accompany degenerative disease processes that primarily affect subcortical structures: **progressive supranuclear palsy, Parkinson's disease** (Chapter 11), **Huntington's disease** (Chapter 12), and **subcortical strokes** (the lacunar state, Chapter 15). Characteristically these patients exhibit slow thought processes, dysarthric speech, lack of mental flexibility, apathy, a tendency for depression, and forgetfulness. Language functions, calculations, and visuospatial skills remain relatively preserved. Specific abnormalities of the motor system occur in each of these conditions. Disease processes in subcortical structures probably do not account for these mental changes in themselves. Rather, it is thought that there is a disruption of cortico-subcortical relationships, particularly with the frontal lobe. The prefrontal cortex projects heavily onto the caudate nucleus, which is damaged in Huntington's disease. Abnormal activity in basal ganglia circuits in Parkinson's disease projects onto premotor and supplementary cortex. Cognitive and behavioral symptoms of diseases that primarily affect the frontal lobes or basal ganglia structures overlap because they are functionally interconnected.

Lewy Body Dementias

With the development of immunohistochemical stains for ubiquitin and neurofilament proteins, it has become relatively easy to search for cytoplasmic inclusions in degenerative diseases. Lewy bodies, prominent in substantia nigra, have now been found in the cortex of demented patients with Parkinson's disease as well as typical Alzheimer's disease. The latter condition has been called the "Lewy body variant" of Alzheimer's disease. At present it is not clear whether cortical Lewy bodies signify a separate, specific disease process or abnormalities of specific cell types undergoing the degeneration process of Parkinson's disease and Alzheimer's disease. Advances in molecular biology and neurochemistry will clarify these issues.

Prion Diseases

Human prion diseases are uncommon dementing disorders that cause neuronal loss, gliosis, vacuolar-spongiform changes, and deposition of prion protein amyloid in the absence of tissue inflammation. The most frequently encountered is **Creutzfeldt-Jakob disease** (CJD), which is characterized by rapidly progressive dementia, focal neurological signs, myoclonus, and death in 3–12 months. There are characteristic changes on the EEG reflecting aggressive pathology in the cerebral cortex. The **Gerstmann-Straussler-Scheinker** (GSS) **syndrome** and **fatal familial insomnia** are two other forms of human prion disease. These latter two are genetically transmitted, while 10–15% of CJD is also familial. Both CJD and GSS syndrome have been experimentally transmitted to various animal species, and horizontal human-to-human transmission of CJD has been documented in cases of corneal transplants, contaminated surgical instruments, and the therapeutic use of human pituitary growth hormone.

The mechanisms underlying the inheritability and infectivity of prion diseases are still being worked out. CJD is the only example of an infectious human disease that can be transmitted by a protein alone. The pathogenetic mechanism of transmission is thought to be related to the structural properties of the protein itself. The prion protein contains 253 amino acids, coded by 759 base pairs from a single exon of the prion protein gene (PRNP). The function of the protein is unknown. In the native state, it exists in an α-helix configuration. In causing disease it comes out of this formation and forms β-pleated sheets that aggregate into insoluble amyloid. Prion protein amyloid plaques are found in these diseases. This abnormal isoform of the protein (called PrP^{Sc} after the infectious agent isolated from scrapie disease of sheep) seems to act as a nidus for amyloid accumulation as well as a stimulus for inducing normal cellular prion protein (PrP^{C}) to undergo formation of β-sheets. The propensity of prion proteins to undergo this pathogenetic conformational change—PrP^{C} to PrP^{Sc}—is at least partly related to rare genetically transmitted amino acid substitutions among nonconserved sites in the protein. GSS syndrome and the inherited form of CJD are linked to several different substitutions in the protein in different families. In addition, codon 129 appears particularly important in conferring susceptibility to sporadic and iatrogenic disease. If there is homozygosity for the alleles, either valine-valine or methionine-methionine, there is increased risk for CJD compared to the heterozygous condition, valine-methionine.

These studies of the rare prion protein disease have provided new insights into disease mechanisms. Simple amino acid substitutions in a protein can confer hereditary susceptibility for amyloid formation in prion disease, Alzheimer's disease (APP717), hereditary cerebral hemorrhage with amyloidosis (APP618), and familial amyloid polyneuropathy (Chapter 9). The discovery of specific wild-type alleles that confer vulnerability for sporadic illness in the prion diseases raises the question whether similar mechanisms might underlie more common types of degenerative disease.

SUMMARY

Dementia is an endemic disorder in the elderly. When it is first encountered, physicians must search for treatable causes of mental impairment associated with concurrent systemic diseases, medications, endocrine and vitamin deficiencies, infections, and tumors. Cerebrovascular disease is a cause of dementia that might be prevented by careful control of risk factors. Alzheimer's disease is the most common cause of dementia and seems to be in part the consequence of abnormal metabolism of the amyloid precursor protein in the neuronal membrane. The presence of ApoE4 is a major risk factor. Experiments focused on understanding and controlling APP metabolism will likely yield new, perhaps primary, forms of therapy.

Selected Readings

Bennet, D. A., R. S. Wilson, D. W. Gilley, and J. H. Fox. Clinical diagnosis of Binswanger's disease. J Neurol Neurosurg Psychiatry 53:961–965, 1990.

Elby, E. M., I. M. Parhad, D. H. Hogan, and T. S. Fung. Prevalence and types of dementia in the very old. Neurology 44:1593–1600, 1994.

Games, D., et al. Alzheimer's-type neuropathology in transgenic mice overexpressing V717F β-amyloid precursor protein. Nature 373:523–527, 1995.

Gibb, W.R.G., M. M. Esiri, and A. J. Lees. Clinical and pathological features of diffuse cortical Lewy body disease (Lewy body dementia). Brain 110:1131–1153, 1985.

Lampe, T. H., T. D. Bird, D. Nochlin, et al. Phenotype of chromosome 14–linked familial Alzheimer's disease in a large kindred. Ann Neurol 36:368–378, 1994.

Ma J., A. Yee, H. B. Brewer, Jr., et al. Amyloid-associated proteins α_1-antichymotrypsin and apolipoprotein E promote assembly of Alzheimer β-protein into filaments. Nature 372:92–94, 1994.

McKhann, G., D. Drachman, M. Folstein, et al. Clinical diagnosis of Alzheimer's disease. Neurology 34:939–944, 1984.

Neary, D., J. S. Snowden, B. Nothen, and P. Goulding. Dementia of the frontal lobe type. J Neurol Neurosurg Psychiatry 51:353–361, 1988.

Pruisner, S. Human prion diseases. Ann Neurol 35:385–395, 1994.

Roman, G. C., et al. Vascular dementia: Diagnostic criteria for research studies. Neurology 43:250–260, 1993.

Sherrington, R., et al. Cloning of a gene bearing missense mutations in early-onset familial Alzheimer's disease. Nature 375:754–760, 1995.

Smith, M. A., S. L. Siedlak, P. L. Richey, et al. Tau protein interacts with the amyloid β-precursor: Implications for Alzheimer's disease. Nature Medicine 1:365–369, 1995.

Terry, R. D., E. Masliah, D. P. Salmon, et al. Physical basis of cognitive alterations in Alzheimer's disease: Synapse loss is the major correlate of cognitive impairment. Ann Neurol 30:572–580, 1991.

INDEX

Note: Page numbers in italics indicate figures; those with a t indicate tables; those with a b indicate boxes.

A

Abducens nerve, 15–16
Absence seizure, 151, *151*
Acalculia, defined, 73b
Accessory nerve, 16
Acetaminophen, 45t
Acetylcholine receptor, *99,* 102–103
Achromatopsia, defined, 50
Acoustic nerve. *See* Vestibulocochlear nerve.
Acoustic neuroma, 53t, 53–54
Acquired immunodeficiency syndrome (AIDS), cytomegaloviral infections in, 115–116
    Guillain-Barré syndrome with, 116
    herpes zoster in, 116
    neuropathy in, 115–116
    polymyositis syndrome in, 86t, 94
Action tremor, 33–35
Adrenal transplant, for parkinsonism, 137
Aging, Alzheimer's disease and, 191
    dementia and, 185
    disease risks with, 5
    hearing loss and, 50t
    transient global amnesia and, 79
Agnosia, 73b
Agraphesthesia, 41
Agraphia, alexia without, 73, 73b
    Broca's aphasia with, 72
AIDS. *See* Acquired immunodeficiency syndrome (AIDS).
Akinesia, in parkinsonism, 128
Akinetic mutism. *See* Persistent vegetative state.
Alcohol, headaches and, 44, 45t
    myopathy with, 86t
    neuropathy from, 4, 109t
    nystagmus and, 55t
    seizures with, 149t
    stroke and, 176
    tremor with, 12
    vertigo with, 53t
Alexia, 73, 73b

Allergic encephalomyelitis, 164, 165b
ALS. *See* Amyotrophic lateral sclerosis (ALS).
Altered consciousness, 57b
Alzheimer's disease, 185–192. *See also* Dementia.
    amyloid hypothesis of, 187–188, 188b–189b
    anterior horn cell degeneration in, 120
    apraxia in, 74
    depression in, 191
    diagnosis of, 190t, 190–192, 191t, *192*
    Down syndrome and, 188b–189b
    early description of, 185b
    genetic factors in, 4, 187t, 187–188
    head trauma and, 188
    hippocampus, *190*
    language in, 186, *187*
    neurofibrillary tangles in, 188–189, *190*
    parkinsonism and, 186
    pathophysiology of, 188–190, *190*
    presentation of, 185b, 185–186
    risk factors for, 186–188, 188b
    senile plaques in, 189–190, *190*
    treatment of, 192
Amantadine, for multiple sclerosis, 170t
Amaurosis fugax, 175
Aminoglycoside antibiotics, myasthenia and, 104
Amitriptyline, for pain syndromes, 45t
Amnesia. *See also* Memory.
    anterograde, 78
    causes of, 77t
    from head trauma, 77t, 79
    hippocampus and, 77t, 80b
    retrograde, 78
    transient global, 79
Amygdala, limbic system and, *71*
Amyloid hypothesis, of Alzheimer's disease, 187–188, 188b–189b
Amyloid polyneuropathy, 115
Amyotrophic lateral sclerosis (ALS), 118–125
    diagnosis of, 119t, 123–124, *124*
    genetic factors in, 4, 120

Amyotrophic lateral sclerosis (ALS) *(Continued)*
    pathology of, 120–123, *121, 122*
    patient survival in, 119, *120*
    presentation of, 118b, 118–120, 119t, *121,* 121b
    treatment of, 124–125, 125b
    variability in, 121b
Anatomical localization, of symptoms, *10,* 13
Aneurysm, pupil response with, 58
    saccular, 182
Angelman syndrome, 8
Anhedonia, in depression, 79
Anosognosia, in parietal lobe syndrome, 74
Anoxic seizure, 150
Anticholinesterase drugs, for myasthenia, 104, 105t
Anticipation phenomenon, in myotonic dystrophy, 89
Anticonvulsant drugs, 153t
Antidepressant drugs, 80, 145t
Aphasia, agraphia with, 72
    Broca's, 68b, 71–72, *72*
    conduction, 72–73, 73b
    global, 72, 73b
    types of, 71–73, 73b
    Wernicke's, 72, 73b
Aphemia, 68b
Apnea, sleep, 61
Apraxia, 73b, 73–74
    defined, 31
Archaeocerebellum, 33
Arnold-Chiari malformation, 55t
Arteriovenous malformations (AVMs), 182
Aspirin, 45t
Astereognosis, defined, 41
    in parietal lobe syndrome, 74
Ataxia, hereditary, 146t, 146–147
    chorea with, 143
Athetosis, 32
Atrophies, multiple system, 134–135, 134t
Attention, impaired, 14
Attentional systems, *74,* 74–75

Aura, in epilepsy, 153
Autonomic disorders, 63–64
AVMs (arteriovenous malformations), 182
Azathioprine, 105t
AZT (zidovudine) myopathy, 86t, 94

B

Baclofen, 30t, 124, 170t
Basal ganglia, anatomy of, 31, 31–32
    in Huntington's disease, 145
    in parkinsonism, 129
    infarction of, 143
    oculomotor disorders and, 36t
Behavior. See also specific types, e.g., Manic-
        depressive behavior.
    circuit-specific, 75
    neurobiology of, 69–71
Benign familial tremor, 33
Benign positional vertigo, 54–55
    test for, 56
Benign prostatic hypertrophy, 63
Benign senile chorea, 143
Berry aneurysm, 182
Binswanger's disease, 191–192, 193
Bipolar disorders, 80. See also Manic-
        depressive behavior.
Bladder, spastic, 63–64
Blindness. See also Visual impairment.
    cortical, 73b
Botulism, myasthenia gravis vs., 103
Bradykinesia, in parkinsonism, 32, 128
Bradyphrenia, in parkinsonism, 130
Brain. See also specific part, e.g.,
        Cerebellum.
    biochemistry of, 178b–179b
    blood flow to, 177–178
Brain death, 57b
Brain stem, hearing loss and, 50t
    infarction of, 58t
    tumor in, 53t
    vestibular pathways of, 54
Brain-derived growth factor, 125, 125b
Broca's aphasia, 68b, 71–72, 72
Brodmann's map, of cerebral cortex, 67, 69
Bruxism, trigeminal neuralgia from, 43
Bulbar palsy, progressive, 118, 119t
Buspirone, 145t

C

Caffeine, migraines and, 12, 44
Carbamazepine, for manic-depressive
        behavior, 145t
    for pain syndromes, 45t
    for seizures, 153t
    for tremor, 170t
Carcinomatous meningitis, 50t
Cardiac emboli, causes of, 181t
    heparin for, 181t
    stroke from, 173t, 180
Carotid stenosis, stroke and, 176
Carpal tunnel syndrome, 109t, 110, 111
Cataplexy, clomipramine for, 64
    symptoms of, 61–63
Cataracts, 47t
Caudate nuclei, adrenal transplant to, 137
    atrophy of, 144
        Huntington's disease and, 144
    manic-depressive behavior and, 80
Causalgia, 43
Cerebellar gait, 15
Cerebellar tremor, 33
Cerebellum, anatomy of, 33–35, 34

Cerebellum (Continued)
    vestibular pathways of, 54
Cerebral circulation, functional anatomy of,
        174
    neurovascular syndromes and, 175t
Cerebral cortex, behavior and, 69–71
    Brodmann's map of, 67, 69
    subdivisions of, 66–67
Cerebrospinal fluid (CSF), in multiple
        sclerosis, 169
    radiographic density of, 18
Cerebrovascular disease, 173–182. See also
        Stroke.
    epidemiology of, 5t
Cervical spine, examination of, 15
    pain syndromes in, 4t, 46, 46t
Chagas' disease, 115
Charcot-Marie-Tooth disease, diabetic
        neuropathy vs., 5
    genetic factors in, 7
    nerve conduction studies for, 113b
    neuropathies with, 114–115, 115t
Chorea. See also Huntington's disease.
    benign senile, 143
    causes of, 143
    defined, 32
    Huntington on, 140b
Choreoathetosis, 32
    gait in, 15
    paroxysmal, 143
Chronic inflammatory demyelinating
        polyneuropathy, 107, 109t, 112, 114
Ciliary neurotrophic factor, for amyotrophic
        lateral sclerosis, 125, 125b
Cingulate gyrus, limbic system and, 71
Circuit-specific behaviors, 75
Clomipramine, for cataplexy, 64
Clonazepam, for sleep disorders, 61
    for tremor, 170t
Clonidine, for spasticity, 30t, 170t
Clonus, 151–152, 152
    motor neuron syndromes with, 25t
Clostridium botulinum, 103
Club foot, Charcot-Marie-Tooth disease and,
        114
Cluster headaches, 46. See also Headaches.
Cocaine, intracranial hemorrhage from, 182t
    seizures with, 149t
Color discrimination, 50
Coma, altered consciousness and, 57b
    causes of, 58t
    defined, 57b
    evaluation of, 55–59, 58t
    Glasgow scale for, 57, 58t
    pupil response in, 58–59, 60–61
    treatment of, 59
    vigil. See Persistent vegetative state.
Compound muscle action potential, 113b
    in nerve conduction studies, 28
Computed tomography (CT), applications
        of, 7t
    for neurological examination, 18, 19
    of stroke, 177
Concussion, 57b
Conduction aphasia, 72–73, 73b
Consciousness, altered, 57b
    disorders of, 55–59
Convolution, Broca's, 68b
Coordinative movements, examination of,
        16
Cortical blindness. See Visual agnosia.
Corticosteroids, for muscular dystrophy, 89
    myopathy from, 86t, 94–95
Cranial nerves. See also specific nerves, e.g.,
        Vestibulocochlear nerve.
    examination of, 15–16

Cremasteric reflex, 25t
Creutzfeldt-Jakob disease, 193
    anterior horn cell degeneration in, 120
    chorea with, 143
    transmission of, 7
CSF. See Cerebrospinal fluid (CSF).
CT. See Computed tomography (CT).
Cutaneous nerve distribution, 39
Cyclobenzaprine, 45t
Cytomegalovirus (CMV) infection, 115–116

D

Dantrolene, 30t, 170t
Daytime sleepiness, 61–63
Deafness, causes of, 50, 50t
    Meniere's disease and, 55
Death, brain, 57b
Delirium, defined, 57b
Dementia, 192–194. See also specific types,
        e.g., Alzheimer's disease.
    brain, 57b
    diagnosis of, 190t, 190–192, 191t, 192
    epidemiology of, 5t
    frontal lobe, 192–193
    in Huntington's disease, 193
    in parkinsonism, 130, 131, 193
    Lewy body, 193
    multi-infarct, 191
    subcortical, 193
Deoxyribonucleic acid (DNA),
        mitochondrial, 92
    tests with, 19
Depression. See also Manic-depressive
        behavior.
    anhedonia in, 79
    as altered consciousness, 57b
    drugs for, 80, 145t
    electroconvulsive therapy for, 80
    in Alzheimer's disease, 191
    in Huntington's disease, 139
    in parkinsonism, 130
    neurobiology of, 80
    prefrontal-limbic system and, 80
    stroke and, 80
    symptoms of, 79–80
Dermatomes, 39
    cervical, 46t
    herpes zoster and, 110
Dermatomyositis, 86, 86t, 94
Diabetes mellitus, oculomotor disorders in,
        36t
    peripheral neuropathy from, 109t, 112
        Charcot-Marie-Tooth disease vs., 5
    stroke and, 176
Diazepam, for spasticity, 30t, 170t
Dideoxycytidine neuropathy, 116
Diencephalon, amnesia and, 77t
Diet, headaches and, 12, 44, 45t
Dihydroergotamine mesylate, 45t
Disability status scale, 160t, 169
Dizziness, 53. See also Vertigo.
DNA (deoxyribonucleic acid),
        mitochondrial, 92
    tests with, 19
Doll's eye maneuver, 59, 62
Dopamine synapse, parkinsonism and,
        136–137
Down syndrome, Alzheimer's disease and,
        188b–189b
Drug interaction(s), myasthenia gravis and,
        104
Dysdiadochokinesia, 33
Dyskinesia, from levodopa, 135
Dysmetria, 33

Dystonia, defined, 32
  gait in, 15
Dystrophin, genetic alterations to, 7
  in muscular dystrophy, 87–88, *88*

E

Ear, Meniere's disease and, 55
  trauma to, 50, 50t
Eaton-Lambert syndrome, 103–104
Edinger-Westphal nucleus, *35*
  pupillary light reflex and, *60–61*
Edrophonium test, 101b, 103
EEG. *See* Electroencephalography (EEG).
Elderly clients. *See also* Aging.
  disease risks in, 5
  transient global amnesia in, 79
Electroconvulsive therapy, 80
Electroencephalography (EEG), 18, 149t,
  155–156
  interictal spikes on, *155*
  of absence seizure, *151*
  of tonic-clonic seizure, *152*
Electromyography (EMG), for amyotrophic
  lateral sclerosis, *124*
  for motor neuron syndromes, 25t, 26–27,
    124
  for myasthenia gravis, 103, *104*
  for peripheral neuropathy, 18
Electrophysiological test, for myasthenia
  gravis, 103, *104*
EMG. *See* Electromyography (EMG).
Emotions, language and, 79
Encephalitis, coma from, 58t
  herpes simplex, 77t
  Rasmussen's, 149t
Encephalomyelitis, 164, 165b
Encephalomyopathies, mitochondrial, 86t,
  91–94, *92, 93*
Encephalopathy, hepatic, 58t
Endolymphatic hydrops, Meniere's disease
  and, 55
  vertigo with, 53t
Entrapment neuropathies, *110*, 111–112
Enuresis, imipramine for, 59
Epilepsy, 149–157. *See also* Seizures.
  aura in, 153
  defined, 149
  diagnosis of, 149t, 155–156
  drugs for, 153t
  electroencephalography for, 18, 149t, *151,*
    152, 155, 155–156
  epidemiology of, 5t
  hippocampal sclerosis and, 153–154, *154,*
    156b–157b
  Jackson on, 10
  juvenile myoclonic, 149t, 151
  kindling phenomenon and, 155
  pathophysiology of, 154–155, *155*
  syndromes, 149t, 150–151
  temporal lobe, 153–154, *154,* 156b–157b
  treatment of, 153t, 156–157
Essential tremor, 33
Evoked potential studies, for multiple
  sclerosis, 168–169
Extrapyramidal system, spasticity and, 28
Eyes. *See also* Visual impairment.
  disorders of, movement, *35*
  examination of, 15–16

F

Faces, identification of, 50
Facial nerves, 16, *44*

Facies, in myasthenia gravis, 97
  in myotonic dystrophy, 90
  in parkinsonism, 129
Facioscapulohumeral dystrophy (FSHD),
  86t, 89
Fainting, blood flow and, 177–178
  evaluation of, 53
  from orthostatic hypotension, 54, 64, 130
  seizure vs., 150, 156
Falx, meningioma of, 64
Familial amyloid polyneuropathy, 115
Familial periodic paralysis, 86t, 91
Familial tremor, 33
Fascia dentata, hippocampal sclerosis and,
  157b
Fasciculations, fibrillations vs., 27
  in amyotrophic lateral sclerosis, 119
  motor neuron syndromes and, 25, 25t
  myopathy and, 86
Fatal familial insomnia, 193
Febrile seizures, 150
Festination, in parkinsonism, 130
Fibrillations, fasciculations vs., 27
Fight-or-flight reaction, hypothalamus and,
  63
Fine movements, examination of, 16
Flocculonodular lobe, of cerebellum, 33, *34*
Fluoxetine, 80, 145t
Footdrop, diagnosis of, 24
  gait with, 15
  peripheral neuropathy and, 116
Fornix, limbic system and, *71*
Fractured somatotopy, 31
Fragile X syndrome, 8
Frontal lobe, dementia involving, 192–193
  functions of, 75
FSHD (facioscapulohumeral dystrophy), 86t,
  89

G

Gag reflex, 16
Gait, 15
  in multiple sclerosis, 161b
  in muscular dystrophy, 87
  in parkinsonism, 129–130
  waddling, 87
Gaze centers, *35. See also* Visual fields.
General practitioners, referrals to, 4t
  role of, 6
Genetic factors, in muscular dystrophy, 7, 87
  in narcolepsy, 63
  in neurological disease, 4–5, 7–8
Genetic imprinting, in myotonic dystrophy,
  90
Gerstmann syndrome, 73
Gerstmann-Straussler-Scheinker syndrome,
  193
Giant cell arteritis, cluster headache with, 46
Glasgow Coma Scale, 57, 58t
Glaucoma, 47t
Global aphasia, 72, 73b
Glossopharyngeal nerve, 16
Gower's sign, 87
Grand mal seizure, 151–152, *152*
Graves' disease, 103
Growth factors, for amyotrophic lateral
  sclerosis, 125, 125b
Guillain-Barré syndrome, 26, 112–113, *114*
  AIDS with, 116
  nerve conduction studies for, 27, 113b
  peripheral neuropathy in, 108, 109t
  triggers for, 112
Gunshot wounds, pain syndromes with, 43

H

Haloperidol, for chorea, 145t

Haloperidol *(Continued)*
  for hemiballismus, 33
"Hatchet face," in myotonic dystrophy, 90
Hawking, Stephen, 121b
Head trauma, Alzheimer's disease and, 188
  amnesia from, 77t, 79
  epilepsy and, 153
  incidence of, 4t
Headaches. *See also specific types, e.g.,*
  Migraines.
  cluster, 46
  diet and, 12, 44, 45t
  incidence of, 4t, 43
  nerve pathways for, 43–44
  posttraumatic syndrome with, 79
  tension, 44, 45t
  trigeminal neuralgia and, 43
Hearing loss, causes of, 50, 50t
  from Meniere's disease, 55
Hemiballismus, 32–33
Heparin, for cardiac emboli, 181t
Hepatic encephalopathy, 58t
Hereditary ataxias, 143, 146t, 146–147. *See
  also specific types, e.g.,* Huntington's
  disease.
Hereditary neuropathies, 5t, 114–115, 115t
Herniation, transtentorial, *62*
Herpes simplex encephalitis, 77t
Herpes zoster, in AIDS, 116
  rash of, *110*
  vertigo with, 53t
Hippocampus, amnesia and, 77t, 80b
  in Alzheimer's disease, *190*
  limbic system and, 70–71, *71*
  sclerosis of, 156b–157b
    epilepsy and, 153–154, *154*
    MRI of, *154*
    normal fascia dentata vs., *157b*
Horner's syndrome, 63
Human immunodeficiency virus (HIV)
  infection. *See* Acquired
  immunodeficiency syndrome (AIDS).
Huntington's disease, 139–147, 140b
  chorea in, 32
  dementia in, 193
  depression in, 139
  diagnosis of, 143
  epidemiology of, 5t
  genetic factors in, 8, 139–141, *141,* 142b
  juvenile onset of, 139
  manic-depressive behavior in, 80, 145t
  pathophysiology of, 141–143, *144, 145*
  presentation of, 130, 140b
  test for, 143b
  treatment of, 143–146, 145t
Hydrops, endolymphatic, Meniere's disease
  and, 55
  vertigo with, 53t
Hyperalgesia, defined, 38
Hyperesthesia, defined, 38
Hyperkinetic movement disorders, 32–33.
  See also specific types, e.g.,
  Huntington's disease.
Hypertension, stroke and, 176
Hypoglossal nerve, examination of, 16
Hypoglycemia, 58t
Hypokinetic movement disorders, 32, 128.
  See also specific types, e.g.,
  Parkinsonism.
Hypotension, orthostatic, 54, 63, 130
Hypothalamus, autonomic functions of, 63
  limbic system and, *71*
Hypotonic weakness, 28, 30

I

Ibuprofen, 45t

Ice-water calorics, 59, *62*
Imipramine, for enuresis, 59
Immune-mediated neuropathies, 112–114, 113b, *114. See also specific types, e.g.,* Guillain-Barré syndrome.
Immunosuppression, for multiple sclerosis, 170t, 170–171
Impotence, male, 64
Inclusion body myositis, 86t, 94
Incontinence, drugs for, 170t
    from autonomic disorder, 63–64
    from prostatic hypertrophy, 63
Infectious neuropathies, 115–116
Inflammatory myopathies, 86t, 94
Insomnia, evaluation of, 61
    fatal familial, 193
    sleep disorders and, 59–63
Insulin-like growth factor, for amyotrophic lateral sclerosis, 125
Intention tremor, 33
Interictal spikes, *155*
Intracranial hemorrhage, 181–182. *See also* Stroke.
    causes of, 182t
Intracranial pressure, oculomotor disorders in, 36t
Ischemic stroke, 173–181. *See also* Stroke.

J

Juvenile myoclonic epilepsy, 149t, 151

K

Kearns-Sayre syndrome, genetic factors in, 86t, 92
    heart problems in, 86
    oculomotor disorders in, 36t
    symptoms of, 92
Ketoacidosis, coma from, 58t
Kindling phenomenon, 155
Klüver-Bucy syndrome, 193
Korsakoff's syndrome, 77, 77t
Kuru, transmission of, 7

L

Labyrinth, vestibular pathways of, *54*
Lambert-Eaton syndrome, 103–104
Language, Alzheimer's disease and, 186, *187*
    emotions and, 79
    functions of, 71–74
    mental status and, 15
    stroke and, 175–176
    zone of, 68b, 71, *72*
Learning, declarative, 77
    memory and, 75–77, 76b, 80b
    procedural, 77
    synaptic, 76b
Lennox-Gastaut syndrome, 149t
Levodopa, for parkinsonism, 135, *136*
Lewy bodies, anterior horn cell degeneration and, 120
    dementia and, 193
    parkinsonism and, 130, 134
Light reflex, pupillary, 15, *35*, 58–59, *60–61*
Lightheadedness, 53. *See also* Dizziness.
Limbic system seizures, 153
Limbic-prefrontal system, 70, *70*
Limbic-temporal system, 70–71, *71. See also* Temporal lobe.
Locked-in syndrome, 57b
Lorazepam, for status epilepticus, 153t

Low back syndrome, 15, 46–47, 47t. *See also* Spine.
Lumbar puncture, indications for, 19
Lumbar spine, examination of, 15
    pain syndromes with, 4t, 46–47, 47t

M

Machado-Joseph disease, 141b
Macular degeneration, 47t
Magnetic resonance angiography (MRA), 7t
Magnetic resonance imaging (MRI),
    applications of, 7t
    functional, 7t, 67
    of Binswanger's disease, *193*
    of hippocampal sclerosis, *154*
    of multiple sclerosis, 167–168, *168*
    of neurological examination, 18, *19*
    of stroke, *177*
Magnetic resonance spectroscopy (MRS), 7t
Male impotence, from autonomic failure, 64
Manic-depressive behavior. *See also* Depression.
    caudate nuclei and, 80
    drugs for, 145t
    Huntington's disease with, 80, 145t
Meclizine, for Meniere's disease, 55
MELAS (mitochondrial encephalopathy, lactic acidosis, and stroke-like episodes), 86t, 92–94
Memory. *See also* Amnesia.
    hippocampus and, 80b
    learning and, 75–77, 76b
    mental status and, 15
Meniere's disease, 55
    hearing loss from, 50, 50t
    treatment of, 55
Meningioma, in falx, 64
Meningismus, cluster headache with, 46
Meningitis, carcinomatous, 50t
    coma from, 58t
    lumbar puncture for, 19
    lymphomatous, 116
Mental status examination, 14–15
MEPP (miniature end-plate potential), 97–98, *99,* 100
Meralgia paresthetica, *110,* 111–112
MERRF (myoclonic epilepsy with ragged red fibers), 86t, 94
Metabolic brain disease, causes of, 58t
Metabolic myopathies, 86t, 91
1-Methyl-4-phenyl-1,2,3,6-tetrahydropyridine (MPTP), 134b
Methylprednisolone, for multiple sclerosis, 170t
MGUS (monoclonal gammopathy of undetermined significance), 114
Migraines. *See also* Headaches.
    aura in, 45, *45*
    diet and, 12, 44, 45t
    neurologists for, 4
    photophobia in, 45
    scotoma in, 45, *45*
    seizure vs., 149, 156
    treatment of, 45t, 45–46
    vertigo with, 53
Miller Fisher's syndrome, 113
Miniature end-plate potential (MEPP), 97–98, *99, 100*
Mini-Mental State Examination, 77, 78b
    for Alzheimer's disease, 190
Mitochondrial encephalomyopathies, 86t, 91–94, *92, 93*
Mitochondrial encephalopathy, lactic acidosis, and stroke-like episodes (MELAS), 86t, 92–94

Mitochondrial myopathy, 36t
MMN (multifocal motor neuropathy), 114
Molecular biology, advances in, 7
Monoclonal gammopathy of undetermined significance (MGUS), 114
Mood, depressed. *See* Depression.
    emotion and, 79–81, *81*
Motor cortex, 30
    supplementary, 30
Motor neuron diseases, 25t, 118–125. *See also specific types, e.g.,* Amyotrophic lateral sclerosis (ALS).
    animal models of, 125b
    epidemiology of, 5t
    examination for, 16
    patient survival in, 119, *120*
    types of, 119t
Motor neuron system, diagram of, *24*
    disorders of, 24–36
    lower, 25t, 25–27, *26,* 27t, *28*
    upper, 27–30, *28, 29,* 30t
        hypotonic weakness and, 28, 30
        spasticity with, 27–28
Movements, eye, *35*
    rapid, 59–61
    fine, 16
    hyperkinetic, 32–33
    hypokinetic, 32
MPTP parkinsonism, 134b
MRA (magnetic resonance angiography), 7t
MRI. *See* Magnetic resonance imaging (MRI).
MRS (magnetic resonance spectroscopy), 7t
Multifocal motor neuropathy (MMN), 114
Multi-infarct dementia, 191
Multiple sclerosis, 160–171
    cerebrospinal fluid analysis for, 169
    clinical profile of, 160, 161b, *162*
    diagnosis of, 167–170, *168, 169,* 170t
    disability status scale for, 160t, *169*
    gait in, 161b
    genetic factors in, 160–163, *163*
    hearing loss from, 50t
    incontinence with, 64
    leukoencephalopathy vs., 164
    MRI for, 167–168, *168*
    nystagmus from, 55t
    oculomotor disorders in, 36t
    pathophysiology of, 163–167, 165b, *166, 167*
    symptoms of, 160, 161b, 164t
    treatment of, 170t, 170–171
    vertigo with, 53t
Multiple system atrophies, 134–135
    diagnosis of, 134t
Muscle(s), 16. *See also* Electromyography (EMG).
    atrophy of, 118, 119t
    biopsy of, for mitochondrial myopathy, *93*
        for muscular dystrophy, *88, 89*
    motor neuron syndromes and, 25t
    skeletal, disorders of, 86t
Muscular dystrophy, Becker's, 87–89
    corticosteroids for, 89
    Duchenne's, 87–89, 87b, *89*
    epidemiology of, 5t, 87
    facioscapulohumeral, 86t, 89
    genetic factors in, 7, 8, 87
    myotonic, 86t, 89–91, *90,* 90t
    scoliosis with, 88–89
Mutism, akinetic, 57b
Myasthenia gravis, 97–105
    acetylcholine antibodies in, 102–103
    biopsies for, 101–102, *102*
    diagnosis of, 102–104, *104*
    epidemiology of, 5t

Myasthenia gravis *(Continued)*
  experimental autoimmune, 101b
  Graves' disease vs., 103
  immunopathology of, 100–102, 101b, *102*
  immunosuppression for, 105, 105t
  neuromuscular junction in, 97–98, *99,
    100, 102*
  oculomotor disorders in, 36t
  pathophysiology of, 97–100, *99, 100*
  presentation of, 97, 98b
  stages of, 97t
  thymus in, 98–100
  treatment of, 104–105, 105t
Myocardial infarction, after stroke, 176
Myoclonic epilepsy, juvenile, 149t, 151
Myoclonic epilepsy with ragged red fibers
    (MERRF), 86t, 94
Myogenic lesions, *27*
Myopathy(ies), 86–95, 87b
  corticosteroid, 86t, 94–95
  inflammatory, 86t, 94
  metabolic, 86t, 91
  mitochondrial, 86t, 91–94, *92, 93*
  oculomotor disorders in, 36t
Myositis, inclusion body, 86t, 94
Myotonia, 86
  genetic classification of, 90t
  percussion, 90
Myotonic dystrophy, 86t, 89–91, *90,* 90t
  trinucleotide repeats in, 141b

N

Naproxen sodium, 45t
Narcolepsy, 61–63
  genetic factors in, 63
Neck pain, 4t, 46
  cervical root syndromes with, 46t
  evaluation of, 15
Neocerebellum, 33
Nerve(s), cranial, 15–16
  reinnervation of, 110
  trauma to, 110–111
Nerve conduction studies, for neuropathies,
    113b
  indications for, 27, *28*
Nerve growth factor, 125b
Neuroacanthocytosis, 143
Neurobiology, of behavior, 69–71
Neurofibrillary tangles, 188–189, *190*
Neuroimaging. *See also specific types, e.g.,*
    Computed tomography (CT).
  advances in, 6–7, 7t
  of stroke, *177*
Neurological disease(s). *See also specific
    types, e.g.,* Strokes.
  diagnosis of, *10,* 14–17
  epidemiology of, 4t, 4–5, 5t
  patient history for, *10,* 11–13, *12*
  somatosensory system and, 39t
  temporal onset of, *12*
  trinucleotide repeats in, 142b
Neurological examination, *10,* 14–17
  CT for, 18, *19*
  for Alzheimer's disease, 186, *187*
  for multiple sclerosis, 161b
  for seizures/epilepsy, 150t
  laboratory tests for, 18–19, *19*
  MRI for, 18, *19*
  screening, 17, 17b
Neurologists, consultations with, 4
  demographics of, 6
  medical generalists vs., 4t
  role of, 6, 7b
Neurology, practice of, 4t, 4–8, 5t, 7t

Neurology *(Continued)*
  student education in, 5
  trends in, 6–8, 7t
Neuroma, acoustic, 53t, 53–54
Neuromelanin, in parkinsonism, *132–133*
Neuromuscular junction, in myasthenia
    gravis, 97–98, *99, 100, 102*
Neuronitis, vestibular, 53t, 55
Neuropathy(ies). *See also* Neurological
    disease(s).
  Chagas' disease and, 115
  Charcot-Marie-Tooth disease and, 5, 114–
    115, 115t
  entrapment, *110,* 111–112
  from dideoxycytidine, 116
  hereditary, 114–115, 115t
  immune-mediated, 112–114, 113b, *114*
  infectious, 115–116
  optic, 47t, *48*
  peripheral. *See* Peripheral neuropathy.
Nociception, 41–47
Nonsteroidal anti-inflammatory drugs
    (NSAIDs), 45t
Nortriptyline, 80, 145t
Nutrition, headaches and, 12, 44, 45t
Nystagmus, defined, 36
  evaluation of, 54
  types of, 55t
  vertigo with, 54, *54*

O

Obsessive-compulsive disorder, 80–81
Obtundation, defined, 57b
Oculomotor system, *35,* 35–36, 36t
  examination of, 15–16
Olfactory nerve, 15
Optic chiasm, 47t, *48*
Optic nerve, 15, 47t, *48*
Orientation, mental status and, 14
Orthostatic hypotension, 54. *See also*
    Fainting.
  from autonomic neuropathy, 63
  in parkinsonism, 130
Otitis media, 50t
Otosclerosis, 50t
Oxybutynin, 170t
Oxycodone, 45t

P

Pain syndromes, gunshot wounds and, 43
  in spine, 4t, 15, 46, 46t
  neuropharmacology of, *42,* 45t
  pathways of, 41–47
  treatment of, 45t
Paleocerebellum, 33
Palsy, bulbar, 118, 119t
  peroneal, *110,* 112
  "shaking," 128b
  supranuclear, 135, 193
    cause of, 30t
    diagnosis of, 134t
Papovavirus, demyelination with, 164
Parallel processing, defined, 68
Paralysis, familial periodic, 86t, 91
  Todd's, 150
Paralysis agitans, 128b
Paraplegia, spastic, 15
Paraproteinemia, 114
Parasomnia. *See* Sleep, disorders of.
Paresthesia, defined, 38
  from stroke, 175
Parietal lobe syndrome, *74,* 74–75

Parkinsonism, 128–134, 128b, *129–130,
    132–133,* 134b, 134t
  Alzheimer's disease and, 186
  anterior horn cell degeneration in, 119–
    120
  basal ganglia circuits in, *129*
  bradykinesia in, 32
  dementia in, 130, 131, 193
  epidemiology of, 5t
  gait in, 15
  levodopa for, 135, *136*
  Lewy bodies in, 130, 134
  movement disorders with, 32
  oculomotor disorders in, 36t
  substantia nigra in, *130,* 130–131
  treatment of, 135t, 135–137, *136*
Paroxysmal choreoathetosis, 143
Pathophysiology, evaluation of, 13–14
Patient, history of, *10,* 11–13, *12*
  neurological evaluation of, *10,* 14–17
  perspectives of, 4
Peripheral nerves, anatomy of, *208*
  cutaneous, *39*
  pain in, 43
Peripheral neuropathy, causes of, 111t
  clinical approach to, 107b
  diagnosis of, 109t, 109–110
  electromyography for, 18
  patterns of, *110*
  presentation of, 107–109
  restless leg syndrome vs., 13
  tests for, 111t
  treatment of, 116
Peroneal nerve, *208*
Peroneal palsy, *110,* 112
Persistent vegetative state, 57b
PET. *See* Positron emission tomography
    (PET).
Petit mal seizure, 151, *151. See also*
    Seizures.
Phenobarbital, 153t
Phenytoin, for myotonic dystrophy, 90–91
  for pain syndromes, 45t
  for seizures, 153t
Photophobia, migraines and, 45
Pick's disease, *190*
Pineal tumor, nystagmus from, 55t
  oculomotor disorders with, 36t
Pituitary tumor, 47t, *48*
Plantar responses, 25t
PML (progressive multifocal
    leukoencephalopathy), 164
Polymyositis, 86t, 94
  epidemiology of, 5t
Polyneuropathy. *See also* Neuropathy(ies).
  idiopathic, 116
Pons infarction, 57
Positional vertigo, 54–55
  test for, *56*
Positron emission tomography (PET),
  applications of, 7t
  circuit-specific behaviors and, 75
  of amyotrophic lateral sclerosis, *12*
Posterior fossa lesions, 58t
Posttraumatic syndrome, headaches with, 79
Posture, examination of, 15
  in parkinsonism, 129–130
Prader-Willi syndrome, 8
Prednisolone, for multiple sclerosis, 170t
Prednisone, for myasthenia, 105t
Prefrontal-limbic system, 70, *70*
  depression and, 80
Premotor cortex, 30
Presbycusis, 50t
Primidone, for tremor, 33, 170t
Prion diseases, 193–194

Prion diseases *(Continued)*
transmission of, 7
Procedural learning. *See* Learning.
Progressive bulbar palsy, 118, 119t
Progressive multifocal leukoencephalopathy (PML), 164
Progressive muscular atrophy, 118, 119t
patient survival in, *120*
Progressive supranuclear palsy (PSP), 135, 193
cause of, 30t
diagnosis of, 134t
Propantheline, for incontinence, 170t
Propranolol, for tremor, 33, 170t
Prosopagnosia, defined, 50, 73b
Prostatic hypertrophy, incontinence with, 63
Pseudoathetosis, 107
PSP. *See* Progressive supranuclear palsy (PSP).
Psychomotor epilepsy, 153–154, *154*
Pupillary light reflex, 15, 58–59
pathways for, *35, 60–61*
Putamen, atrophy of, *144*
lesion of, *19*
projection pathways from, *31, 32*
Pyramidal system, spasticity and, 28, *29*
Pyridostigmine, for myasthenia, 105t

R

Ragged red fibers, mitochondrial myopathy and, *93*
myoclonic epilepsy and, 86t, 94
Rapid eye movement (REM) sleep, 59–61
Rasmussen's encephalitis, 149t
Reflex(es), cremasteric, 25t
doll's eye, 59, *62*
examination of, 17
grading of, 17t
ice-water caloric, 59, *62*
pupillary light, 15, *35*, 58–59, *60–61*
segmental, 17t
somatosensory system and, 39t
tendon, 25t
types of, 17t
vestibulo-ocular, 54
Reflex sympathetic dystrophy, 43
REM (rapid eye movement) sleep, 59–61
Repetitive nerve stimulation test, 103, *104*
Reserpine, behavioral retardation and, 80
Restless leg syndrome, 59
clonazepam for, 61
peripheral neuropathy vs., 13
Rigidity, spasticity vs., 32

S

Saccadic dysmetria, 33
Saccular aneurysm, 182
Sarcoidosis, hearing loss from, 50t
Schizophrenia, limbic circuits and, 81
Sciatic nerve, *208*
Scissor gait, 15
Scoliosis, in muscular dystrophy, 88–89
Scopolamine, for Ménière's disease, 55
Scotoma, migraine, 45, *45*
Scrapie, 7, 193–194
Screening neurological examination, 17, 17b
Segmental reflexes, 17t
Seizures. *See also* Epilepsy.
absence, 151, *151*
anoxic, 150
causes of, 149t
defined, 149

Seizures *(Continued)*
diagnosis of, 149–154, 150t
differential, 155–156
drugs for, 153t
during sleep, 12
electroencephalography for, 18, 149t, *151, 152, 155,* 155–156
epidemiology of, 5t
febrile, 150
first, 149–150
kindling phenomenon and, 155
limbic system, 153
partial, 149t, 153
pathophysiology of, 154–155, *155*
stroke vs., 180
tonic-clonic, 151–152, *152*
trauma and, 4
treatment of, 153t, 156–157
Senile plaques, in Alzheimer's disease, 189–190, *190*
Senile tremor, 33
Sensation, disorders of, 38–50
Sensory examination, 16–17
Sensory loss, 38–41, 39t, *39–41*
dissociated, 39
Sensory nerve action potential (SNAP), *28*
"Shaking" palsy, 128b
Shy-Drager syndrome, autonomic failure in, 63
diagnosis of, 134t
Simultanagnosia, defined, 50
Single-photon-emission computed tomography (SPECT), 7t
Skeletal muscles, 86t. *See also* Muscle(s).
Sleep, apnea, 61
disorders of, 59–63, 193
clonazepam for, 61
insomnia and, 61, 193
stages of, 59
SNAP (sensory nerve action potential), *28*
Somatosensory system pathways, 39t, *40–41*
Somatotopy, fractured, 31
Spasmodic torticollis, 33
Spasticity, bladder, 63–64
cause of, 27
drugs for, 30t, 124, 170t
motor neuron syndrome with, 27–28
pyramidal system and, 28, *29*
rigidity vs., 32
SPECT scan. *See* Single-photon-emission computed tomography (SPECT).
Spine, cervical, 4t, 15, 46, 46t
disorders of, 5t
lumbar, 4t, 15, 46–47, 47t
muscular atrophy of, 118, 119t
peripheral nerves of, *208*
scoliosis of, 88–89
Status epilepticus, 152–153, 153t. *See also* Seizures.
Steppage gait, 15
Stereotaxic surgery, for parkinsonism, 135–137
Stroke. *See also* Transient ischemic attack (TIA).
alcohol and, 176
depression after, 80
diabetes and, 176
diagnosis of, 180, 180t
epidemiology of, 5t
from cardiac embolus, 173t, 180, 181t
from carotid stenosis, 176
hearing loss from, 50t
hypertension and, 176
impaired language from, 175–176
MELAS and, 92–94
morbidity/mortality from, 173

Stroke *(Continued)*
myocardial infarction after, 176
neuroimaging of, *177*
nystagmus after, 55
oculomotor disorders in, 36t
pathophysiology of, 177–180, 178b–179b
presentation of, 173t, 173–176, *174,* 175
risk factors for, 176t, 176–177, *177*
seizure vs., 180
subcortical, 193
treatment of, 180–181, 181t
visual impairment from, 47t, 174–175
Stupor, defined, 57b
Subdural hematoma, headache with, 46
herniation from, *62*
Substantia nigra cells, in parkinsonism, *130,* 130–131
transplant of, 137
Sumatriptan, 45t
Supplementary motor cortex, 30
Supramaximal repetitive nerve stimulation test, 103, *104*
Supranuclear palsy, progressive, 135, 193
cause of, 30t
diagnosis of, 134t
Supratentorial mass lesions, 58t
Synaptic learning, 76b. *See also* Learning.
Syncope, blood flow and, 177–178
evaluation of, 53
orthostatic hypotension and, 54, 64, 130
seizure vs., 150, 156
Syphilis, hearing loss from, 50t
neuropathies with, 115–116
vertigo with, 53t

T

Tactile agnosia, 41, 74
Tardive dyskinesia, 143
Temporal lobe, arteritis of, 46
epilepsy, 153–154, *154,* 156b–157b
limbic system and, 70–71, *71*
Temporal onset, of neurological disease, 12
Temporal-limbic system, 70–71, *71*
circuit diagram of, *81*
Tendon jerk, in somatosensory system, 39t
motor neuron syndromes and, 25, 25t, *26*
Tendon reflexes, 25t
Tensilon (edrophonium) test, 101b, 103
Tension headaches. *See* Headaches.
Thiamine deficiency, vertigo with, 53t
Thioridazine, for chorea, 145t
Thrombosis, stroke from, 173t
Thymus, in myasthenia gravis, 98–100, 104–105
TIA. *See* Transient ischemic attack (TIA).
Titubation, defined, 33
Todd's paralysis, 150
Tonic-clonic seizures, 151–152
electroencephalograph of, *152*
Torticollis, spasmodic, 33
Transient global amnesia, 79. *See also* Amnesia.
Transient ischemic attack (TIA). *See also* Stroke.
diagnosis of, 180, 180t
risk factors for, 176–177
seizure vs., 149, 156
treatment of, 180–181, 181t
Transplantation, for parkinsonism, 137
Transtentorial herniation, from subdural hematoma, *62*
pupil response in, 58
Tremor, 33–35
drugs for, 33

Trigeminal nerve, 16
  pain in, 5t, 43, *44*
Trinucleotide repeat disease, 142b
Trochlear nerve, 15–16
Trypanosoma cruzi, 115
Tuberculosis, hearing loss from, 50t

U

Ulnar nerve entrapment, *110,* 111
Unsteadiness, 53. *See also* Vertigo.
Upper motor neuron syndromes, 28, 30
Uremic coma, 58t
Urinary incontinence, drugs for, 170t
  from autonomic disorder, 63–64
  from prostatic hypertrophy, 63

V

Vagus nerve, examination of, 16
Valproic acid, for manic-depressive
  behavior, 145t

Valproic acid *(Continued)*
  for seizures, 153t
Vegetative state, 57b
Vertigo. *See also* Fainting.
  benign positional, 54–55
    test for, *56*
  evaluation of, 53–54
  localization of, 53t
  nystagmus with, 54, *54*
Vestibulocochlear nerve, examination of, 16
  inflammation of, 55
  Meniere's disease and, 53t, 53–54
  neurofibroma of, 50t
  pathways of, *54*
  tumors of, 53t, 53–54
  vertigo and, 53t, 53–54
Vestibulo-ocular reflex (VOR), 54. *See also*
  Reflex(es).
  doll's eye maneuver and, 59, *62*
  ice-water calorics and, 59, *62*
Vision, pathways of, *48*
  peripheral, 50
Visual agnosia, 73b
Visual evoked response (VER), 168–169

Visual fields, examination of, 15
  loss of, 47t
  striate cortex and, *49*
Visual impairment, 47–50, 73b
  evaluation of, 15, 47t, 50
  from stroke, 47t, 174–175
  localization of, 47t
VOR. *See* Vestibulo-ocular reflex (VOR).

W

Warfarin, for atrial fibrillation, 181t
Wasting syndromes, motor neurons in, 25t
Wernicke's aphasia, 72, 73b
Wisconsin Card Sorting Test, 75
  for frontal lobe dementia, 193
  schizophrenia and, 81
Wolf-Hirschhorn syndrome, 143

Z

Zidovudine (AZT) myopathy, 86t, 94
Zone of language, 68b, 71, *72*